Advances in Diagnostic Urology

Edited by C. C. Schulman

With 283 Figures and 45 Tables

Springer-Verlag Berlin Heidelberg New York 1981

Claude C. Schulman, M. D.

Chief of the Department of Urology
Cliniques Universitaires de Bruxelles, Hôpital Erasme
Route de Lennick, 808, B-1070 Bruxelles, Belgium

ISBN-13: 978-3-642-95396-5 e-ISBN-13: 978-3-642-95394-1

DOI: 10.1007/ 978-3-642-95394-1

Library of Congress Cataloging in Publication Data

Advances in diagnostic urology. Based on contributions given during the congress of the European Association of Urology.
Bibliography: p. Includes index.
1. Genito-urinary organs–Diseases–Diagnosis–Congresses. 2. Urology–Congresses.
I. Schulman, C. C. (Claude C.), 1943-. II. European Association of Urology.
RC874.A 38 616.6′075 81-8878 ISBN 0-387-10806-8 (U.S.) AACR2

Softcover reprint of the hardcover 1st edition 1981

Typesetting, printing and bookbinding: Konrad Triltsch, Würzburg
2122/3130-543210

Preface

Accuracy in preoperative diagnosis has always been the basis of success in urology. In the past decade, major advances have been made in diagnostic imaging of the kidney and genitourinary tract. Of the new reliable techniques available, echography, radioisotope studies and computerized tomographic scanning are of the greatest importance in the investigation of renal and urinary tract diseases. These new methods of investigation have led to a radical change in the attitude and practical approach when evaluating a patient presenting with a urologic disorder. The techniques each yield information of a different type and in conjunction with classic radiology must be used safely and with a logical sequence in the investigation of a diagnostic problem. They have greatly increased the available evidence on which diagnosis is based and their use should diminish the number of false diagnoses and ultimately improve treatment. The applications of these recently developed diagnostic methods in urology are reviewed in this book, based on the main contributions given by a wide range of experts in their field during the last Congress of the European Association of Urology, held in Athens in 1980.

Intravenous urography, the first and major step in urologic diagnosis, developed more than half a century ago, can still be improved, as shown by the routine use of early nephrotomography with rapid injection.

The role of varicocele in male infertility has stimulated increased interest in the detection of infraclinical disorders by spermatic phlebography, and the use of nonsurgical methods of treatment has been developed. Thermography and Doppler investigations are also of great interest in the assessment of varicoceles.

Echography has brought about remarkable progress in the diagnosis of urologic diseases. Its application ranges from the diagnosis of the nature of space-occupying lesions of the kidney to antenatal demonstration of urologic malformations in the fetus. Investigations of the bladder and prostate benefit from specially developed devices that allow scanning via the rectum or directly within the bladder to discern extension of neoplastic lesions.

Computerized tomographic scanning provides valuable morphological information on the extension of invasive lesions of the kidney and retroperitoneal structures that can hardly be obtained by other noninvasive techniques in the staging of neoplastic diseases.

Radioisotope studies have opened up a new field in the precise measurement of the separate function of each kidney. This is of foremost importance in the preoperative evaluation of most kidney diseases and is the key factor in the long-term follow up of surgically corrected lesions and in particular of congenital malformations in children. Nuclear medicine can also be used as a dynamic investigation since the need to diagnose even minor degrees of upper urinary tract obstruction accurately has been emphasized in recent years and doubt has been cast on the efficacy of conventional radiology in this respect. Newer methods have thus been developed, such as sophisticated radioisotope studies measuring parenchymal transit times and diuresis renography. Direct measurement of the dynamics of the upper urinary tract by means of pressure-flow studies has its own advantages in this difficult diagnostic challenge.

Urodynamics has not only effected important developments in the diagnosis of equivocal upper urinary tract obstruction but, most importantly, has become a precise and invaluable diagnostic aid in the understanding of incontinence and micturition disorders which should improve our therapeutic results.

This book brings together, in one easily accessible volume, a good deal of work that would otherwise be scattered widely throughout the world literature and provides a useful summary of the current views on recently developed diagnostic methods in urology. Allowing for the fact that new diagnostic methods are undergoing continuous and rapid evolution and that necessity is usually the mother of invention, one should remember that everything born from progress also dies with further progress.

Brussels Claude C. SCHULMAN

Contents

General Radiology

Varicocele Evaluation

Evaluation of Male Impotence

Peroperative Renal Stone Localization

Lymph Node Evaluation

Ultrasounds

Computed Tomography

Nuclear Medicine

Differential Renal Function

Imaging Procedures

Urodynamics

Urodynamics

Upper Urinary Tract

Lower Urinary Tract

Intravenous Nephrourography by Systematic Very Rapid Injection

A. N. Dardenne, P. Bodart, and P. J. Van Cangh

Introduction

In screening the upper urinary tract, a careful analysis of the renal parenchyma is at least as important as that of the collecting system.

Intravenous urography is capable of providing precise information not only on the excretory system, but also a detailed analysis of the renal parenchyma as well as useful data on the renal vessels. In order to achieve these goals, some fundamental technical aspects should be followed. Before reaching the collecting system, the injected contrast medium travels through the vascular spaces of the kidney and through the various segments of the nephron; the vessels and parenchyma can be clearly examined if films are obtained at the exact moment of the passage of the contrast medium in adequate concentration (Bodart et al. 1978).

In 1976 we reported our preliminary experience of 1200 urographies with early nephrography after fast intravenous injection of contrast material (intravenous nephrourography – IVNU) (Dardenne and Bodart 1977 a).

At the present time, we have carried out more than 20 000 examinations. The nephrography obtained with this technique is, at the same dosage of contrast medium, denser than that obtained with a perfusion technique (Saxton 1969). Moreover, it appears successively under two aspects: the first, early and transient – *vascular nephrography* – demonstrates the morphology of the renal vessels as well as the glomerular and medullar compartments of the parenchyma; the second, later and more prolonged – *tubular nephrography* – consists of an homogeneous parenchymal opacification, which is similar to that obtained by perfusion or high-dose, slow injection techniques. Likewise, the quality of the pyelocaliceal opacification is similar to that of classic urography; used with an effective ureteral compression it yields comparable images to those obtained by direct opacification (retrograde or antegrade) as long as renal function is intact and a moderate degree of antidiuresis achieved (van Ypersele et al. 1979).

In many cases, the density of the opaque urine is sufficient to perform a micturating cystourethrogram at the end of the test. The results of 20 000 consecutive IVNUs warrant its continued systematic use.

Technique of Very Rapid Intravenous Injection

The insertion of a wide caliber needle (14 G or 16 G) into a vein of the forearm is indispensable to achieve the very rapid injection (cf. below) (Dardenne and Bodart

1977 b). We use a needle with a Teflon cannula, which remains in the vein until the end of the examination. This allows a further injection of contrast medium if deemed necessary during the examination (e.g., chronic obstructive uropathy, renal failure). It also has the advantage of access to a large intravenous channel should an adverse reaction occur. In more than 90% of the cases, the wide caliber needle can be inserted at the first attempt.

The contrast media are classic triiodinated highly concentrated compounds (Between 35 and 45 g I/100 ml). The amount injected varies according to the weight of the patient and the suspected clinical problem: between 30 and 60ml, the usual dose being 50 ml. The contrast medium is preheated to 37 °C in order to decrease its viscosity; the injection is given without difficulty with a normal syringe at an approximate rate of 10 ml/s. At low injection rates, the quality of early nephrography diminishes markedly.

Following very rapid injection, the patient very often feels a brief sensation of intense warmth in the whole body. The patient should be warned about the possible occurrence of this sensation and be reassured as to its benign nature. After the first films, 10–20 ml normal saline is injected into the vein in order to diminish the possibility of endothelial irritation by stagnation of the contrast medium. Such side effects diminish markedly with less-hypertonic contrast media (nonionic molecules or monoacid dimers). They are, however, not in current use, mainly because of their high cost (Dardenne et al. 1979).

Very rapid intravenous injection causes no more severe reactions than other urographic techniques. It is, however, preferable to avoid its use in cardiac failure or in very anxious patients. However, these cases also constitute a contraindication to urography in general, whatever the technique of injection.

Early Phase Technique (Vascular Nephrography)

With very rapid injection of a concentrated contrast medium, the plasma concentration curve presents an early and an acute peak corresponding to the passage of the opaque bolus (Dardenne and Bodart 1977 b; van Ypersele et al. 1979). The concentration curve decreases rapidly thereafter due to the diffusion of the opaque medium at first in the plasma volume and then in the extracellular space. The concentration peak, which is responsible for the vascular opacification, is therefore very transient. The proper time to take the first film (*arterial phase*) is usually between 10 and 15 s after starting the injection; it depends on the patient's age (Table 1, Fig. 1).

Ingrisch (Ingrisch et al. 1980) has recently suggested a method of improving the timing of the first film by mixing the contrast material with a small amount of radioactive tracer (0.2 of 0.3 $mCi^{99m}Tc$); the film is taken at the moment of detection of radioactivity at an abdominal level. Three films are obtained in fast succession after the first; they record the selective opacification of the glomerular cortex (*cortical nephrographic phase*) (Fig. 2).

This sequence of four films (arterial phase and cortical nephrographic phase) constitutes the early phase, and is carried out using a tomographic technique, which is indispensable for the study of the renal parenchyma, but is rarely indicated for

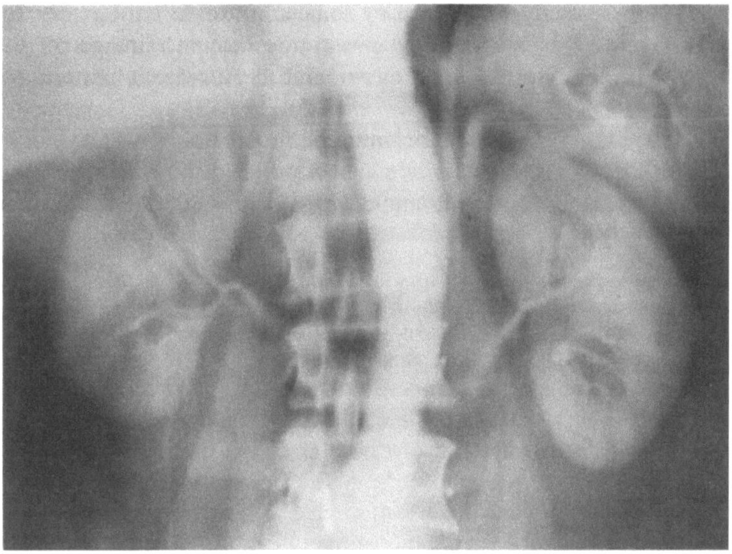

Fig. 1. Arterial phase. Film taken 13 s after the beginning of the injection in a 45-year-old patient. The aorta, as well as the intrarenal arteries are shown.

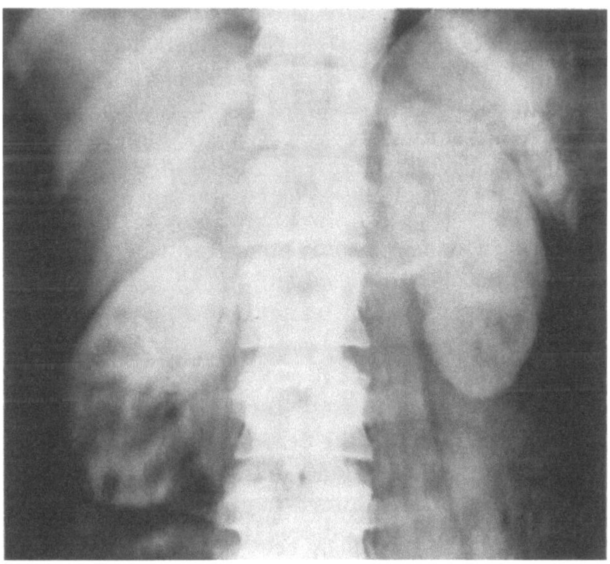

Fig. 2. Cortical nephrographic phase. Dense selective opacification of the glomerular cortex. The renal outline is clearly delineated.

analysis of the excretory system when urinary concentration is satisfactory. In comparison with standard films, tomography gives more accurate images of the renal contours, the homogeneity of the nephrogram, and the absence of anterior or posterior renal masses.

In order to obtain optimal contrast, we recommend the use of a 65–75 kv beam. The first tomogram following the injection is taken in order to show the ramifications of renal artery. It is thicker (swaying angle: more or less 10°) than the three

Table 1. Timing of the first tomogram after starting very rapid intravenous injection, dependent on the age of the patient.

Age (years)	Time of first tomogram after injection (s)
< 20	9 – 11
20 – 30	10 – 12
30 – 40	11 – 13
40 – 50	12 – 14
50 – 60	12 – 14
60 – 70	13 – 15
70 >	14 – 16

subsequent films (swaying angle: more or less 30°) and is situated 1.5 cm in front of the central plane of the renal substance, previously determined by a preliminary tomogram. The subsequent three cuts of the cortical nephrogram are taken 1 cm in front of the central plane of the kidney, in the central plane and 1 cm behind respectively. When the kidneys are located at a different depth or when the long renal axis is horizontal, one or two further tomographic cuts are performed in other planes to study the whole renal parenchyma. If the first arterial tomogram is not satisfactory, it is possible to carry out another arterial phase at a different level or timing (Figs. 7, 11).

Diagnostic Interest of the Early Phase

The essential goal of the early phase is to obtain the densest possible nephrogram during urography (Fig. 3) (Dardenne 1977; Dardenne and Bodart 1977 b). This is the purpose of the three tomographic cuts of the cortical nephrogram following the *arterial phase. The latter* is systematically studied, because it provides useful diagnostic information in more than 70% of cases. It is capable of showing a renal arterial tree regardless of the ultimate excretory function of the kidney. This is particularly useful when the kidney is otherwise "silent". The renal arteries can be located and numbered (Fig. 4).

The arterial origin of some renal pelvic defects, which could otherwise be mistaken for tumor or inflammatory processes, can be ascertained, thereby avoiding retrograde pyelography or arteriography (Fig. 5).

The normal permeability of the arterial midline can be established directly (Fig. 6). In certain cases it is possible to confirm the ischemic origin of an atrophic kidney and to identify the causal lesion. Thus, arterial stenosis (Fig. 7) as well as aneurysmal dilatation (Fig. 8) can be shown. The arterial phase will also disclose the arterial location of central renal calcification. Arterial sinuosities in cases of vascular sclerosis are easily documented. Intraparenchymal branches appear sparse and stretched in hydronephrosis (Fig. 9) and in polycystic kidneys (Fig. 10); they may be deviated in the case of a space-occupying lesion. Hypervascularization so characteristic of most hypernephromas is almost always clearly shown (Fig. 11 a). In pelviureteric obstruction, the arterial phase can demonstrate an accessory polar vessel crossing the junction. The extension of an abdominal aortic aneurysm to the renal arteries may be seen. In renal trauma, the site of a hemorrhage can be demonstrated. When the examination is required as a complementary investigation for studying extrarenal pathology, enlargement of the field can enhance the diagnostic data on the principal pathology, which is often better than that obtained without the vascular phase (e.g., gynecological or hepatic masses, vascular disease; Fig. 12).

Cortical nephrography details the renal contours better than tubular nephrography. Anatomic incisures can be very clearly demonstrated and seen to originate from cortical septa (columns of Bertin). The lightly delineated triangular areas correspond to Malpighi pyramids (Fig. 13). Anomalies of a pathologic contour are much more evident than at the other phases of the examination. Cortical atrophy (normal thickness of the cortex: 0.8 to 1 cm) can be discovered, as well as any modification of the cortex–medulla ratio. Nonperfused cortical zones can be easily recognised. The hypervascular tumors remain clearly impregnated with contrast medium at this stage (Figs. 11 b, 14); they sometimes appear encircled by newly developed vascular venous channels. In the absence of a tumor, such channels may hint at the presence of renal vein thrombosis. Venous structures are easily recognized (Fig. 15). The "pseudotumors" caused by hypertrophy of Bertin's columns are characterized by their nephrographic pattern, which is strictly similar to that of the glomerular cortex in early and delayed films (Fig. 16). These will show that the opacification of the area under suspicion behaves in exactly the same way as the remainder of the renal parenchyma. This is in contrast to vascularized tumors, in which the tumoral tissue quickly becomes relatively hypodense compared with the normal renal parenchyma. A renal cyst is characterized by its rounded or oval shape, and by its homogeneous hypodense content after opacification of the parenchyma. Cysts a few millimeters in diameter can be detected especially when they have a cortical location. The wall of uncomplicated cysts is very thin but cannot be distinguished when the cyst has a central location; in the latter case, it is not possible to establish the true nature of a parenchymal translucency (Fig. 16). The cortical nephrogram, which normally disappears within 1 min after the injection, is more prolonged when there is renal hypoperfusion such as in narrow arterial stenosis or in hypotension. In acute renal failure, the cortical nephrogram is usually nonspecific, the corticomedullary junction being frequently ill defined. In the study of "silent kidney," congenital absence of kidney has to be differentiated from a nonfunctioning kidney secondary to chronic disease. In cases of agenesis, the absence of the renal silhouette is associated with absence of the renovascular pedicle.

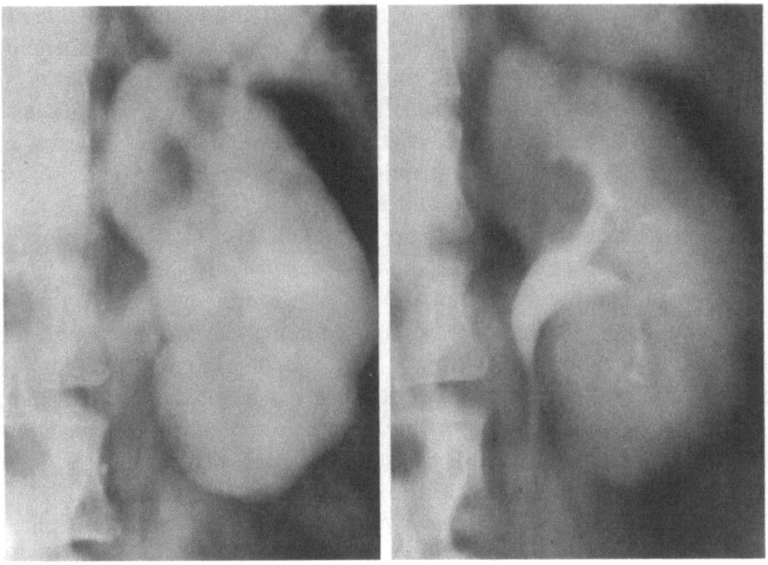

a b

Fig. 3a, b. Nephrography. **a** Early nephrogram. **b** Late tubular nephrogram. Parenchymal opacification is denser in **a** and the renal outline better delineated.

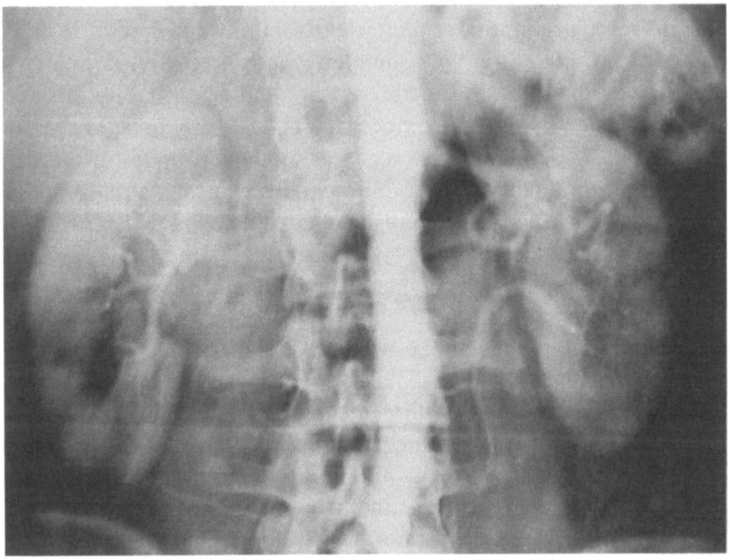

Fig. 4. Multiple renal arteries. Arterial phase demonstrating two left renal arteries as well as the level of their origin.

Fig. 6. Renal transplantation. Arterial phase. Normal arterial anastomosis demonstrated a few days after transplantation. The *arrows* indicate surgical drains.

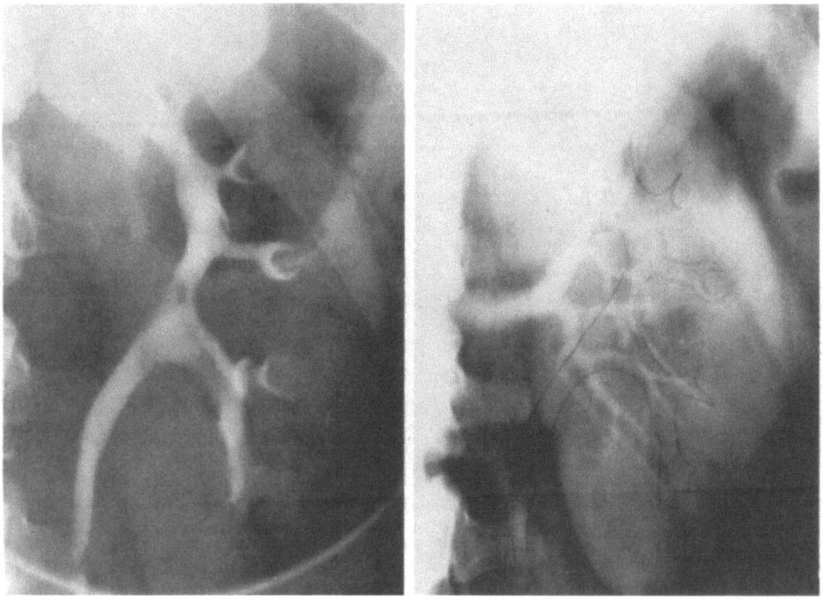

a b

Fig. 5a, b. Renal pelvic lacuna. **a** Pyelogram with central triangular filling defect. **b** Arterial phase: the superimposition of the pyelogram indicates the vascular origin of the pelvic lacuna, which therefore is not pathologic.

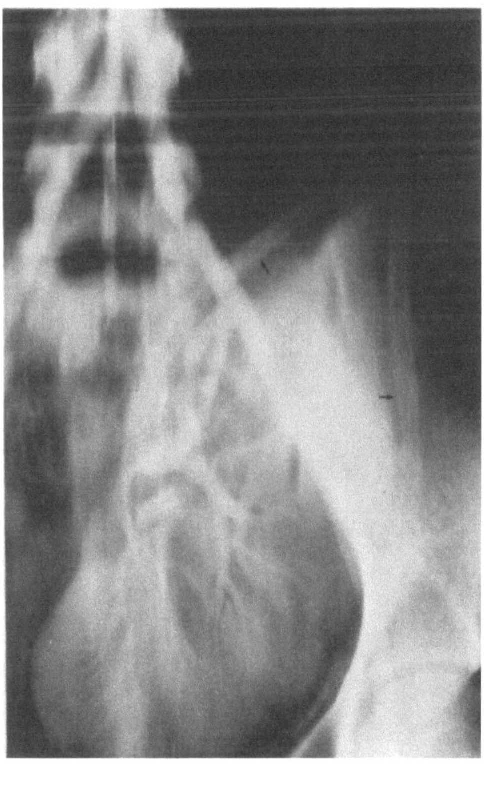

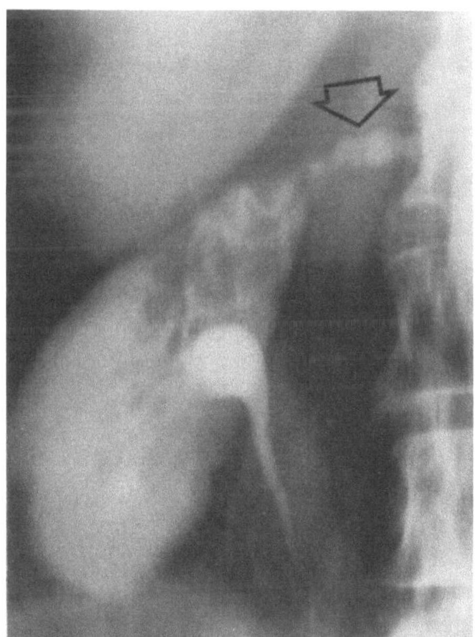

▲

Fig. 7. Arterial stenoses. Second arterial phase performed at the end of an examination. Moniliform aspcct of right distal renal artery typical of fibromuscular dysplasia (*arrow*).

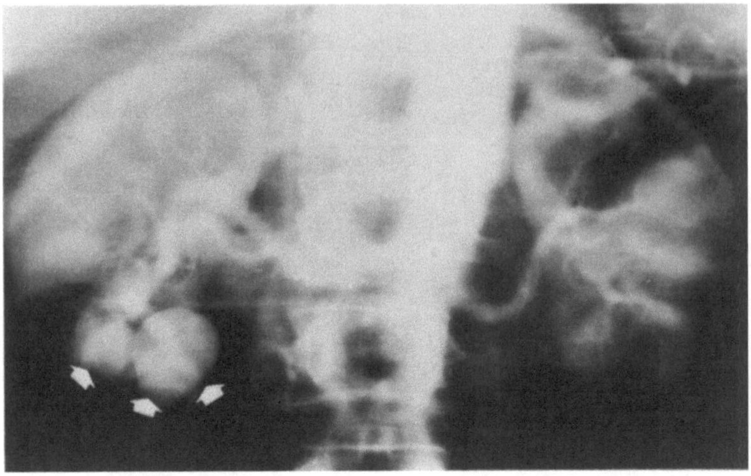

Fig. 8. Aneurysmal lesion of the right lower pole (*arrows*). Arterial phase (Courtesy of Dr. F. de Fays).

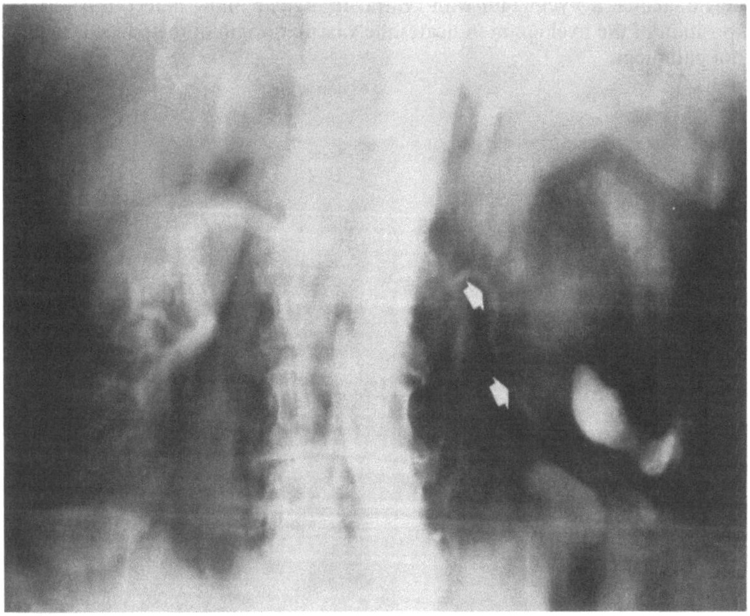

Fig. 9. Left chronic hydronephrosis with stones. Arterial phase. Atrophic left renal artery with sparse intrarenal branches (*arrows*).

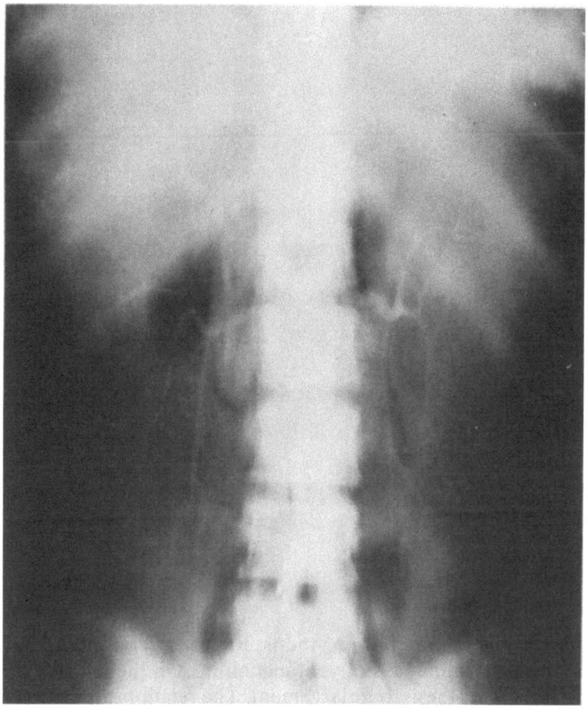

Fig. 10. Polycystic kidneys. Arterial phase. Stretching of the arterial tree.

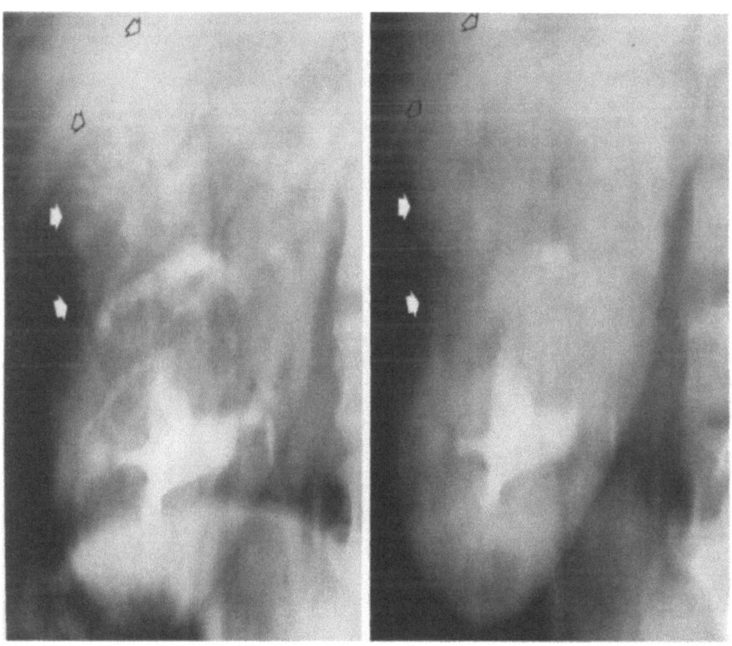

a b

Fig. 11 a, b. Hypernephroma. Repeat early arterial phase performed at the end of the examination. **a** Arterial phase demonstrating an irregular, highly vascularized tumor in the right upper pole (*arrows*). **b** Cortical nephrographic phase: persistent staining of the tumor (*arrows*).

a
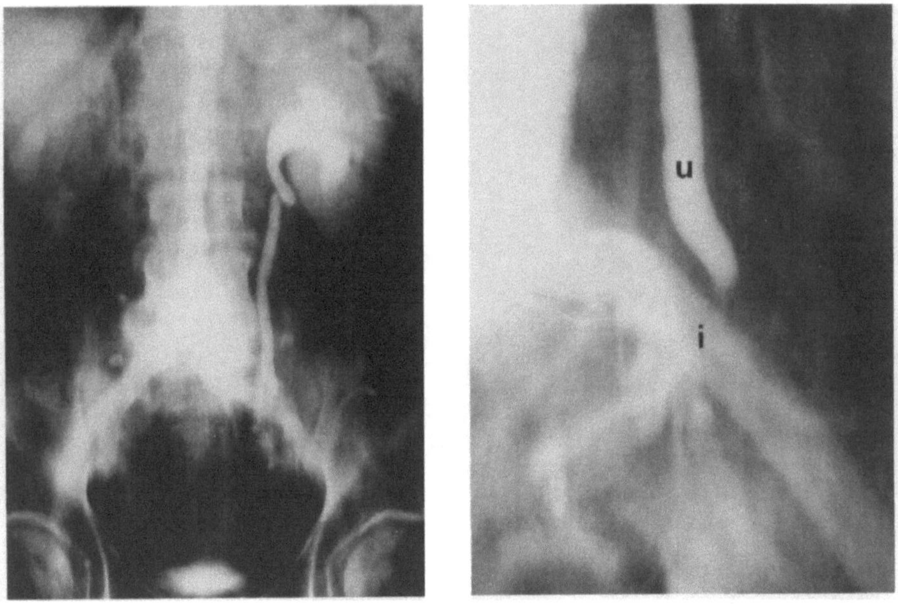

b

Fig. 12 a, b. Left ureteric obstruction by dacron arterial prosthesis. Repeat arterial phase performed during the examination. **a** The right kidney is not yet functioning. On the left side the ureter is dilated above the left limb of the prosthesis. **b** Enlargement. The relationship between the opacified arterial graft (*i*) and the dilated ureter (*u*) is clearly shown.

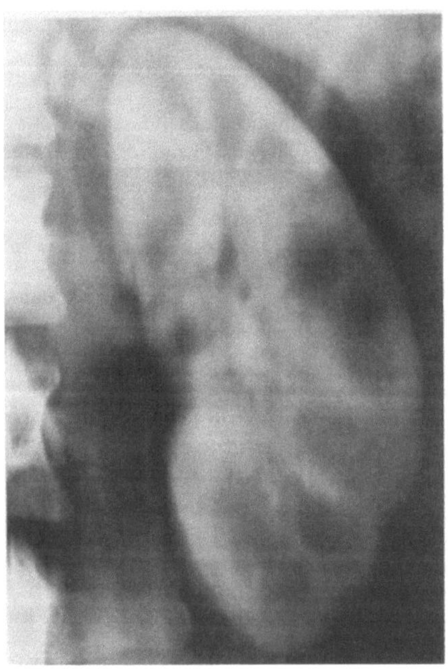

Fig. 13. Normal cortical nephrographic phase. Opacified columns of Bertin and translucent triangular medullary areas.

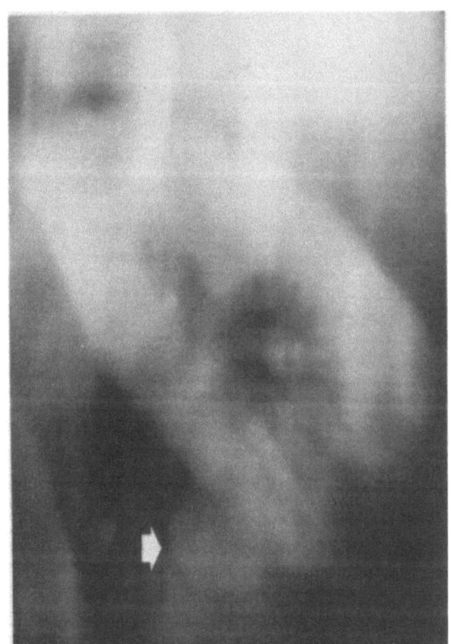

Fig. 14. Small hypernephroma (*arrow*). Cortical nephrographic phase.

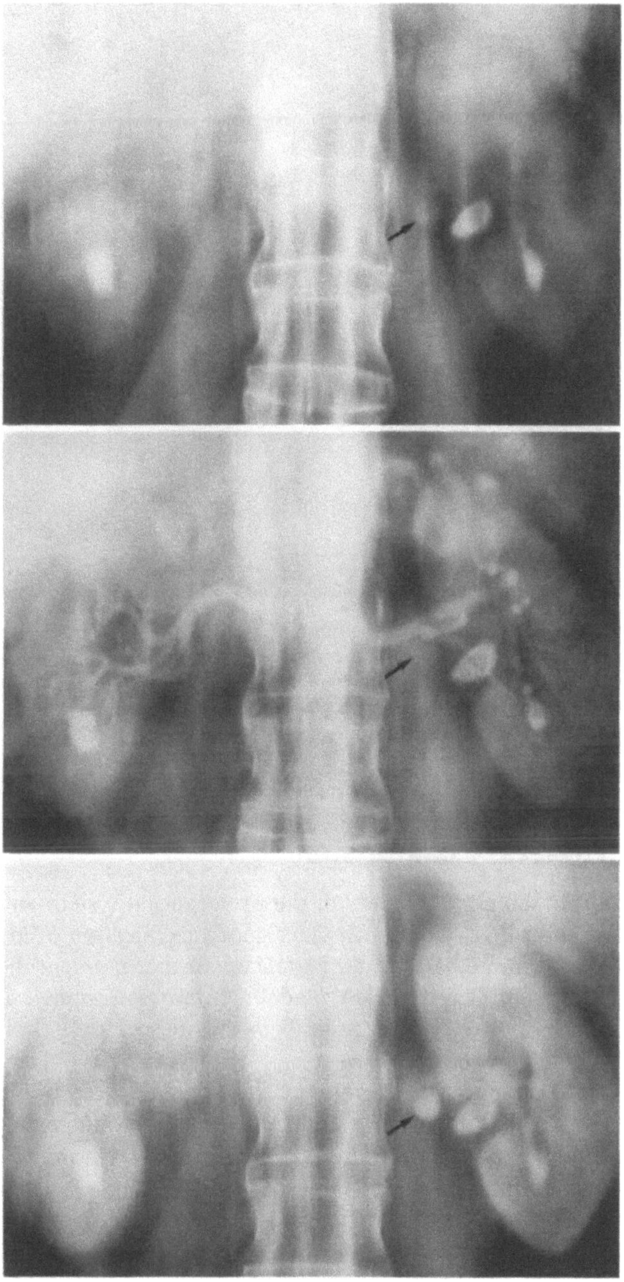

a

b

c

Fig. 15a–c. Venous opacity. **a** Preliminary tomogram. Bilateral opaque stones. There is a small rounded opacity in the hilar area (*arrow*). **b** Arterial phase. No enhancement of the opacity (*arrow*). **c** Cortical nephrographic phase and venous return. Enhancement of the opacity showing it to be a venous structure (*arrow*).

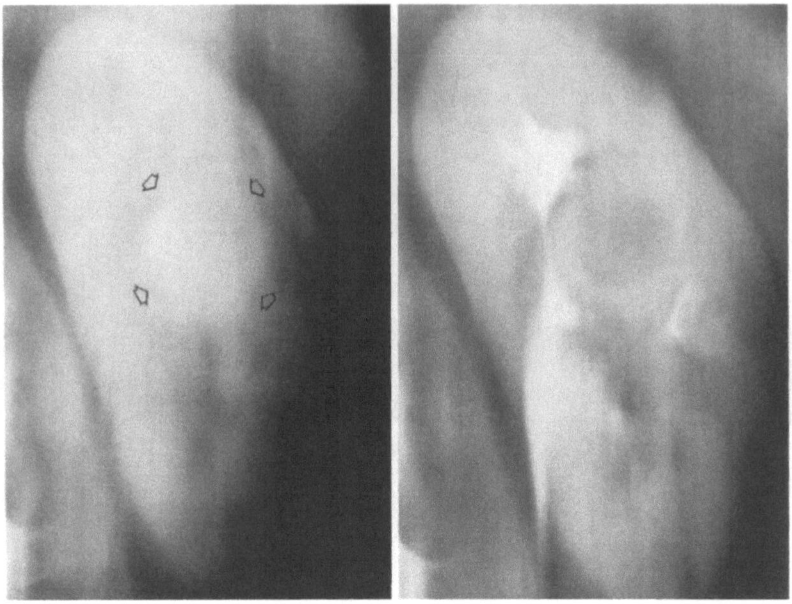

a b

Fig. 16a, b. Pseudotumor and cyst. **a** Cortical nephrographic phase. Rounded area (*arrows*) with a nephrographic pattern similar to that of the glomerular cortex. **b** Tubular nephrography. The nephrographic pattern at the periphery of the rounded area is similar to that of the adjacent parenchyma. Using ultrasonography, the central sharply delineated round translucency proved to be a benign cyst in the pseudotumor.

Urographic Phase – Ureteral Compression

Ureteral compression is indispensable in the study of the pyelocaliceal system and the proximal ureters (Bodart et al. 1978). It also provides good opacification of the distal ureters if a film is obtained immediately after its release; at that moment the accumulated opaque urine flows abundantly to the bladder. It must be applied at the precise point where the posterior skeletal wall is at its most anterior, which is at the entry to the pelvic inlet.

Ureteral compression should not be started before the functional integrity of the excretory system has been established: in normal studies, after one film obtained at 4 min has demonstrated the permeability of the ureters; in obstructive syndromes, only if it is necessary to study further the aspect of an obstructive factor located above the compression site.

Ureteral compression is the only adequate means of excluding or documenting abnormal filling defects of the excretory system.

Micturating Cystourethrography

The micturating cystouretrogram is frequently performed at the end of nephro-urography, especially when the examination of the upper tract has not documented the origin of the pathology (e.g., hematuria), or as the main part of the examination when symptoms suggest a lower tract pathology, the study of the upper tract then being part of a global evaluation of the urinary system. It is essentially the same technique as the voiding phase of other cystographies (retrograde or by a suprapubic puncture). It is performed in the upright position: in man, at a 45° oblique incidence with a 15° ascending beam; in women, in a strictly lateral position. One or two films are sufficient to reveal the urethral morphology. When voiding cystourethrography is desirable, an additional dose of contrast medium (40–100 cc) is frequently added to the initial rapid injection during the examination of the upper urinary tract. The study is performed when the patient has a voiding sensation. There is usually an interval for eating and drinking before the completion of the last part of the study.

Conclusion

The study of renal parenchyma and the upper and lower urinary tract is necessary in the evaluation of many diseases of the nephrourologic system. Intravenous nephrourography constitutes an important tool in the study of the entire urinary tract. The systematic use of this technique is justified in view of the quality of the information provided and in view of the fact that there is no increase in the risk, number, or intensity of side effects and no increase in the technical burden of the study. The three fundamental aspects of this detailed radiologic analysis are, in addition to the plain film, the very rapid injection of the contrast medium, the performance of tomograms to study the renal parenchyma at the early phase, and ureteric compression. Using these three principles, accurate investigation of the whole urinary system, between the renal arteries, and the urethral meatus becomes possible with only one radiologic investigation.

Acknowledgment. We are indebted to Dr. Pierre-Marie Bouloux for his invaluable assistance in the translation of the original French manuscript.

References

Bodart P, Dardenne AN, Claus D (1978) Radiodiagnostic – Haut appareil urinaire. Eléments de sémiologie. C.I.B. Bruxelles

Dardenne AN (1977) Nephrourography by rapid intravenous injection. Medicamundi 22: 26–29

Dardenne AN, Bodart P (1977a) La néphrotomographie de principe dans l'urographie intraveineuse. J Radiol Electrol Med Nucl 58:327

Dardenne AN, Bodart P (1977b) Fast injection intravenous nephrourography. Technique and results. J Belge Radiol 60:239–248

Dardenne AN, Bodart P, van Ypersele Ch, Van Changh P (1979) La néphro-urographie (N.U.I.V.). Trois ans d'expérience. J Belge Radiol 62:311

Ingrisch H, Holzgreve B, Sommer K, Westerburg KW, Frey KW (1980) Technik der Nierenarteriendarstellung in Rahmen des Ausscheidungsurogrammes Bolustechnik – Zeitbestimmung – Simultantomographie. Fortschr Röntgenstr 132, 4:422–427

Saxton HM (1969) Urography. Br J Radiol 42:321–346

van Ypersele Ch, Bodart P, Dardenne AN (1979) General techniques in clinical nephrology. In: Hamburger J, Crosnier J, Grünfeld JP (eds) Nephrology. Wiley, West Sussex

Contribution of Phlebography to the Diagnosis of Nonfunctioning Kidneys

H. U. Braedel, E. Schindler, and N. Papandreou

The diagnostic workup of urographically non functioning kidneys includes a series of procedures: retrograde and antegrade pyelography, sonography, computerized tomography (CT), and arteriography as an invasive method.

If the renal artery is not contrasted or if in spite of sufficient filling of the arterial branches a definite diagnosis cannot be made, retrograde phlebography is suggested as another helpful adjunct within an angiographic investigation.

Phlebography is performed:

1) In suspected renal agenesis or dysgenesis;
2) in obstruction of the renal artery (thrombosis, after embolism or trauma);
3) for differentiating malignant diseases from chronic inflammations (urothelial tumors, tumors of renal bed, retroperitoneal fibrosis, xanthogranulomatous pyelonephritis, abscesses).

Eight cases are presented to demonstrate the efficacy of selective renal phlebography in some of these entities.

Case Reports

Agenesis/Dysgenesis

Case 1 (W. H.). A 65-year-old male was hospitalized for evaluation of hypertension. An IVP revealed nonvisualization of the right kidney with hypertrophy of the left organ and a suspected mass in its middle portion. Sonography failed to demonstrate a kidney on the right side. At cystoscopy, two orifices were present. Blood pressure was measured at 160/100 mm Hg on medication. Angiography demonstrated a lateral cyst with a diameter of 5 cm in the middle part of the left kidney. A right renal artery could not be identified. Phlebography (Fig. 1) exhibited a venous convolution in the area of the kidney. Renal vein angiotensin I was 0.3 ng/ml per hour on the right side and 2.0 ng/ml per hour on the left. The cyst was removed surgically. Postoperative blood pressure remained normal off medication.

Case 2 (M. E.). A 32-year-old female suffered from right-sided flank pain for 5 years. Appendectomy had been performed 10 years previously. An IVP did not visualize the right kidney and ring-shaped calcifications were seen in the right upper abdomen. At cystoscopy, two orifices were found. A retrograde ureterogram showed a ureter of normal caliber ending at the os sacrum level. Sonography and

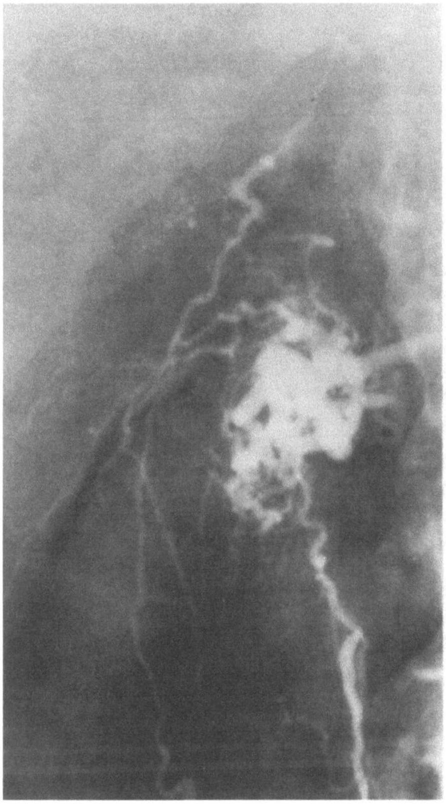

Fig. 1. Right-sided renal phlebogram: venous plexus at the level of the right kidney.

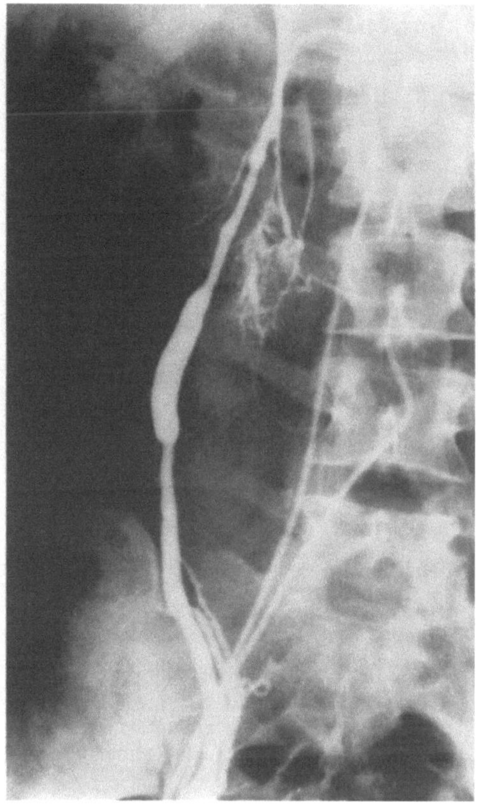

Fig. 2. Right-sided phlebogram: venous convolutions draining into the right ovarian vein. Lateral subtle arcuate veins deriving from an area of fine calcifications.

CT failed to identify a right kidney. A renal scan revealed absence of renal function on the right side. Phlebography (Fig. 2) showed tender vessels running from the right ovarian vein to the annular calcified structure; additionally, there was a venous convolution, medial to the ovarian vein, suggesting a dysgenic kidney.

Obstruction of the Renal Artery

Case 3 (G. A.). A 69-year-old female was admitted for a non functioning left kidney and hypertension. Arteriography could only demonstrate a small arterial bud on the left side. At phlebography (Fig. 3), there was a massive thrombosis in the preaortal portion of the renal vein and its intrarenal branches. The retroaortal portion of the renal vein was patent. Nephrectomy was performed. Histology revealed a subtotal infarction of the kidney, older anemic areas, thrombi in the renal veins, and an almost entire occlusion of the renal vein by a thrombus; a blood clot was found in the renal artery (Reported by Prof. Dr. Seeliger, Institute of Pathology).

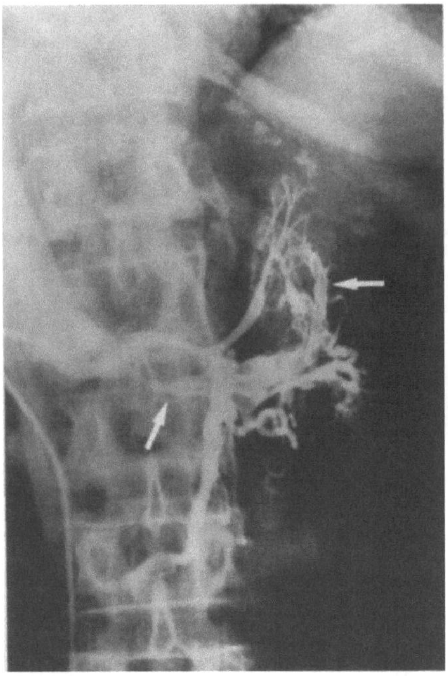

Fig. 3. Left-sided phlebogram: reduced venous system of the left kidney with thrombi in larger veins and the preaortal portion of the main renal vein (*arrows*). Normal adrenal veins.

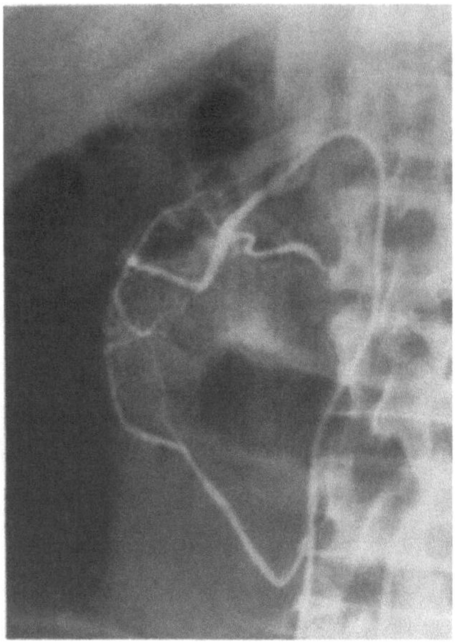

Fig. 4. Right-sided phlebogram: contrasting of exorenal arcade (Braedel et al. 1976).

Case 4 (S. E.). A 46-year-old male had been crushed between two railway cars 20 years previously. Blood pressure was measured at 160/100 mm Hg. Urinalysis was normal. Excretory urography revealed a nonvisualizing right kidney with calcifications in its area. There was a left-sided ureteropelvic junction obstruction. At arteriography, a medial right adrenal artery with a rich network of collaterals was encountered but no renal artery. Phlebography (Fig. 4) demonstrated the exorenal venous arcade; the renal vein could not be cannulated.

Differentiation of Malignant Disease from Chronic Inflammation

Case 5 (S. I.). A 49-year-old female had been treated with insulin for diabetes mellitus for 11 years. She was admitted for obesity, hypertension (210/110 mm Hg), and renal insufficiency due to Kimmelstiel-Wilson syndrome. She reported loss of weight, weakness, and nausea. A palpable mass in the right upper abdomen and a nonfunctioning right kidney at urography suggested a renal tumor. Examination showed microscopic hematuria. Creatinine was 3.6 mg% with severe metabolic acidosis. The erythrocyte sedimentation rate was 145/150 mm/h. A renal scan failed to delineate a kidney on the right side. A retrograde pyelogram was attempted, but the renal pelvis could not be visualized. At angiography (Fig. 5 a), a peripheral vessel rarefaction was encountered together with numerous renal pelvic

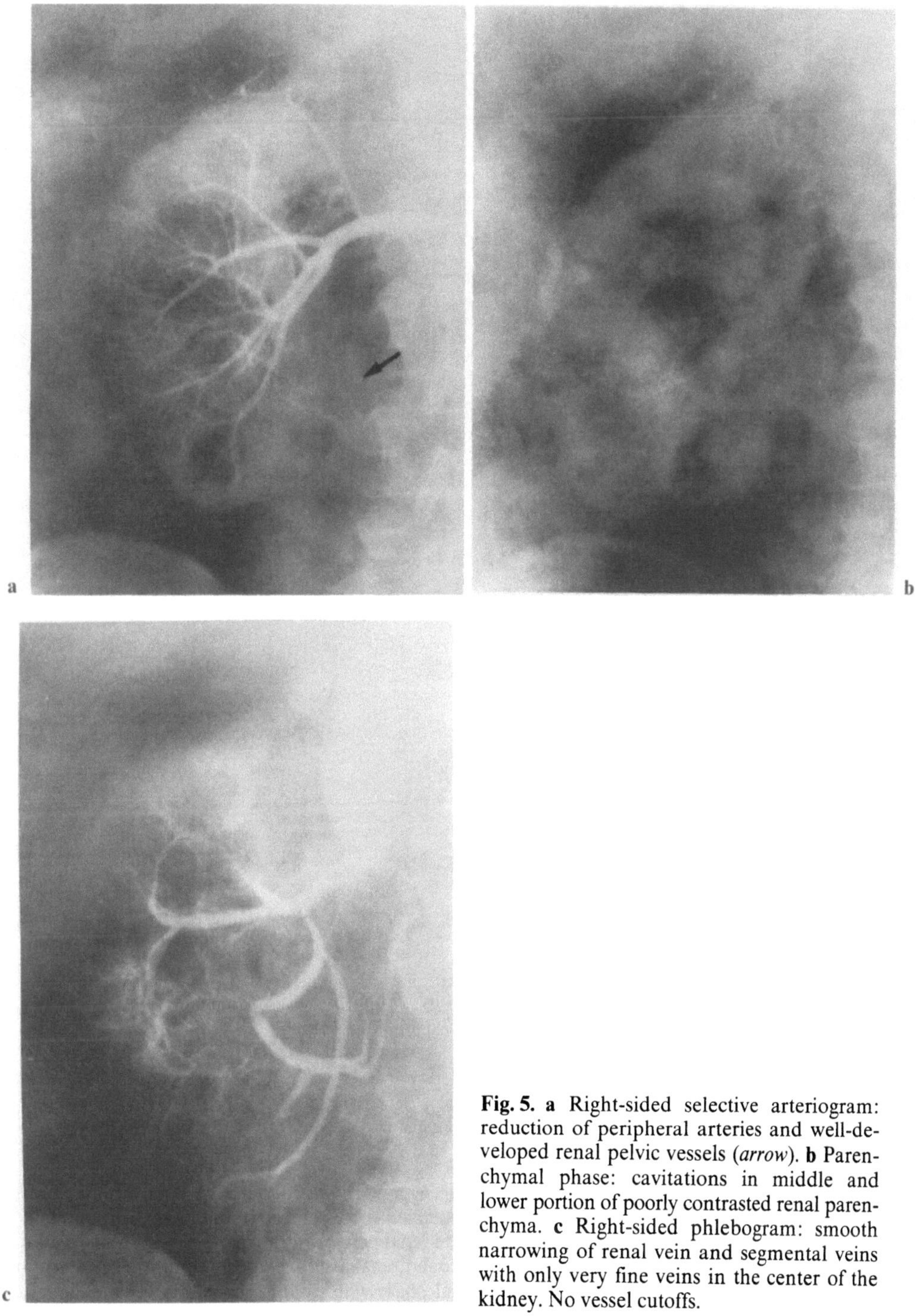

Fig. 5. a Right-sided selective arteriogram: reduction of peripheral arteries and well-developed renal pelvic vessels (*arrow*). **b** Parenchymal phase: cavitations in middle and lower portion of poorly contrasted renal parenchyma. **c** Right-sided phlebogram: smooth narrowing of renal vein and segmental veins with only very fine veins in the center of the kidney. No vessel cutoffs.

a b c

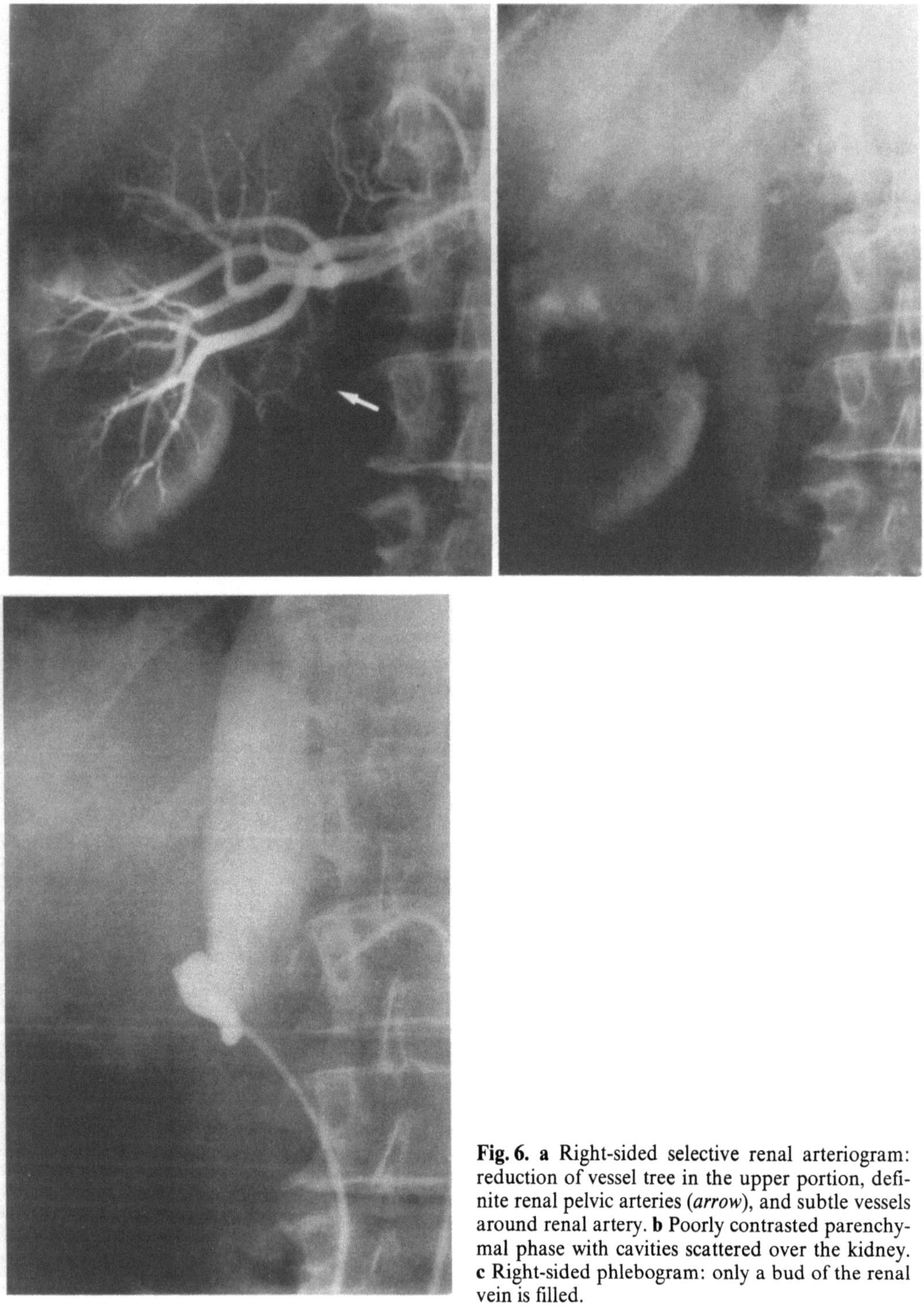

Fig. 6. a Right-sided selective renal arteriogram: reduction of vessel tree in the upper portion, definite renal pelvic arteries (*arrow*), and subtle vessels around renal artery. **b** Poorly contrasted parenchymal phase with cavities scattered over the kidney. **c** Right-sided phlebogram: only a bud of the renal vein is filled.

arteries. At the time of the parenchymal phase (Fig. 5 b), cavitations in the middle and lower portion were seen. Phlebography (Fig. 5 c) revealed a distinct narrowing of the main and larger segmental renal veins with only some fine vessels in the center of the organ. At nephrectomy, parahilar and paracaval hazelnut-sized lymph nodes were removed. Histology showed a severe destructive granulomatous pyelonephritis with unspecific lymph node reaction (Reported by Prof. Dr. Dhom, Institute of Pathology).

Case 6 (A. J.). A 64-year-old male was admitted for painless gross hematuria. RBC's were too numerous to count. ESR was 55/85 mm/h. The right kidney did not visualize on IVP. Sufficient filling of the right renal pelvis was not accomplished by a retrograde pyelogram. At selective angiography (Fig. 6 a, b), a vessel rarefaction in the area of the upper pole was encountered. There were well-developed pelvic arteries, in addition to fine arteries around the main trunk of the renal artery. Several larger defects were seen scattered over the right kidney. At retrograde phlebography (Fig. 6 c), only a stump of the right renal vein could be contrasted. Nephrectomy was performed. Histology showed a papillary urothelial carcinoma grade III (Reported by Prof. Dr. Dhom, Institute of Pathology).

Case 7 (H. K.). A 59-year-old male was treated for hypertension. The left kidney did not visualize on IVP and the left orifice could not be cannulated. At selective arteriography (Fig. 7 a; Dr. W. Herbig, Dr. P. Nödl, Kaiserslautern), well-developed renal pelvic arteries suggested a renal pelvic carcinoma. The patient was admitted for nephrectomy. Creatinine was 1.9 mg% and ESR was 101/113 mm/h. Left-sided renal phlebography (Fig. 7 b) revealed a definite concentric narrowing of the renal vein with a rich capsular venous network. Intrarenal veins were not contrasted and left adrenal veins were normal. Radiology continued to suggest a renal pelvic carcinoma. At nephrectomy, a small contracted hydronephrotic kidney was encountered with an ectatic proximal ureter, which was compressed by a dense fibrous tissue in its distal portion. Histology demonstrated retroperitoneal fibrosis with chronic destructive pyelonephritis and renal contraction (Reported by Prof. Dr. Dhom, Institute of Pathology).

Case 8 (S. H.). A 53-year-old male was admitted for a nonvisualizing left kidney, thrombosis in his left leg, and left-sided flank pain. A retrograde pyelogram showed complete obstruction of the left ureter at the L-4 level. ESR was 13/27 mm/h. Left-sided selective renal arterpography (Fig. 8 a) demonstrated a distinct development of capsular arteries and some tortuous vessels in the hilar region with normal intrarenal vessel tree and parenchyma. At the time of a left-sided pharmaco phlebogram (Fig. 8 b), an almond-sized thrombus within a somewhat narrow left renal vein was seen with a reduction of the intrarenal venous system in the upper portion and distinct capsular veins. Radiologic diagnosis was tumor in the left renal hilar region. At surgical exploration, the entire hilum was infiltrated with firm tumorous tissue, which caused the complete obstruction of the upper ureter. A radical nephrectomy was accomplished and histopathologic diagnosis was well-differentiated adenocarcinoma (Reported by Prof. Dr. Städtler, Institute of Pathology). To date, no primary tumor has been found.

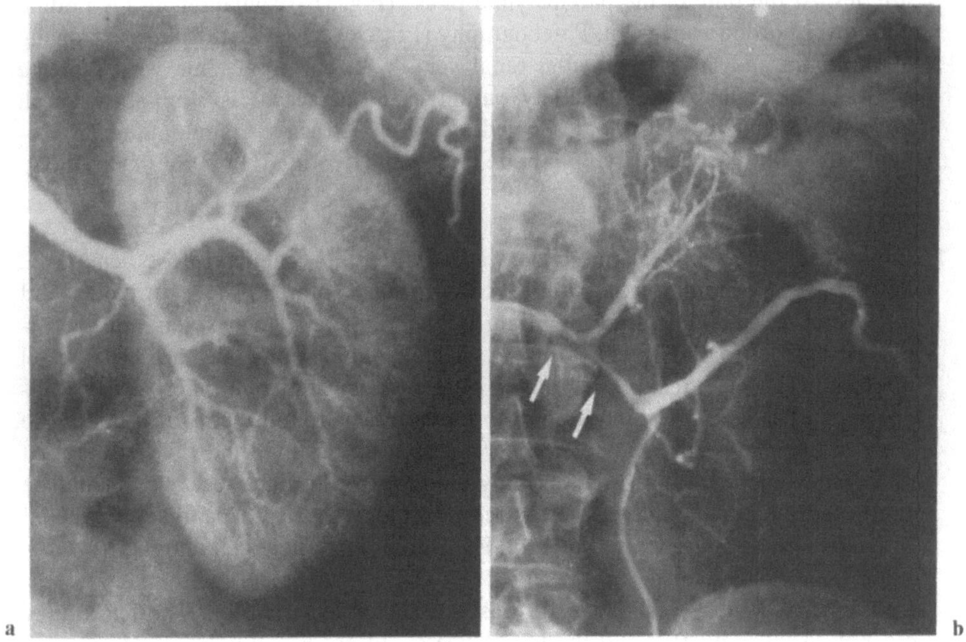

Fig. 7. a Left-sided selective arteriogram: marked renal pelvic arteries with otherwise normal vessel tree (Braedel et al. 1979). **b** Left-sided phlebogram: explicit concentric narrowing of left renal vein (*double arrow*). Rich capsular venous network with no intrarenal veins contrasted. Normal left adrenal venous system (Braedel et al. 1979).

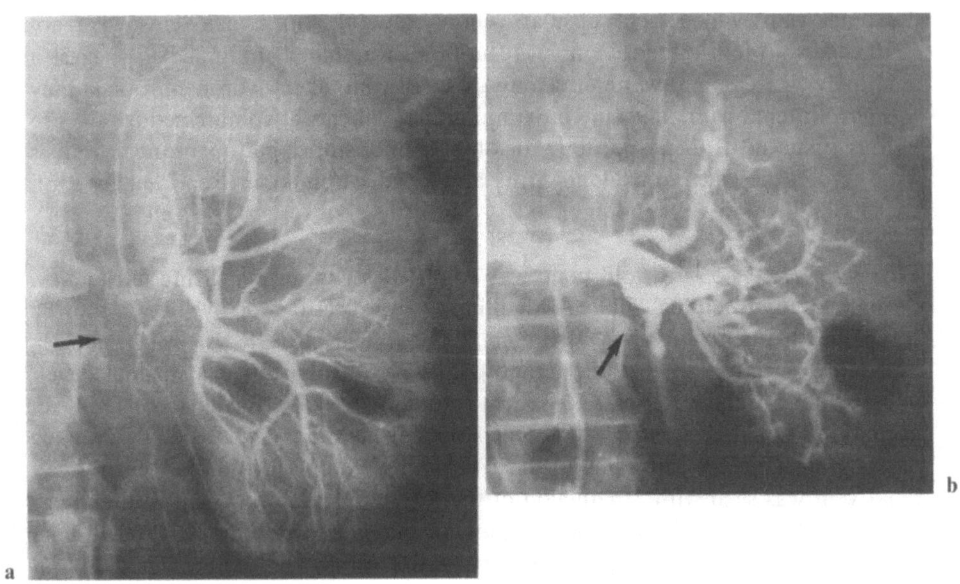

Fig. 8. a Left-sided selective renal arteriogram: normal intrarenal vessel tree and development of capsular arteries with tortuous course in hilar region (*arrow*) (Braedel et al. 1979). **b** Left-sided pharmacophlebogram: almond-sized tumor thrombus in narrowed renal vein (*arrow*). Reduction of intrarenal venous system in upper portion. Marked capsular veins (Braedel et al. 1979).

Discussion

Renal agenesis and dysgenesis are often incidentally discovered during routine investigations. IVP and cystoscopy may provide some diagnostic hints, but the renal parenchyma cannot even be judged by retrogade pyelography in the presence of a blind-ending ureter. Nuclear medicine is not very helpful either. Sonography and CT cannot always give a definite diagnosis, as demonstrated by our cases. At aortography, the small arteries of a dysgenetic kidney often are not sufficiently visualized. Selective arteriography is usually not feasible and entails the danger of inadvertent cannulation of a lumbar artery with a possible spinal cord lesion (Broy 1971).

Renal phlebography offers the following advantages (Athanasoulis et al. 1973; Itzchak et al. 1974; Braedel et al. 1976): The larger caliber of the renal veins allows for an easy catheterization, especially on the left side, where, due to embryology, a renal vein is always developed, although in cases of renal agenesis the main renal vein on this side is thinner than normal. On the right side, cannulation of the small renal vein of a dysgenetic kidney is more difficult, but is much easier than, for example, the catheterization of the right adrenal vein. If a renal vein cannot be demonstrated on the right side, a renal vein or a small parenchymal nubbin cannot be absolutely excluded, but the failure rate is low. A rudimentary pelvic kidney probably cannot even be demonstrated by phlebography. The necessity for a complete diagnostic workup of a suspected dysgenetic kidney, however, will largely depend upon the clinical symptomatology, above all on the presence of hypertension or a suspected malignancy (Hynes et al. 1970). In renal artery obstruction, phlebography remains the only angiographic diagnostic method (Athanasoulis et al. 1973; Itzchak et al. 1974; Braedel et al. 1976).

Diagnostic difficulties are sometimes encountered in the differentiation of hypovascular tumors from inflammatory diseases (Caplan et al. 1967; Michel et al. 1975; Barth et al. 1976; Morehouse et al. 1978). Lang (1973) and Levin et al. (1976) underline the fact that, above all, narrowings and indentations of arteries as well as distinct contrasting of pelviureteric and capsular vessels can be seen both in chronic inflammatory and tumorous disease.

Sudden cutoffs of renal veins, especially in larger vessels and irregular wall indentations, and possibly also in the presence of thrombi, are in favor of a tumor (Boijsen and Folin 1961; Renert et al. 1972; Rösch et al. 1975; Smith et al. 1975). On the other hand, filiform narrowings of intrarenal veins are said to be characteristic of inflammatory changes (Braedel et al. 1978, 1979; Goldman et al. 1978; Pingoud et al. 1979).

Summary

Retrograde renal phlebography is a valuable diagnostic adjunct in cases of urographically nonvisualizing kidneys that cannot be sufficiently evaluated by other investigative methods, including arteriography. Main indications are renal dysgenesis, obstruction of the renal artery, and differential diagnostic problems with hypovascular tumors and chronic inflammatory processes. Case reports demonstrate the importance of this method.

References

Athanasoulis CA, Brown B, Baum S (1973) Selective renal venography in differentiation between congenitally absent and small contracted kidney. Radiology 108:301–305

Barth KH, Lightman NJ, Ridolfi RL, Catalona WJ (1976) Acute pyelonephritis simulating poorly vascularized renal neoplasm. Non-specificity of angiographic criteria. J Urol 116:650–652

Boijsen E, Folin J (1961) Angiography in carcinoma of the renal pelvis. Acta Radiol [Diagn] (Stockh) 56:81–93

Braedel HU, Schindler E, Moeller JF, Polsky MS (1976) Renal phlebography: an aid in the diagnosis of the absent or non-functioning kidney. J Urol 116:703–707

Braedel HU, Schindler E, Polsky MS (1978) Séminologie radiographique, et en particulier angiographique, des affections suppurées du rein. J Radiol Electrol Med Nucl 59: 141–148

Braedel HU, Schindler E, Polsky MS, Papandreou N (1979) Differentialdiagnostische Gesichtspunkte bei der Angiographie stummer Nieren. Fortschr Röntgenstr 131:9–16

Broy H (1971) Die Querschnittslähmung, eine fatale angiographische Komplikation, Kasuistik und Übersicht. Fortschr Röntgenstr 114:353–366

Caplan LH, Siegelmann SS, Bosniak MA (1967) Angiography in inflammatory space-occupying lesions of the kidney. Radiology 88:14–23

Goldman ML, Gorelkin L, Rudé III JC, Sybers RG, O'Brien DP (1978) Epinephrine renal venography in severe inflammatory disease of the kidney. Radiology 127:93–101

Hynes DM, Watkin EM (1970) Renal agenesis – roentgenologic problem. AJR 110:772–777

Itzchak Y, Adar R, Mozes M, Deutsch V (1974) Renal venography in the diagnosis of agenesis and small contracted kidney. Clin Radiol 25:379–383

Lang EK (1973) Roentgenographic assessment of asymptomatic renal lesions. An analysis of the confidence level of diagnoses established by sequential roentgenographic investigation. Radiology 109:257–269

Levin DC, Gordon D, Kinkhabwala M, Becker JA (1976) Reticular neovascularity in malignant and inflammatory renal masses. Radiology 120:61–68

Michel JR, Vital JL, Moreau JF, Affre J (1975) Le diagnostic radiologique des tumeurs pyélo-calicielles, accent mis sur l'interêt de l'arteriographie surtout après épreuve à l'angiotensine. J Radiol Electrol Med Nucl 56:875–886

Morehouse HT, Panchacharam P, Friedenberg RM, Biuse ThJ (1978) Arterial encasement in xanthogranulomatous pyelonephritis. Radiology 128:617–618

Pingoud EG, Osher Pais S, Glickman M (1979) Epinephrine renal venography in acute bacterial infection of the kidney. AJR 133:665–669

Renert WA, Rudin LJ, Casarella WJ (1972) Renal vein thrombosis in carcinoma of renal pelvis. AJR 114:735–740

Rösch J, Antonovic R, Goldman ML, Dotter CT (1975) Epinephrine renal venography. Fortschr Röntgenstr 123:501–515

Smith JC jr, Rösch J, Athanasoulis CA, Baum S, Waltman AC, Goldman M (1975) Renal venography in the evaluation of poorly vascularized neoplasm of the kidney. AJR 123: 552–556

Spermatic Phlebography in Cryptorchidism

J. F. Jiménez Cruz, I. Perez-Bustamante, S. Zubicoa Espeleta, S. Navío Niño, J. F. García Alonso, and C. Romero Aguirre

The incidence of clinically impalpable testes is approximately 20% in an undescended testes population (Levitt et al. 1978). When a testis is not palpable it may be absent or it may be located anywhere along the course of its embryologic descent from the level of the renal fossa to its exit from the inguinal canal. Different methods have been employed for the preoperative localization of these testes: pneumoperitoneography (Lunderquist and Rafstedt 1967), herniogram (Dwoskin and Kuhn 1973), selective testicular arteriography (Ben-Menachen et al. 1974), selective testicular phlebography (Jacobs 1969; Weiss et al. 1979), and sonography (Madrazo et al. 1979). For the last 3 years we have been using spermatic phlebography in cases of nonpalpable undescended testes.

Before spermatic phlebography is recommended, the patient undergoes a physical examination on at least three different occasions, by more than one specialist. If both testes are nonpalpable, we first perform HCG stimulation tests (LH-RH). If these are positive we recommend phlebography.

Radiologic Technique

We use the Seldinger technique in the femoral vein. Numbers 5 F–7 F catheters are employed according to the age of the patient. For catheterization of the right spermatic vein, we use a double curved catheter while the left spermatic vein requires a J-shaped single curved catheter. We inject manually 8 ml contrast medium at 60%, with a flux of 2 ml/s. A series of X-rays is taken at a frequency of one shot per second, for 10 s.

In children under 10 years old, the examination is carried out during anesthesia. In older children and adults, an anesthetic is not necessary.

Results

We have performed 21 spermatic phlebographies in 15 patients, six with bilateral and nine with unilateral *nonpalpable undescended testes.* Of the unilateral, five were left and four were right sided. Seven patients were under 7 years old and six were adults. We obtained four different radiographic patterns (Table 1). No complications were observed.

Pattern I. In ten cases, complete or partial filling of the pampiniform-like plexus was achieved. The filling was sufficiently demonstrative of the presence of testes (Fig. 1). On occasions it may appear that there is no pampini-form-like plexus, as

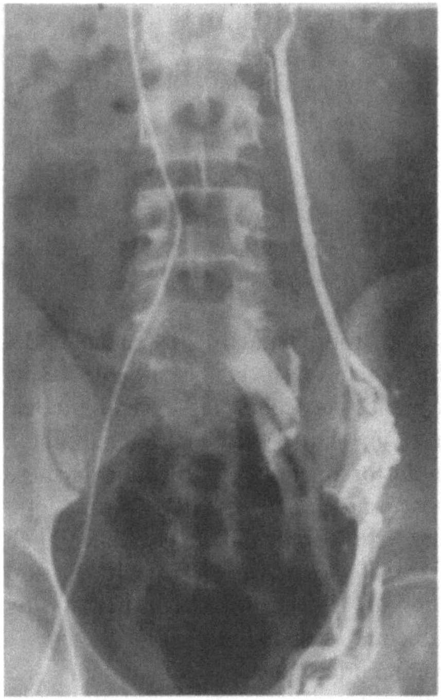

Fig. 1. Complete filling of pampiniform-like plexus: Intraabdominal testis.

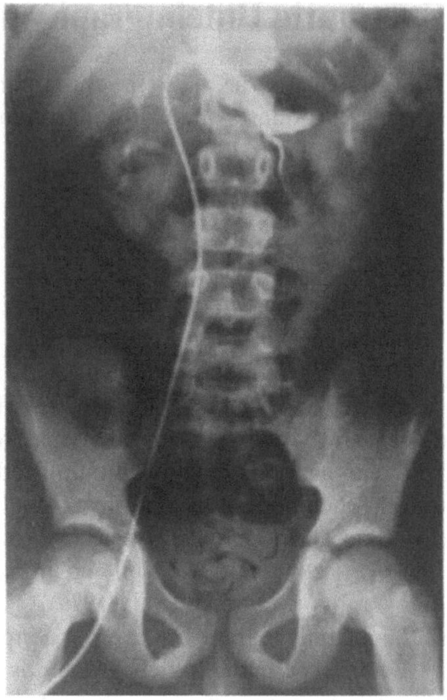

Fig. 2. Filling of a short segment of spermatic vein, tapering to a blind ending.

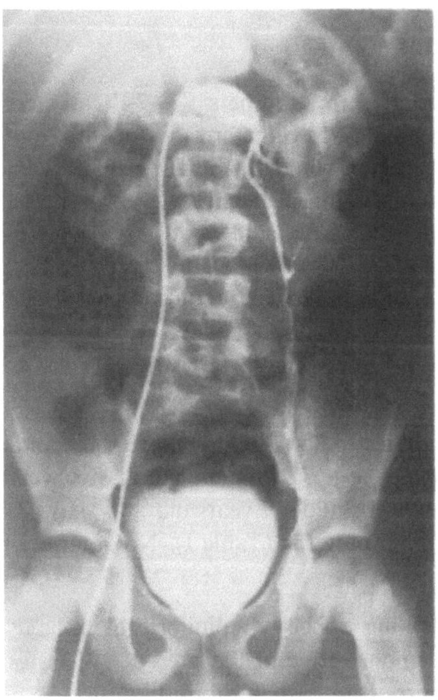

Fig. 3. The same case as in Fig. 2. With a Valsalva maneuver, complete filling of spermatic vein and pampiniform plexus was obtained. Inguinal testis.

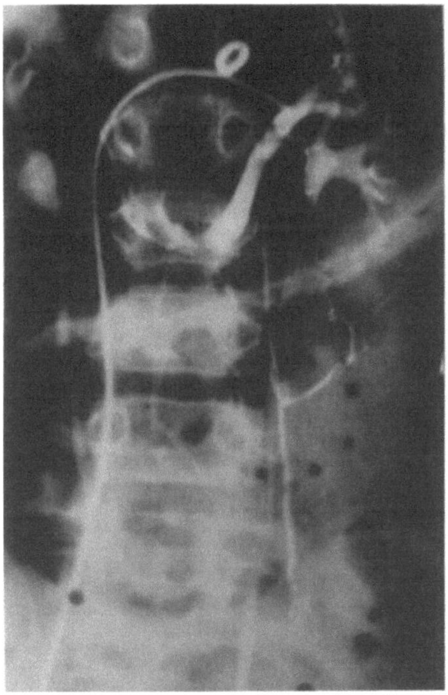

Fig. 4. Spermatic vein ending in three branches (brush-like image). Intraabdominal testis.

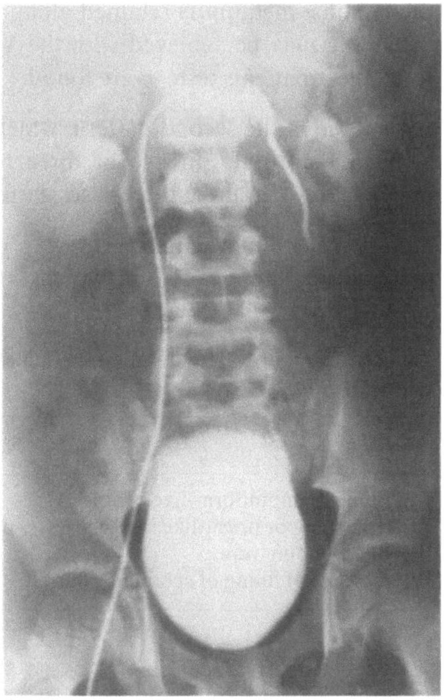

Fig. 5. Filling of the short vein tapering to a blind ending. No testis was found at surgery.

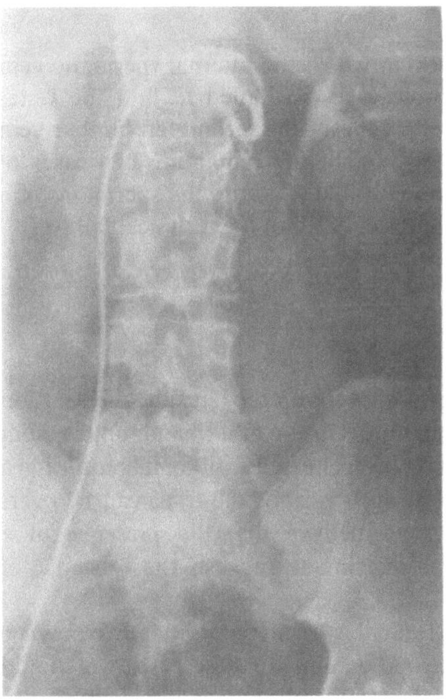

Fig. 6. Absence of internal spermatic vein. Filling of the second lumbar vein. No testis was found at surgery.

the contrast medium is retained along the spermatic vein (Fig. 2). In certain cases, the filling may be achieved with the Valsalva or other similar maneuvers (Fig. 3). In all these patients testes were found.

Pattern II. In the second pattern, which was obtained in three cases, the spermatic vein ends abruptly, in two or three branches, occasionally forming a brush-like image (Fig. 4). In these three cases, testes were found.

Pattern III. Blind-ending vein was observed in the third pattern, which was presented in three cases. In two cases we found a short vein, tapering to a blind ending (Fig. 5). In these cases no testes were found. In one adult the spermatic vein ended in a saccular dilatation. During surgery it was found that this was caused by the transection of the spermatic vessels in the course of a previous operation that failed to locate the testes. This was found, atrophied, in an ectopic transpubic position.

Table 1. The four different patterns of phlebography in nonpalpable testes.

Pattern	Number of cases
I. Filling pampiniform-like plexus	10
II. Branching or brush-like image	3
III. Blind-ending vein	3
IV. Absence of filling of spermatic vein	5

Pattern IV. This group consisted of five cases, in which the internal spermatic vein was not identified phlebographically. In three cases we failed to find the testes during surgery. In two of these cases, with left agenesis, the second left lumbar vein was filled in the course of phlebography (Fig. 6). In the remaining two cases of nonpalpable undescended right testis, we were unable to locate the spermatic vein in spite of the existence of the testis. These represent 9.5% of the technical failures.

Discussion

Because of the anatomic situation of the spermatic vein on the left side, the location is technically easy and sure and requires little time. On the other hand, on the right side, because of anatomic variations, it may be technically difficult, requiring a lengthy examination before location and even on occasions the testis can be overlooked as occurred in two of our cases. We believe that the presence of a pampiniform-like plexus, branches, or brush-like image suggests the existence of the testis.

The blind-ending vein is suggestive of testicular agenesis although it may be caused by the incomplete filling of the spermatic vein. In these cases we should suspect the presence of valves or technical defects. For this reason it is necessary to employ the Valsalva or similar maneuver before completing the examination. On the left side the filling of the second lumbar vein, in the absence of the internal spermatic vein, is suggestive of testicular agenesis, but further data is required to confirm this deduction. At present the finding of blind-ending vein or failure to locate the vein does not eliminate the need for surgery. In the case of blind-ending vein or of an image demonstrative of the presence of the testis the surgical exploration must be directed to the place indicated by phlebography. Thus, phlebography facilitates surgery as it enables the surgeon to plan his procedure, above all in cases of intraabdominal testis. In this way morbidity is reduced as well as the possibility of overlooking the testes.

References

Ben-Menachen Y, De Berardinis MC, Salinas R (1974) Localization of intraabdominal testes by selective testicular arriography: A case report. J Urol 112:493–494

Dwoskin JY, Kuhn JP (1973) Herniograms in undescended testes and hydroceles. J Urol 109:520–523

Jacobs J (1969) Selective gonadal venography. Radiology 92:885–888

Levitt SB, Kogan SJ, Engel RM, Weiss RM, Martin DC, Ehrlich RM (1978) The impalpable testis: A rational approach to management. J Urol 120:515–520

Lunderquist A, Rafstedt S (1967) Roentgenologic diagnosis of cryptorchidism. J Urol 98:219–223

Madrazo BL, Klugo RC, Parks JA, Diloreto R (1979) Ultrasonographic demonstration of undescended testes. Radiology 133:181–L183

Weiss RM, Glickman MG, Lytton B (1979) Clinical implications of gonadal venography in the management of the non-palpable undescended testis. J Urol 121:745–749

Scrotal Thermography in Subfertile Males

W. F. Hendry and C. H. Jones

Summary

Twelve fertile and 40 subfertile males with possible varicoceles have been studied clinically and by scrotal thermography. In ten fertile subjects with no clinical evidence of varicocele, the scrotal temperature was 29.5–31.5 °C on anterior view, and 29.6–32.2 °C on underview, after 10 min equilibration with an ambient temperature of 19 °C. Two fertile controls and 23 subfertile patients had thermographic abnormalities associated with the presence of a varicocele. Seventeen subfertile males suspected of possible varicocele were thermographically normal and were therefore not operated on. Scrotal thermography provides objective evidence of increased scrotal temperature associated with varicocele, which is clinically valuable in the subfertile patient with doubtful clinical findings, in defining whether the varicocele is unilateral or bilateral, and in assessing the results of surgery. Several subfertile patients appeared to derive benefit from reoperation for residual or recurrent varicocele associated with persistent thermographic abnormality.

Introduction

In man, as in many other mammals, the testes are situated in the scrotum apparently to maintain their temperature from 2 °C to 7 °C lower than core body temperature. There are powerful physiological mechanisms for maintaining this differential, particularly by countercurrent heat exchange between venous blood leaving the scrotum and arterial blood entering the testis. If this normal temperature gradient is abolished, for example by heating or insulating the scrotum or by returning the testes to the abdominal cavity, spermatogenesis is depressed and may eventually cease (for a comprehensive review, see Setchell 1978). Varicocele is caused by reversal of blood flow in the internal spermatic vein (Ahlberg et al. 1966; Brown et al. 1967); this interferes with the normal circulation of blood in the scrotum and produces an increase in temperature, the extent of which depends on the severity of the varicocele (Kormano et al. 1970). This condition is very common, affecting about 10% of young men (Johnson et al. 1970), and it occurs in about 20% of subfertile males (Hendry et al. 1973), when it may be associated with a variable degree of impaired spermatogenesis (Fritjofsson and Ahren 1967; MacLeod 1969; Dubin and Hotchkiss 1969).

There have been many reports of improvement in seminal analysis in about 70% of men following ligation of varicocele, with pregnancies in up to 55% of the wives (Dubin and Amelar 1977). In practice, however, there may be difficulties in the clinical diagnosis of the presence or extent of a varicocele. In some patients it may be difficult to be sure whether there is a varicocele or not, even with coughing, or a Valsalva manoeuvre. It may not be clear whether the varicocele is unilateral or bilateral and this may be important – for example, Dubin and Amelar (1977) described bilateral ligation in 15% of 986 cases. Finally, there may be a few residual dilated veins after operation, and if the sperm count fails to improve it will be important to define whether the veins are significant or not. In order to clarify situations such as these, objective measurement of the effects of the varicocele on the scrotum and its contents is required.

Thermography provides a satisfactory methof of measurement of scrotal surface temperature, and the absence of subcutaneous fat allows accurate assessment of the temperature of the underlying testes. Kormano et al. (1970) used thermography to show that varicocele increased the temperature of the left side of the scrotum, and Comhaire et al. (1976) showed that thermographic abnormality correlated well with the presence of internal spermatic vein reflux demonstrated by retrograde caval venography. The non-invasive nature of thermography makes it preferable to phlebography for routine investigation and, because it involves no radiation hazard, it can be repeated as often as necessary in sequential studies on an individual patient before and after treatment.

Patients and Methods

Forty subfertile males with possible varicoceles and 12 fertile control subjects were examined clinically, and studied by scrotal thermography. The methods of clinical management and details of the thermographic techniques have been described previously (Hendry et al. 1973; Jones and Hendry 1979). The scrotal temperature was measured with the Rank Thermographic System or the 680 AGA Medical Thermovision after 10 min equilibration with an ambient temperature of 19 °C. The subjects stood in front of the thermography camera with legs slightly apart and penis held out of the field of view. The anterior view was supplemented by an underside or posterior view obtained with the aid of a narrow polished aluminium mirror supported at an angle of 45° beneath the scrotum (see Fig. 1).

Forty subfertile males were examined thermographically for the following reasons:

Group 1 – In 12 patients a small varicocele was suspected but the clinical findings were too indefinite to allow a firm conclusion to be reached.

Group 2 – In seven patients there was doubt as to whether a varicocele was unilateral or bilateral.

Group 3 – Twenty-one patients had had ligation of the internal spermatic vein by an inguinal approach at least 3 months previously, and it was clinically uncertain whether the varicocele had completely disappeared or not. Several of these patients were studied on more than one occasion, before and after reoperation on the varicocele, usually by the suprainguinal approach (Palomo 1949).

Twelve medical students who were known to be fertile because they had provided sperms for successful donor insemination were also examined. Ten appeared clinically normal and two had obvious varicoceles.

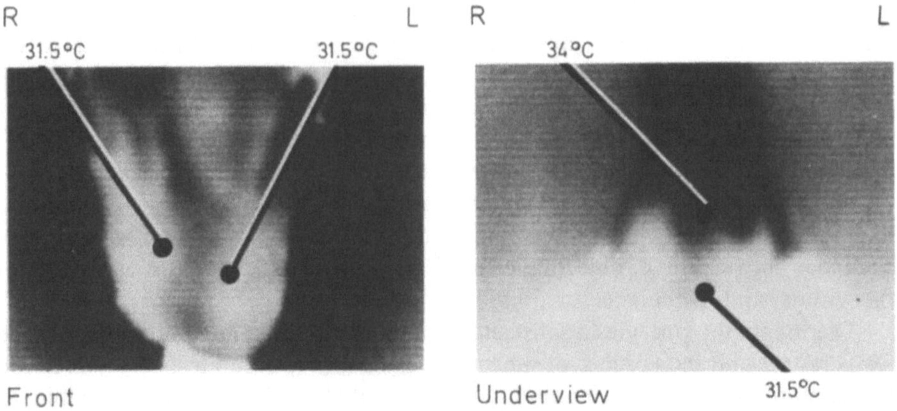

Fig. 1. Anterior and underview thermograms in subfertile male with doubtful clinical findings; normal anterior findings, but markedly raised temperature on left side posteriorly.

Results

Normal Controls. The results in the ten fertile control subjects with no clinical evidence of varicocele are shown in Table 1. All had scrotal temperatures of 29.5–31.5 °C (mean 30.4 °C) measured from the front, and 29.6–32.2 °C (mean 30.7 °C) measured from below. The maximum temperature difference between the two sides was 0.3 °C. The two fertile control subjects with varicoceles had scrotal temperatures as follows:

Subject 1 – 29.8 °C (right) and 34.1 °C (left) on anterior view, 30.4 °C both sides on underview;

Subject 2 – 31.8 °C both sides anterior view, 35 °C both sides on underview.

Subfertile Males. In the subfertile patients, the thermograph was considered to be abnormal if the scrotal temperature exceeded 32 °C, or if there was a difference between the two sides of more than 1 °C. The results in the 12 men with possible varicoceles (group 1) are shown in Table 2. Thermographic abnormality was demonstrated in five patients, four of whom had scrotal temperatures above 32 °C; the abnormality was only detected on the underview in one patient (Fig. 4.1) and was bilateral in one case. In one patient the left side was 31.5 °C, the right side 29 °C; giving an abnormal temperature differential of 2.5 °C. All five patients with thermographic abnormalities had ligation of varicocele, while the seven patients with normal thermograms were not operated on.

Table 1. Scrotal thermographic findings in ten fertile control subjects with no clinical evidence of varicocele (range and mean). Maximum difference between the sides was 0.3 °C.

	Anterior	Underview
Right	29.5 – 31.2 °C (mean 30.4)	29.6 – 32.2 °C (mean 30.7)
Left	29.5 – 31.5 °C (mean 30.5)	29.6 – 32.2 °C (mean 30.7)

In the seven patients with possible bilateral varicoceles (group 2), elevated temperatures on both sides of the scrotum were observed in four cases, although in only one was there a temperature difference between the two sides of more than 1 °C (Table 3). All four patients had bilateral ligation of varicoceles (see Fig. 2). In the remaining three patients the thermographic findings were normal and no surgery was done.

Table 4 shows the results in the 21 patients (group 3) who had had a varicocele ligated 3 months or more previously, and in whom there was doubt on clinical examination whether or not the varices had gone completely. Seven were normal and no further surgery was considered. In 14 patients, however, there were persistent thermographic abnormalities in the scrotum. In six patients the left side was more than 1 °C warmer than the right indicating persistent left-sided varicocele. In a further six patients, the *right* testis was warmer than the left, probably

Table 2. Results of scrotal thermography in 12 subfertile males with possible small varicocele (group 1).

Number of patients	Temperature > 32 °C		Temperature difference > 1 °C	Normal
	Left	Right		
12	4	1	4	7

Table 3. Results of scrotal thermography in seven subfertile males with possible bilateral varicocele (group 2).

Number of patients	Temperature > 32 °C		Temperature difference > 1 °C	Normal
	Left	Right		
7	4	4	1	3

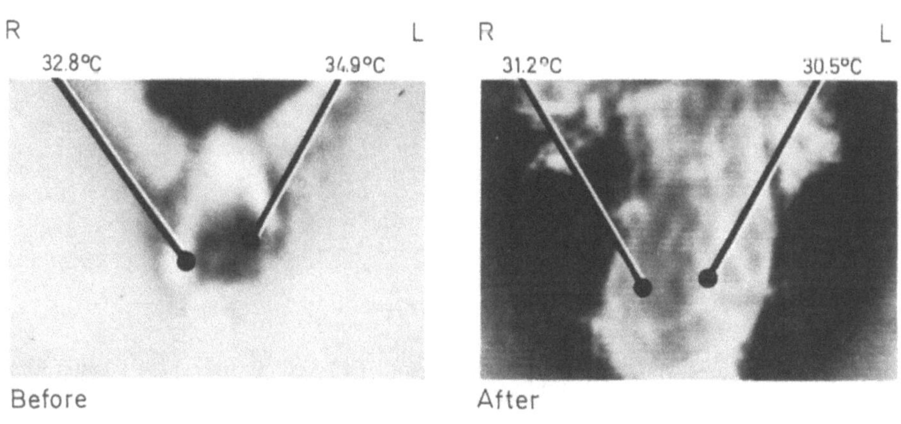

Fig. 2. Bilateral varicoceles, before and after surgical correction.

Table 4. Results of scrotal thermography in 21 subfertile males with possible residual or recurrent varicoceles, 3 months or more after surgical ligation (group 3). Five produced pregnancies after re-operation.

Number of patients	Temperature > 32 °C		Temperature difference > 1 °C		Normal
	Left	Right	L>R	R>L	
21	8	8	6	6	7

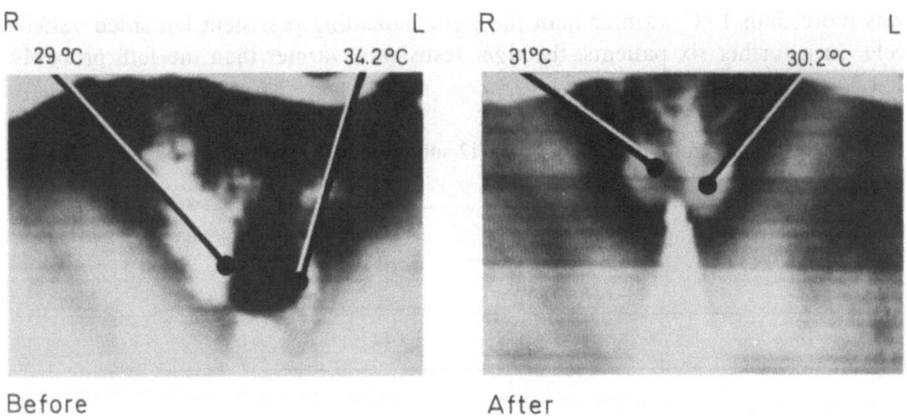

Fig. 3. Thermographic findings in subfertile male after previous high ligation of varicocele. Note persistence of raised temperature on left side, corrected by re-operation.

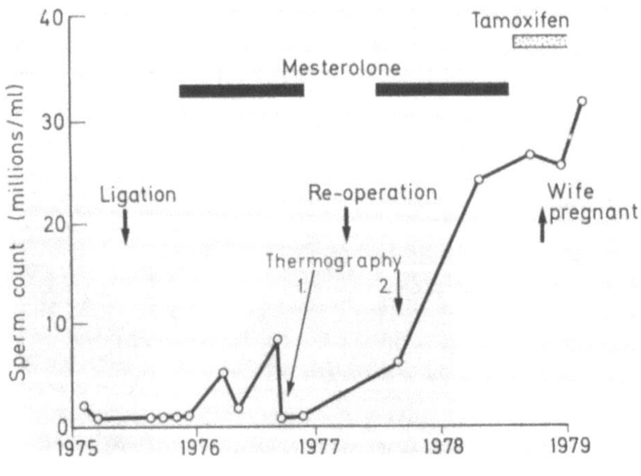

Fig. 4. Subfertile male who had abnormal thermogram (left 32.5 °C, right 30.9 °C) after ligation of varicocele, subsequently corrected (28.8 °C and 28 °C) by re-operation. Note that sperm count did not improve to satisfactory levels, even with medical therapy, until the thermographic abnormality was corrected.

indicating unrecognised bilateral varicoceles that were only partially corrected by ligation on the left side only. Following re-operation on left, right, or both sides the thermographic findings were rechecked in five patients: These were normal in all cases (Fig. 3). In these cases improvement in sperm count did not occur until the varicocele was completely corrected, despite supplementary medical therapy (see Fig. 4). Five pregnancies were produced following re-operation on these residual or recurrent varicoceles.

Discussion

It may be very difficult to decide upon the presence or absence of a varicocele on clinical examination, even with the patient standing in good light, and it is even more difficult to be sure whether the abnormality is unilateral or bilateral. Scrotal thermography offers a painless, non-invasive objective test which can confirm or refute the diagnosis of varicocele associated with significant alteration in scrotal temperature, and also define the extent of the venous abnormality. This information is of real help to the surgeon who must decide whether or not to recommend operative correction of the varicocele, and then undertake either unilateral or bilateral surgery.

The results of ligation of varicocele are not uncommonly disappointing, and few surgeons can match the excellent results such as those reported by Dubin and Amelar (1977). Our limited experience with thermography so far has indicated that clinical judgement alone gives a false impression of the existence and extent of varicocele in up to one-third of cases. Furthermore, critical examination of selected post-operative patients has indicated that persistence of thermographic abnormality is not uncommon, and that this may affect either the left or right side. Sequential studies in a few patients have indicated that the anticipated improvement in sperm count may not be obtained in such cases until the varicocele is completely corrected by reoperation and that, once a normal temperature has been achieved, pregnancy in the spouse may then follow. Thermography provided an objective test for the critical assessment of the results of varicocele surgery, and unsatisfactory results were then detected with increasing frequency. Reoperation for persistent thermographic abnormality has been recommended without hesitation, and it is estimated that about 5% of varicocele operations have required further surgery since thermography has been used to check all possibly unsatisfactory results.

The findings in the fertile control patients were of considerable interest. The values obtained in the 10 normal men without evidence of varicocele showed a comparatively narrow range of normality of 29.5–31.5 °C (anterior view) after 10 min equilibration at 19 °C. These results are roughly in accordance with those reported in 171 normal men by Fornage and Lemaire (1979) who found mean ($\pm$SD) values of 29.33 ± 0.18 °C; we found a rather broader range of normality, and believe that our upper limits of normal of 32 °C or a differential of more than 1 °C between the two sides are reasonable and probably a little conservative.

The observation of varicoceles with grossly abnormal thermographic findings in two of our fertile control subjects was of considerable interest, and confirmed the well-known fact that varicocele does not necessarily interfere with fertility. Two recent, controlled trials have shown no difference in the pregnancy rates of infertile couples when the male partner had a varicocele, irrespective of whether it was ligated or not (Rodriguez-Rigau et al. 1978; Nilsson et al. 1979). It would be easy to conclude that varicocele *never* needs ligation in a subfertile man. This would be at variance with previously reported experience, and would deny the individual patient with an abnormal sperm count the chance of improvement in seminal characteristics that may occur following surgical correction, after which additional medical or other therapy can be given if necessary (see Fig. 4).

Experience derived from this study has clarified several points about the management of varicocele to us. The mere existence of a varicocele is not by itself an indication for surgery if other findings are normal. Clinical diagnosis of the presence and extent of varicocele is imprecise, whereas thermography can provide accurate objective evidence of disturbed scrotal temperature which may be important in a subfertile man with evidence of impaired spermatogenesis. The results of surgery are not uniformly good, and improvement in semen quality and pregnancy in the spouse may not occur until the temperature abnormality has been corrected, which may require reoperation. We believe that thermography adds a degree of precision to the diagnosis of varicocele which is of considerable value in the management of the subfertile male. The nature of the abnormality in the testis produced by varicocele is complex and imperfectly understood, and there is evidence that intratesticular Leydig's cells function may be disturbed (Weiss et al. 1978). It is possible that these or other factors may require attention, in addition to surgical correction of the venous abnormality. Thermography, by measuring the basic scrotal abnormality produced by the varicocele, provides a baseline for diagnosis and assessment of results of treatment, onto which can be added further studies of the underlying biochemical or pathological abnormalities of spermatogenesis produced by the varicocele.

References

Ahlberg NE, Bartley O, Chidekel N, Fritjofsson A (1966) Phlebography in varicocele scroti. Acta Radiol [Diagn] (Stockh) 4:517–528

Brown JS, Dubin L, Hotchkiss RS (1967) The varicocele as related to fertility. Fertil Steril 18:46–56

Comhaire F, Montyene R, Kunnen M (1976) The value of scrotal thermography as compared with selective retrograde renography of the internal spermatic vein for the diagnosis of sub-clinical varicocele. Fertil Steril 27:694–698

Dubin L, Amelar RD (1977) Varicocelectomy: 986 cases in a twelve-year study. Urology 10: 446–449

Dubin L, Hotchkiss RS (1969) Testis biopsy in subfertile men with varicocele. Fertil Steril 20:51–57

Fornage B, Lemaire Ph (1978) La thermographie du scrotum. 2nd European Congress of Thermography, Barcelona

Fritjofsson A, Ahren C (1967) Studies on varicocele and subfertility. Scand J Urol Nephrol 1:55–62

Hendry WF, Sommerville IF, Hall RR, Pugh RCB (1973) Investigation and treatment of the subfertile male. Br J Urol 45:684–692

Johnson DE, Pohl DR, Rivera-Correa H (1970) Varicocele: An innocuous condition? South Med J 63:34–36

Jones CH, Hendry WF (1978) Thermographic examination of the scrotum. Acta Thermogr 4:38–43

Kormano M, Kahanpaa K, Svinhufvud U, Tahti E (1979) Thermography of varicocele. Fertil Steril 21:558–564

MacLeod J (1969) Further observations on role of varicocele in human male infertility. Fertil Steril 20:545–563

Nilsson S, Edvinsson A, Nilsson B (1979) Improvement of semen and pregnancy rate after ligation and division of the internal spermatic vein: fact or fiction? Br J Urol 51:591–596

Palomo A (1949) Radical cure of varicocele by a new technique: Preliminary report. J Urol 61:604–607

Rodriguez-Rigau LJ, Smith KD, Steinberger E (1978) Relationship of varicocele to sperm output and fertility of male partners in infertile couples. J Urol 120:691–694

Setchell BP (1978) The scrotum and thermoregulation. In: The mammalian testis. Elek, London, pp 90–108 and 360–361

Weiss DB, Rodriguez-Rigau LJ, Smith KD, Steinberger E (1978) Leydig cell function in oligospermic men with varicocele. J Urol 120:427–430

The Doppler Investigation of Varicocele

J. P. Pryor

The importance of varicocele ligation in the treatment of the male partner of an infertile marriage is at present the subject of debate. There is no agreement on the mechanism whereby a varicocele might impair fertility and much current research is being given to this aspect of infertility.

The use of the Doppler principle in the evaluation of varicocele was described by Greenberg et al. (1977) and this chapter is a summary of the experience of the technique at the Institute of Urology over the past 3 years.

The ultrasonic Doppler blood flow detector consists of a device which transmits a narrow beam of ultrasound with a frequency of 2–10 MHz. The ultrasound is reflected by the tissue interfaces and may be picked up by an appropriately positioned receiver. When the ultrasound is reflected by moving particles, for example red blood cells, the received signal frequency differs from that of the transmitted signal. This is the Doppler shift in sound frequency and it is proportional to the component of the velocity of the moving particles along the ultrasound beam. It is possible to detect this effect audibly or it may be recorded on a chart recorder. A fuller description of ultrasound techniques may be found in the article of Roberts (1976).

In clinical practice a Doppler probe is applied to the unshaved scrotum with gel contact and the pulsations of the testicular artery are readily identified. A nearby hum of venous flow is then sought and confirmation that the probe is over a vein may be obtained by gently compressing the scrotal contents to increase venous flow. The initial studies were conducted with the patient supine and standing; recordings were made over the inguinal canal, the root of the scrotum and over the lower pole of the testis. The Doppler examination is now carried out with the patient standing and breathing quietly. The Valsalva manoeuvre is often used to increase the venous flow and in our studies we have standardised this by asking the patient to blow into an anaesthetic flow limiter (AGA) set to a pressure of 25 cm water. The Doppler examinations have been carried out using the portable Sonicaid 7.7 MHz cardiovascular unit (Sonicaid), or with the larger Sonicaid BV 380 machine for recording the directional traces. Over 500 men have been studied and a more full description of the results may be found in two articles published in *The British Journal of Urology* (Hirsh et al. 1980 a, b).

Using the portable Doppler probe it was found that the incidence of a clinical varicocele and of valsalva-induced venous flow was similar in 44 fertile and 107 infertile men. The presence or absence of Valsalva-induced venous flow depended solely upon the presence or absence of a clinical varicocele (Table 1). Left-sided Valsalva-induced venous activity was always detected in the presence of a clinical varicocele, but was present even in 70% of men without a varicocele and in 49% on the right side. This high incidence of Valsalva-induced venous activity reflects the lack of specificity of the portable Doppler probe to determine the direction of blood flow and merely reflects the movement of blood in the cremasteric venous plexus. It should be noted that a certain minimum flow of blood is required in order to detect flow by the Doppler technique and it has been estimated (Setchell 1978) that the total flow from one testis in man is only 3.5 ml/min. This is the net outflow of blood from the venous channels in the cremasteric plexus.

Table 1. The incidence of Valsalva-induced reflux using the pocket Doppler apparatus.

Group	Number	Right reflux	Left reflux
A. Clinical varicocele	33	25 (76%)	33 (100%)
Fertile	10	9 (90%)	10 (100%)
Infertile	23	16 (70%)	23 (100%)
B. No varicocele	118	70 (59%)	98 (83%)
Fertile	34	21 (62%)	28 (82%)
Infertile	84	49 (58%)	70 (83%)

In the subsequent studies a directional Doppler probe was used and the waveform characteristics were recorded from patients in the erect position. Examination of the traces from 111 patients suggested that there were seven reproducible velocity wave forms. The characteristics of these were as follows:

Pattern 0 – No venous activity was recorded and, as the position of the probe over a vein was easily confirmed by scrotal compression, this signified the absence of sufficient venous flow to be recorded by the Doppler technique.

Pattern 1 – No venous activity was detected by the Doppler technique during quiet respiration, but during a valsalva manoeuvre there was an initial period of retrograde flow followed by absence of any apparent flow. On cessation of the Valsalva manoeuvre there was a short period of forward flow along the vein. This type of trace is interpreted as showing a competent valve in the internal spermatic vein.

Pattern 2 – This showed no spontaneous venous activity, but venous reflux occurred throughout the Valsalva manoeuvre and this was followed by a short trough representing forward venous flow on cessation of the Valsalva. This pattern represents Valsalva-induced reflux.

Pattern 3 – This showed intermittent venous refluß a variation in the intervals between spontaneous venous activity. This reflux was sometimes related to respiration, but sometimes occurred for as long as 30 s and it was usually increased during a Valsalva manoeuvre.

Pattern 4 – This showed continuous venous reflux during normal respiration which was augmented during a Valsalva manoeuvre.

Pattern 5 – This showed continous venous reflux which did not differ significantly during the Valsalva manoeuvre.

Pattern 6 – This pattern was only recognised over the inguinal canal in patients with a varicocele and it is thought to represent a forward flow of blood during quiet respiration which ceased during the Valsalva manoeuvre. It is thought this pattern might represent the flow of blood in the cremasteric veins.

The incidence of these wave-form patterns in patients with and without a varicocele is shown in Table 2. This shows that in the 45 patients with a left-sided varicocele, wave forms 3, 4 or 5 were seen in 89% of the spermatic cords where there was clinical evidence of a varicocele. Wave-form patterns 3, 4 or 5 were only seen in eight spermatic cords of patients without clinical varicocele. These patients are considered to have sub-clinical varicoceles.

In the assessment of a varicocele it would seem more practicable to grade spontaneous venous activity of the spermatic cord, recorded in the erect position and with quiet respiration, as either absent (i.e. too low to be recorded), intermittent (pattern 3) or continuous (patterns 4 and 5). Furthermore it is possible to categorise patients in this manner without the need of a directional flow meter. Table 3 is the Doppler classification of the varicocele of 39 fertile and 57 infertile men. This shows that the incidence of grade 1 varicoceles was higher in the men of proven fertility, whereas the grade 3 varicoceles were more common in the men of infertile marriages.

In 17 patients the Doppler grades were correlated with the presence or absence of internal spermatic vein reflux at its junction with the left renal vein. Internal spermatic vein reflux was demonstrated in the one patient with a grade 1 varicocele and in all four patients with the grade 3 varicocele. Internal spermatic vein reflux was only demonstrated in 5 of the 12 patients with grade 2 reflux. These findings show that all patients with clinical varicoceles do not have internal spermatic vein reflux due to an incompetent valve at its junction with the left renal vein. This may be of importance in our understanding of the relationship between a varicocele and infertility, as the mean sperm density of those with demonstrable internal spermatic vein reflux on venography was 4.8 m/ml whereas in those without reflux it was 47.6 m/ml. The decision to perform venography was based solely on the clinical diagnosis of a varicocele in the male partner of an infertile marriage.

The relationship between the Doppler grades and thermography was studied in a group of 37 patients. There was a trend towards increased scrotal temperatures with the higher Doppler grades of varicocele but this was only significant in respect to the left-sided temperature elevation in men with grade 3 varicoceles (Table 4).

The Doppler technique has been utilised in the post-operative assessment of the effectiveness of surgical treatment. Five men in a post-operative group of 22 patients were found to have a persistence of spontaneous venous activity. Four had only intermittent venous reflux and only the patient with clinical evidence of a persistent varicocele was found to have continuous venous reflux. Perrin et al. (1980) in their studies with the Doppler technique also found it to be useful in the post-operative assessment of patients. In a group of 20 patients whom they studied before and after operation with the Doppler technique, they found that 11 patients with doubtful clinical varicoceles, with a positive Doppler examination, were cured by the operation both clinically and by Doppler examination. Of the nine patients with a definite clinical varicocele five were cured both clinically and by negative Doppler examination. There were two clinical failures of the operation to cure the

Table 2. The incidence of Doppler wave-form patterns in the spermatic cord of 84 men.

Wave-form pattern (Grade)	Total number	No varicocele	Varicocele	Percent with varicocele
0 (1)	16	16	–	–
1 (1)	40	40	–	–
2 (1)	62	57	5	8%
3 (2)	33	7	26	79%
4 (3)	10	1	9	90%
5 (3)	5	–	5	100%

Table 3. The distribution of Doppler grades in the varicoceles of men from fertile and infertile marriages.

Group	Number	Doppler grade		
		1	2	3
Fertile	39	18 (46%)	14 (36%)	7 (18%)
Infertile	57	7 (12%)	29 (51%)	21 (37%)

Table 4. The relationship between the average computed scrotal temperature and the Doppler grade of varicocele.

Group	Doppler grade	Number	Average scrotal temperature (°C)	
			Right	Left
No varicocele	1	12	30.5	30.3
Varicocele	1	4	29.9	29.9
	2	15	30.2	30.2
	3	8	31.2	32.3

varicocele and these showed a persistent positive Doppler examination, as did two other patients who had no clinical evidence of a persistent varicocele.

The Doppler technique appears to be a useful and non-invasive technique for detecting blood movement in the cremasteric venous plexus. The significance of Valsalva-induced blood flow is questioned since it was so readily detected by a non-directional machine in all groups of patients. Using a directional Doppler machine it was possible to study the pattern of blood flow in the spermatic cord. The presence or absence of spontaneous venous flow in the erect position during quit respiration would appear to be a useful method of categorising patients and has the advantage that it does not require the use of sophisticated instruments. It is to be hoped that the application of Doppler grading of venous activity in the spermatic cord will be a useful technique that will allow us to categorise the different types of varicocele and determine which are of clinical significance with regard to the treatment of an infertile man.

References

Greenberg SH, Lipshultz LI, Morganroth J, Wein AJ (1977) The use of the Doppler stethoscope in the evaluation of varicoceles. J Urol 117:296–298

Hirsh AV, Cameron KM, Tyler JP, Simpson J, Pryor JP (1980a) The Doppler assessment of varicoceles and internal spermatic vein reflux in infertile men. Br J Urol 52:50–56

Hirsh AV, Kellett MJ, Robertson G, Pryor JP (1980b) Doppler flow studies, venography and thermography in the evaluation of varicoceles of fertile and subfertile men. Br J Urol 52:560–565

Perrin P, Rollet J, Durand L (1980) The Doppler stethoscope in the diagnosis of subclinical varicocele. Br J Urol 52:390–391

Roberts VC (1976) Ultrasound in the assessment of vascular function. Med Prog Technol 4:3–10

Setchell BP (1978) The mammalian testis. Elek, London, p 120

The Anatomy of Varicocele
The Role of Venography

N. A. Green and J. T. Hill

Introduction

The success of operations on varicosities of the lower limb requires the understanding of the anatomical disposition of involved veins and a knowledge of the location of competent or incompetent valvular mechanisms. In the case of varicocele, simple ligation of the internal spermatic veins at or above the internal inguinal ring or ligation of the cremasteric veins through the scrotum may both be effective. It is our view that recurrent varicocele can be prevented by an anatomical approach to the surgical management of the condition, and a simplistic surgical view may not be appropriate in all cases.

Retrograde blood flow may occur in the internal spermatic veins and the cremasteric veins may be involved secondarily because of this. Alternatively, the cremasteric veins within the cremasteric muscle sleeve may be primarily involved and the valves in this system may be incompetent. Communications do exist between both these sets of veins and other systems, for example the superficial external pudendal vein to the long saphenous and femoral veins and, indeed, through the contralateral veins both within the scrotum, the inguinal canal and at a much higher level in the retro-peritoneal area.

An adequate evaluation of varicocele which allows for an anatomical approach to the surgery of the condition is advisable. We therefore performed a series of radiological studies, having ascertained (Hill and Green 1977) that classification of varicocele by ascending operative venography did not allow for a full determination of the anatomy of the condition, a biased classification resulting therefrom.

Patients and Methods

In 25 patients in whom a left-sided varicocele was detected clinically, and in whom there was significant right-sided component in two cases, the following investigations were performed:

1) Pre-operative left renal venogram;
2) per-operative ascending venography through scrotal and/or inguinal approach;
3) retrograde venography of the cremasteric vein exposed through an inguinal incision at the back of the inguinal ligament.

Renal Venography. This was performed by percutaneous puncture of the femoral vein under local anaesthesia using a Gray Odman catheter and 20 ml or more of 45%. Hypaque was injected under vision-intensifier control. The renal vein was

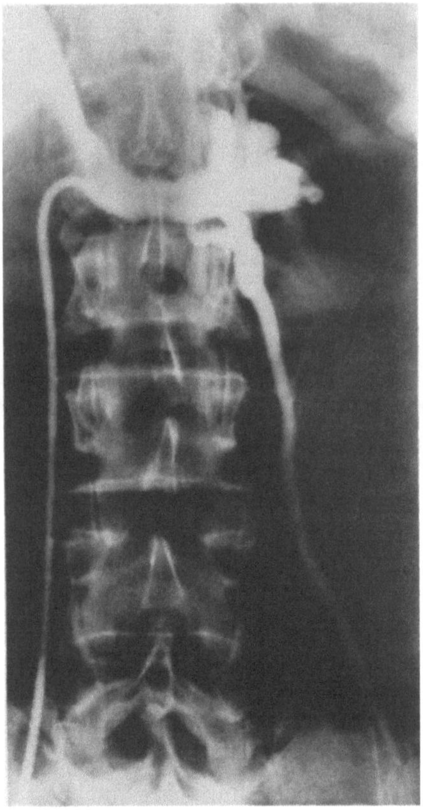

Fig. 1. Left renal venogram showing reflux down internal spermatic vein.

outlined and any reflux occurring, of the contrast into the internal spermatic vein, was noted together with the presence of valves and collateral circulation at various levels by representative radiographs which were taken (Fig. 1).

Peroperative Venography. At operation the varicocele was exposed by routine inguinal approach or scrotal incision and ascending venography was performed (Fig. 2) by 10 ml 45%. Hypaque, injected through a Portsmouth cathether or Medicut cannula. The definitive cremasteric vein was catheterised also when possible at the back of the inguinal ligament, dye being injected towards the scrotum under X-ray control. The presence of an incompetent valvular mechanism was assumed in the cremasteric system when contrast medium flowed freely into the scrotum.

Varicoceles were classified into four groups as a result of these investigations (Table 1).

Where internal spermatic reflux was demonstrated to a significant degree on left renal venography, confirmed on peroperative ascending venography and in the absence of any cremasteric reflux, a pure internal spermatic varicocele was assumed: Ten such cases were noted in a series of 25 patients. In five patients no evidence of reflux into the internal spermatic vein was demonstrated, but in five patients only the cremasteric system was involved, reflux occurring into the scrotum

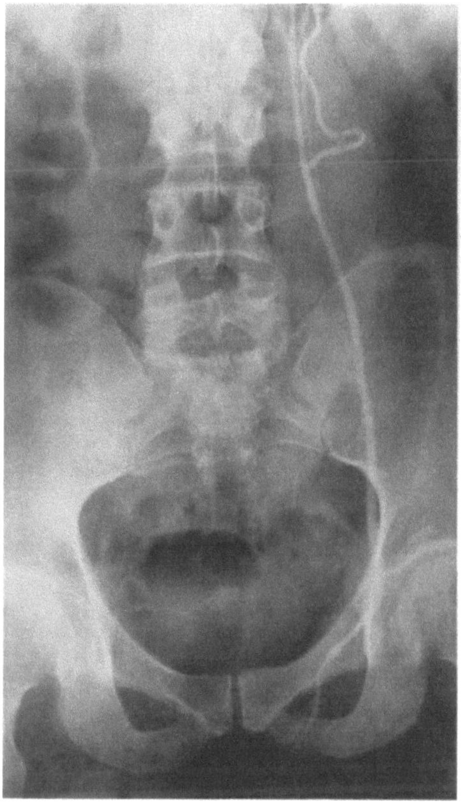

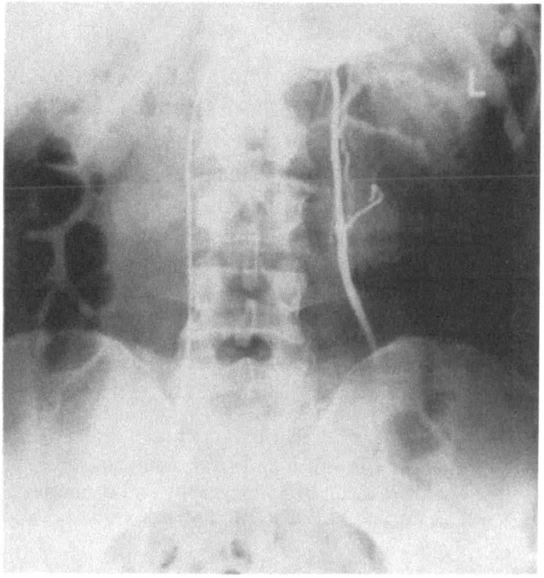

Fig. 3. Left renal venography showing communicant branches.

◀ **Fig. 2.** Ascending peroperative venogram showing perirenal communication.

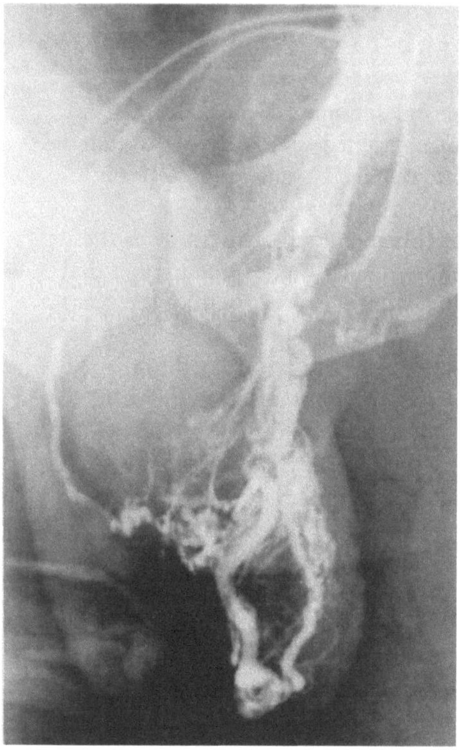

Fig. 4. Demonstration of collateral vessels and communications within the scrotum, inguinal and femoral regions.

on retrograde injection of dye through the involved vein. In three patients incompetence in both systems was demonstrated on both pre-operative and operative venography, in seven patients there was no evidence of reflux and dilatation of the veins was noted in seven patients, mainly in the cremasteric system. In 20 of the 25 cases one or more communicating or collateral veins was noted. Typical examples (Fig. 3) show perirenal veins noted or actual second communications were seen between the renal vein and the internal spermatic veins. In the scrotum and inguinal canal communications were demonstrated into the opposite side and with the femoral vein by the superificial external pudendal vein (Fig. 4).

Table 1. Classification of varicocele using left renal venography, per-operative ascending venography and cremasteric venography.

Type	Number
Internal spermatic	10
Cremasteric	5
Combined internal spermatic and cremasteric	3
Venous dilatation	7
Total	25

Conclusion and Discussion

We have demonstrated a larger number of internal spermatic varicosities existing as a sole abnormality, but also the presence of combined internal spermatic and cremastic varicosities with incompetence in both systems. A smaller 20% (5 out of 25 cases) of patients had pure cremasteric varicosities existing.

Whilst it can be argued that the number of investigations carried out in these patients was excessive for what is a simple condition, equally it can be argued that by so doing the correct surgical approach resulted from the assessment of the veins involved.

In the case of cremasteric varicocele, ligation of these varicosities through the scrotum was advocated by Hanley (1966) and may be appropriate, but we have demonstrated that it is possible to dissect the cremasteric vein from its entrance into the inferior epigastric vein down into the scrotum, securing communicating branches en route: By dislocating the testicle into the wound, radical operation can be performed through the inguinal canal. The advantage of this approach is that it allows for assessment of the internal spermatic veins and the fact that they do not appear to be involved at the time of surgery. Many internal spermatic varicoceles may involve just one or two veins in the inguinal canal and it is possible to ligate these at the internal ring without damaging the internal spermatic artery and dissect these down towards the scrotum securing branches with other systems.

Where internal spermatic reflux is seen and many collateral or communicant branches are noted on the posterior abdominal wall a higher retroperitoneal approach is recommended.

It can be argued that the performance of cremasteric venography necessitates the ligature of this vein whether it is involved or not. The presence of free communication between the normal cremasteric system of veins, the pampiniform plexus in the spermatic cord and neighbouring superficial vessels such as the superficial external pudendal vein is well documented (Hanley and Harrison 1962), and thus alternative routes for return of blood are available.

Where a plexiform arrangement of veins is noted throughout the whole of the inguinal canal, simple ligation at the internal inguinal ring, or by the Palomo approach, should be performed avoiding damage to the internal spermatic artery.

References

Hanley HG (1966) The results of surgical treatment in varicocele. Proc R Soc Med 59: 767–769

Hanley HG, Harrison RG (1962) The nature and surgical treatment of varicocele. Br J Surg 50:64–67

Hill JT, Green NA (1977) Varicocele: A review of radiological and anatomical features in relation to surgical treatment. Br J Surg 64:747–752

Palomo A (1949) Radical cure of varicocele by a new technique. Preliminary report. J Urol 61:604–607

Spermatic Phlebography
Diagnostic and Therapeutic Method

J. Struyven, J. P. Brion, A. Unglik, and C. C. Schulman

Spermatic phlebography was first described by Ahlberg et al. in 1965. Since then, few publications have been related to this technique. Spermatic phlebography is useful for detecting a clinically suspected varicocele and providing a preoperative phlebogram. Recent developments in interventive radiology have introduced a therapeutic side to the method.

Material and Method

We studied 150 patients, age ranging from 5 to 41 years (mean 24 years). Of these patients, 4% were studied for impalpable testis, 23% for painful syndrome related to a clinical varicocele, 7% for postoperative recurrence of varicocele, and 66% for infertility. Both spermatic veins are catheterized using the right femoral vein Seldinger technique. After catheterization of the left renal vein, via the inferior vena cava, the tip of a Cobra polyethylene catheter is introduced into the outlet of the left spermatic vein located on the inferior wall of the left renal vein. During a Valsalva maneuver, 10 to 30 ml contrast media is injected in 2–6 s using a hand injector (Cordis).

The opacification is fluoroscopically monitored (spotfilms 105 mm technique) until the varicocele is visible. The Valsalva maneuver sometimes has to be released to prevent a blockage of the spermatic vein in the inguinal canal. The outlet of the right spermatic vein is usually located on the anterior wall of the inferior vena cava beneath the right renal vein.

The right spermatic vein is usually catheterized with the Cobra catheter or in case of failure with a short curved red Kifa catheter. The radiologic information is recorded on 105 mm spotfilms at the rate of one picture per second during 10–15 s.

Results

Successful catheterization was obtained in 97.4% of cases for the left side and in 91% of cases on the right side. In the last 50 patients the examination was successful in nearly all cases for both sides.

Anatomy

The testicular veins may be subdivided into two groups: a deep group and a superficial network component. The deep system comprises the pampiniform plexus: it

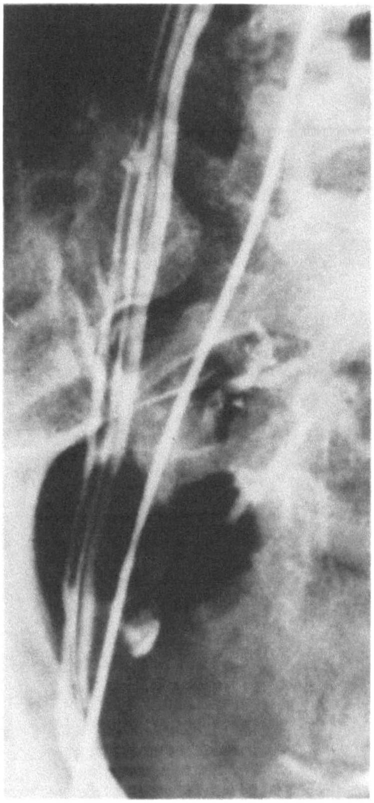

Fig. 1. Example of multiple right spermatic veins.

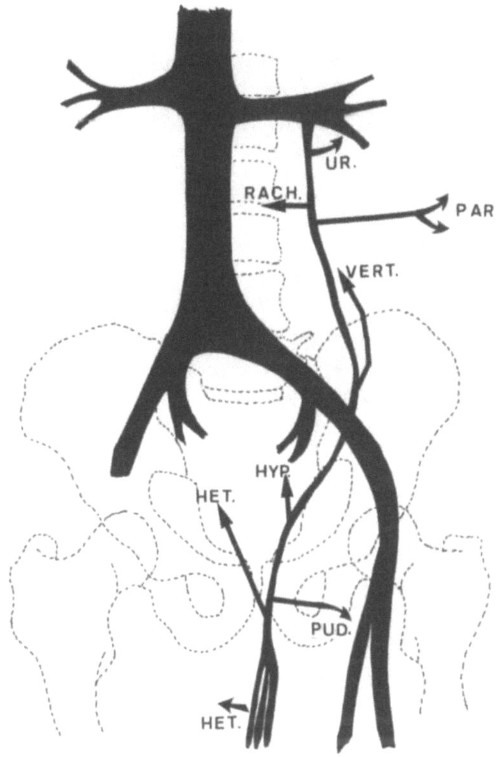

Fig. 2. Schematic representation of tributary veins.

consists of a network of veins which originate in the testis and epididymis. It is drained by the anterior and posterior spermatic plexus and by the ductus deferens veins. The anterior spermatic plexus continues past the left and right spermatic veins. The posterior spermatic plexus ends in the epigastric vein. The ductus deferens veins follow the ductus deferens through the inguinal canal and empty via the vesical veins into the internal iliac vein. The superficial venous system consists of the anterior and posterior scrotal veins. The outlet of the left spermatic vein is always located on the inferior wall of the renal vein. The right spermatic vein usually terminates in the anterior wall of the inferior vena cava below the right renal vein. In 3% of our cases, the outlet of the right spermatic vein was on the inferior wall of the right renal vein.

It is interesting to point out that in our series, in a case with a left inferior vena cava, without situs inversus, the outlet of the left spermatic vein was located on the anterior wall of the inferior vena cava and the right outlet on the right renal vein.

It should be stressed that the spermatic veins may divide into several ramifications and that number of veins has to be carefully evaluated, keeping in mind the expected levels of ligation (inguinal and iliac) (Table 1, Fig. 1). Multiple anasto-

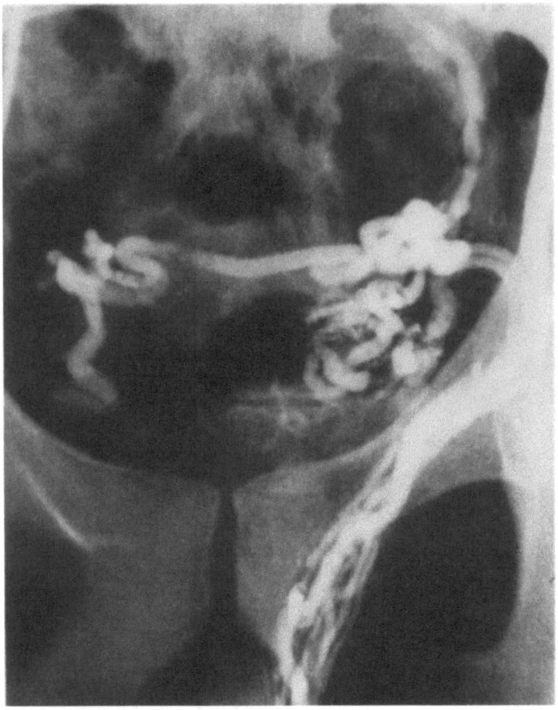

Fig. 3. Dilatation of the vesicoprostatic plexus opacified via the deferential veins, tributaries to a left varicocele.

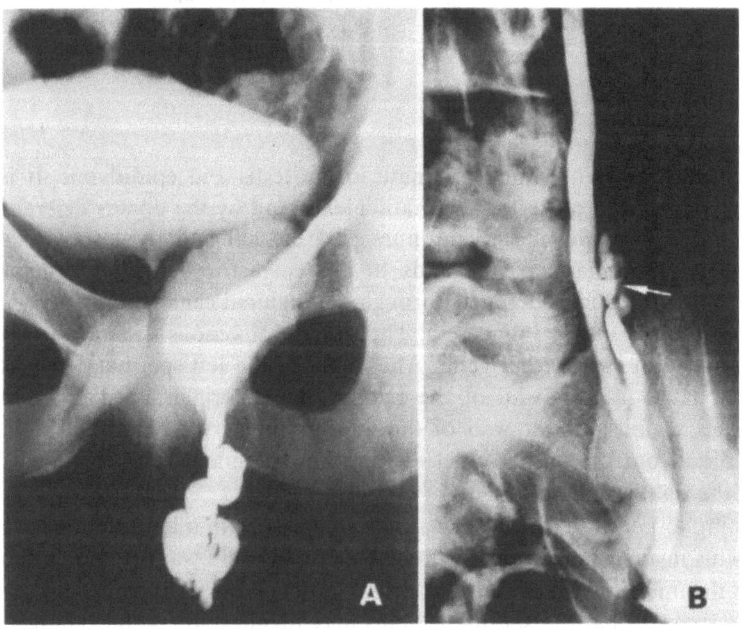

Fig. 4 A, B. Recurrence of varicocele induced by incomplete ligation of spermatic vein. **A** Non-ligated. **B** A vein (*arrow*) is responsible for the recurrence.

Table 1. Anatomy: Number of spermatic veins at various levels.

	Left spermatic vein		Right spermatic vein	
	Single trunk	Two or more trunks	Single trunk	Two or more trunks
Lumbar part	75%	25%	81%	19%
Iliac part	44%	56%	37%	63%
Crural part	14%	86%	7%	93%

Table 2. Distribution of anastomoses in spermatic veins.

Fillling of tributary veins		
Types of anastomosis	Left spermatic vein	Right spermatic vein
I Urinary	37%	29%
II Parietal	28%	22%
III Rachidian	23%	3%
IV Heterolateral	18%	7%
V Hypogastric	16%	11%
VI External pudental	13%	3%
VII Vertical anastomosis	8%	33%

moses exist between the spermatic veins and the lumbar, renal, ureteral, iliac, and parietal veins. These anastomoses do not have a pathologic significance except for vertical spermatic–spermatic anastomosis. The types and importance of anastomoses are illustrated in Table 2 and Figs. 2–4.

Varicoceles

Varicoceles are a pathologic alteration of the venous circulation of the testis due to the absence or incompetence of the valvular system.

In this series, absence of valves was observed on the left side in 50% of cases and on the right side in 32% of cases (2/1 ratio) and incompetence of valves was noted in 8% and 4% at the left and right side respectively. According to the anatomic studies of Ahlberg et al. (1965), 64% of the competent valves were found in the right spermatic vein. Competent valves were found in 33% of the cases on the left side. Considering all the patients, 67% of the varicoceles were found on the left side and 33% on the right in discordance with most published series (80% on the left side for Bigot et al. (1979) to 98% on the left side for Brown et al. (1967)). This can be explained by our high rate of right spermatic vein catheterization, which has not been routinely performed by other authors (Comhaire and Kunnem 1976; Lien and Kolbenstvedt 1977).

The importance of the varicocele is graded from 1 to 4 (Fig. 5). Table 3 shows the distribution. Of the 150 patients of this series, 73 are unselected infertile patients referred for phlebography on the basis of abnormal spermogram only. Clinical examination revealed a varicocele in 45% of the patients but radiology was positive in 55% of the patients, including 31% with left varicocele, of which 9% were on the right side, and 15% with bilateral varicocele. In 12% of additional patients, the phlebography demonstrated reflux without varicocele. No complications occurred in our series.

Table 3. Distribution of varicoceles.

Total	Catheterization	Left side	97.4%			
		Right side	91.5%			
	Varicocele	Left – right ratio = 3/1				
		Grade	1	2	3	4
		Left	16%	29%	35%	20%
		Right	46%	51%	3%	

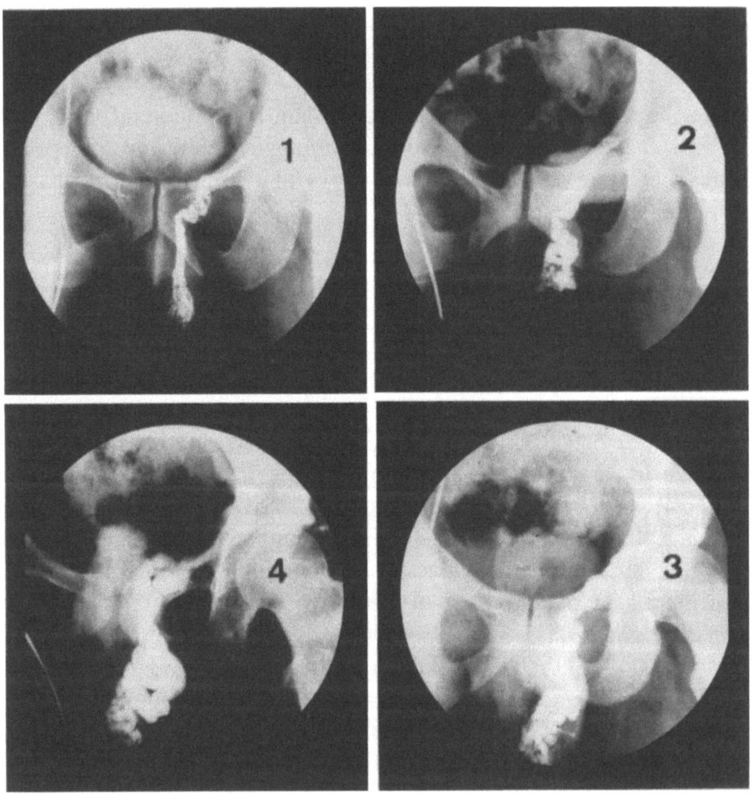

Fig. 5. Grading of varicoceles (1–4) by size.

Interventional Phlebography

Percutaneous treatment following diagnostic phlebography is possible in selected patients (Fig. 6A). The diagnostic catheter is withdrawn and exchanged for a balloon catheter to prevent outflow of the drug. Using a "superselective" wire guide, the tip of the ballon catheter is positioned in the spermatic vein, at the level of L3. After occlusive inflation of the balloon, 2–6 cc sclerosing agent (Aethoxy-

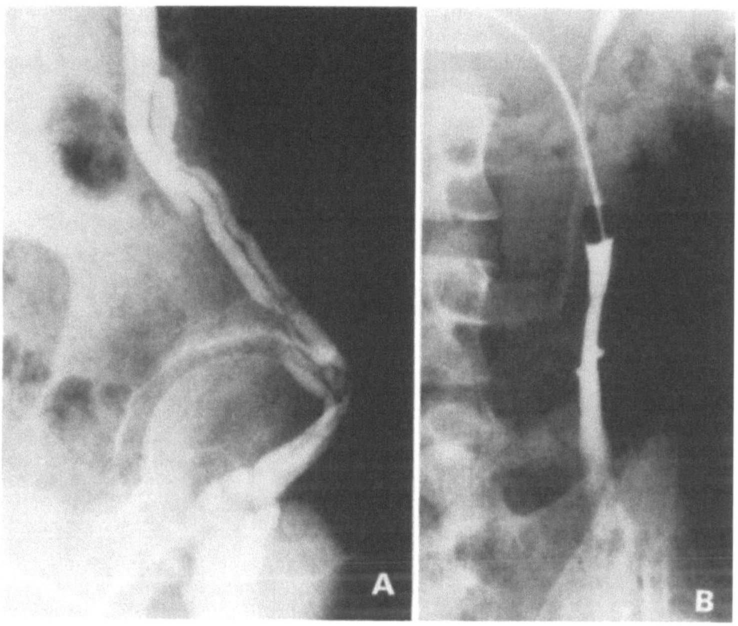

Fig. 6. Example of sclerosis of the left spermatic vein. **A** Patient of 21 years with postoperative recurrence. **B** The balloon catheter is positioned in the left spermativ vein and a sclerosing agent is injected under fluoroscopic control.

sklerol 3%, Hydroxypolyethoxydodecane) is injected at intervals of 5 min (Fig. 6B). The results are documented by a control phlebogram. This method can be easily performed on the left side but is difficult on the right side because of the sharp angle between the inferior vena cava and the spermatic vein. Patients whose phlebogram shows significant anastomosis with another venous system are rejected because of risk of extensive sclerosis.

Conclusion

Spermatic phlebography is a safe and reliable method for detecting and evaluating varicoceles. Data obtained by this examination are essential for correct surgical management. Interventive phlebography is a valuable alternative to surgical treatment.

References

Ahlberg NE, Bartley O, Chidekel N (1965) Retrograde contrast filling of the left gonadal vein. Acta Radiol [Diagn] (Stockh) 3:385

Bigot JM, Chatel A, Dectot H, Helenon CH (1979) Phlebographie spermatique retrograde. Technique et anatomie radiologique à propos de 152 explorations. Ann Radiol (Paris) 21:7, 515

Brown JS, Dubin L, Hotchkiss RS (1967) The varicocele as related to fertility. Fertil Steril 18:46

Charny CW (1962) Effect of varicocele on fertility. Results of varicocelectomy. Fertil Steril 13:47

Comhaire F, Kunnen M (1976) Selective retrograde venography of the internal spermatic vein: a conclusive approach to the diagnosis of varicocele. Andrologia 8:11

Lien HH, Kolbenstvedt A (1977) Phlebography of left renal and left testicular veins. Acta Radiol [Diagn] (Stockh) 18:321

A New Classification of Left-Sided Varicoceles Based on Venography

B. Coolsaet

Introduction

The significance of a varicocele in male infertility has yet to be accurately determined since results of varicocelectomy on proved fertility are inconclusive. Although conception rates of 40%–50% have been reported (Macleod 1969; Brown 1976), Nilsson et al. (1979) were unable to demonstrate an increased pregnancy rate after surgery, which might be due to irreversible damage of testicular function. Generally accepted standardized parameters both from testicular biopsies and semen analysis are required to make a useful comparison of results.

We found it necessary to investigate a group of patients with left-sided varicocele thoroughly in order to determine whether or not all the varicoceles were similar, as regards hemodynamic criteria (Coolseat 1980). The results were very surprising and should be taken into consideration when fertility studies are performed. Whether or not the varicocele should be treated in order to treat male infertility cannot be answered so far. Some authors have suggested that fertility disorders might be prevented by early detection and treatment of the varicocele (Steeno et al. 1976; Lipshultz and Corriere 1977). Results will have to be analyzed carefully in a large group of patients to avoid useless operations and to spare the patient anxiety about his fertility and sexual potency (Steeno et al. 1976). Since varicoceles have been related to sexual inadequacy (Comhaire and Vermeulen 1975) as well as to impotency, it should be clearly indicated which type of varicocele is related to hormonal and sexual dysfunction.

Patients and Method

It is generally accepted that varicoceles are found after puberty (Steeno et al. 1976). However, in one group of radiologically well-documented patients, five children under the age of 10 were found to have a distinct varicocele (Fig. 1) although Øster (1971) found no varicoceles in a study of 1073 Danish boys below this age.

Method

The transfemoral venography technique was used (Seldinger 1953), the patient being in the standing position, and 20 ml 64% urografin was rapidly injected into the left renal vein through a SPE-6.7/65-15-CII catheter. The renal vein, the internal spermatic vein (ISV), and the left common iliac vein were investigated in sequence by selective catheterization.

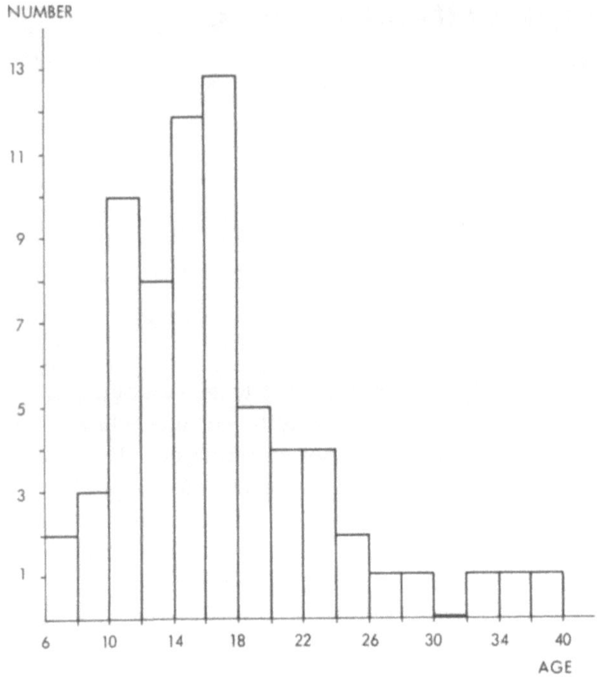

Fig. 1. Age distribution of a group of 67 patients.

Fig. 2 a–c. Varicoceles: **a** grade I, **b** grade II, **c** grade III.

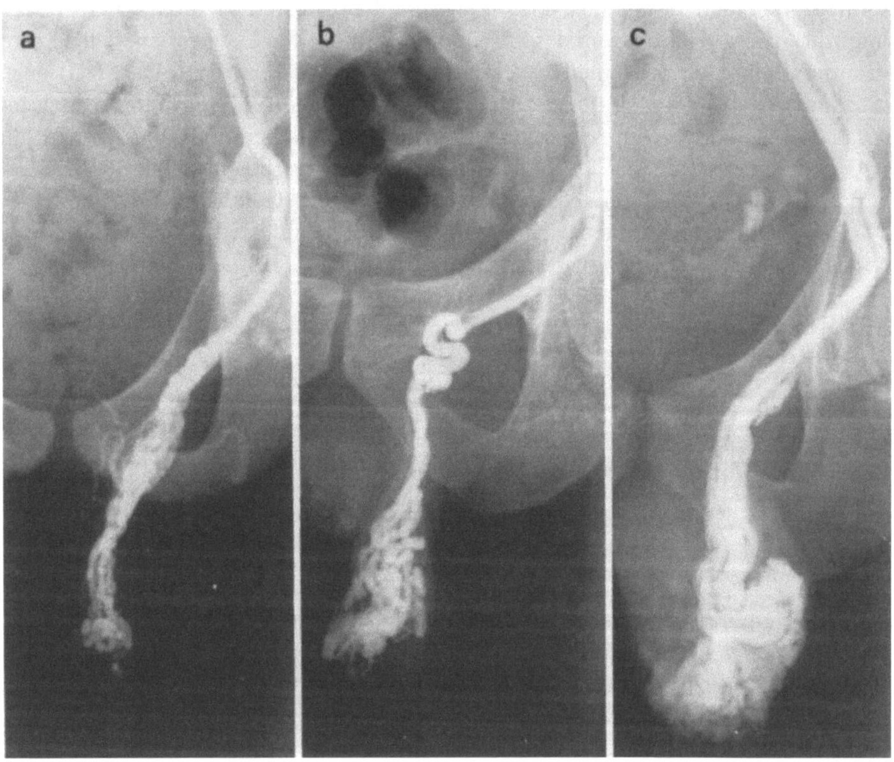

Results

Grading of Varicoceles

In the current literature varicocels have been distinguished solely according to their clinical grade (Steeno et al. 1976), grade I being a palpable scrotal varicosity less than 1 cm in diameter and with no reflux during the Valsalva maneuver. Grade II is a varicocele between 1 and 2 cm in diameter, while in grade III the diameter of the vein measures more than 2 cm and blows up during the Valsalva maneuver.

Although a classification of varicoceles based on this apparently quantitative measurement appears very scientific, clinicians will agree that differences of 0.2 cm are rather difficult to measure. Even during venography (Fig. 2), the differentiation into three groups still allows space for subjective interpretation, despite the possibility of more quantitative measurement. As will be pointed out below, some varicoceles drain through a varicose vein complex. In those cases it is very difficult to measure the dimensions of the varicocele.

Left Renal Vein

The left renal vein was examined for various phenomena. Normally the vein is clearly visible throughout its entire length with an unobstructed efflux of contrast medium from it into the vena cava. The intrarenal veins are only partially filled and there is no collateral circulation. In 25% of our patients the renal vein was obviously obstructed at the point where it crossed the aorta, with delayed flow into the vena cava and more pronounced filling of the intrarenal veins combined with a collateral circulation (Fig. 3 a). In another 23% of patients these phenomena were visible but less marked. Compression of the left renal vein at the bifurcation of the aorta and the superior mesenteric artery (Fig. 3 b) has been described as the "Nutcracker" phenomenon (El-Sadr and Mina 1950; Chait et al. 1971; De Schepper 1972; Coolseat 1978, 1980). A difference in pressure between the renal vein and the vena cava could be measured in some patients but not in others. Probably pressure differences depend on the extent to which a collateral circulation has developed. The better the collateral circulation the smaller the differences in pressure. There are a variety of ways in which a collateral circulation can be formed, e.g., via splenorenal anastomoses, the renoazygomal canal, the gonadal veins, the ascending lumbar vein, and what we have named the renogonadal canal (Coolsaet 1978). Other anomalies of the renal veins, such as double pre- and retroaortic branches can easily be demonstrated. In about 50% of the cases in which retrograde flow was detected in the ISV, an obstruction or an anomaly of the left renal vein was the cause.

Study of passive reflux in the ISV, which is the generally accepted cause of a varicocele (Verstoppen and Steeno 1977), gave surprising results. Twenty percent of cases showed no passive reflux in the standing position while in 8% of cases only partial filling of the ISV was seen. Therefore, while the assertion that "varicoceles are characterized by retrograde flow in the testicular veins" (Verstoppen and Steeno 1977) applies to the majority of cases, it does not apply to every case. Hence we must clearly distinguish between varicoceles with and without compression of the renal vein and varicoceles with and without passive ISV reflux. Other causes of

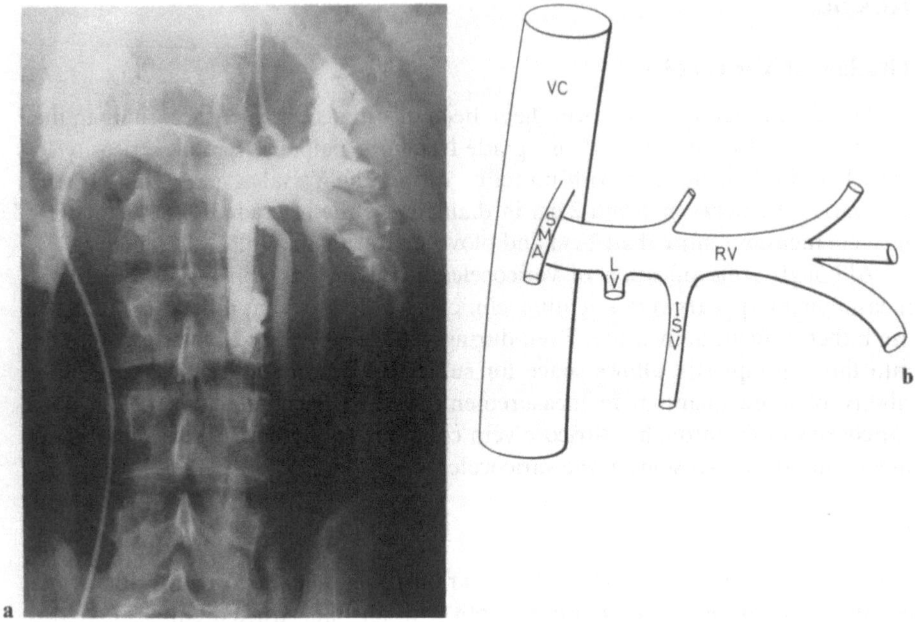

Fig. 3. a Nutcracker phenomenon with pronounced filling of the intrarenal veins, collateral circulation via lumbar, splenorenal, and the ISV. **b** Drawing of the nutcracker phenomenon, with compressing of the renal vein (*RV*) between the aorta and the superior mesenteric artery (*SMA*). *VC*, Vena cava; *LV*, lumbar vein.

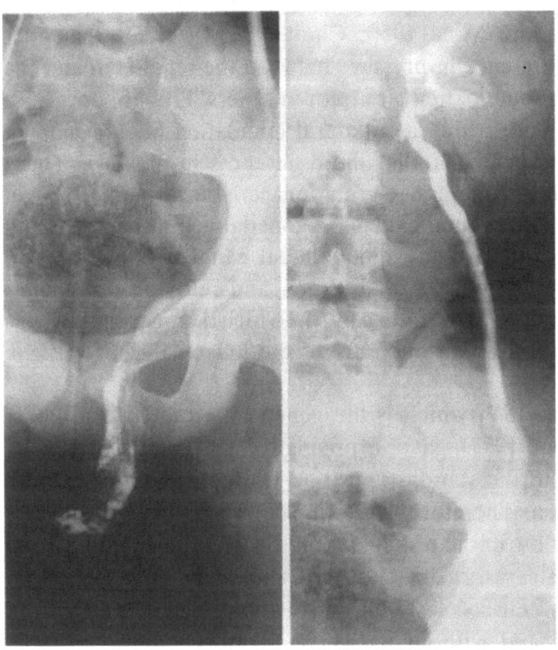

Fig. 4. Short renogonadal canal bypassing a proximal competent ISV and causing a varicocele.

varicoceles demand further differentiation. In about 8% of cases a competent proximal portion of the ISV is bypassed by a renogonadal canal, which usually connects a distal branch of the renal vein with the ISV somewhere along its course. This renogonadal canal, which is normally present in some people, can dilate and be responsible for a large volume of retrograde flow into the ISV, which is dilated distal to the anastomosis (Fig. 4). In only about half of these cases could a renal vein obstruction be shown to be the cause. The ISV can normally vary from a single vessel to a network of veins on either side and duplicate and triplicate veins are often seen in varicocele patients.

Internal Spermatic Vein

Investigation of the ISV disclosed a variety of shunts both proximally and distally within the area of reflux. Proximal shunts have no effect on the diameter of the ISV distal to them but distal shunts are of hemodynamic significance. A high proportion of the blood flow drains into the pelvic venous system, the diameter of the ISV distal to the shunt being noticeably less than the proximal diameter. That the reflux in the ISV due to these shunts affects testicular function is easily understood.

Varicocele Outflow Obstructions

Although the cause of a varicocele is obvious in the majority of cases, there remains a group comprising about 15% of cases in whom neither a direct nor an indirect total reflux in the ISV can be demonstrated. Although some authors claim a 100% cure after suprainguinal ligation of the ISV (Palomo 1949; Ivanessevich 1960),

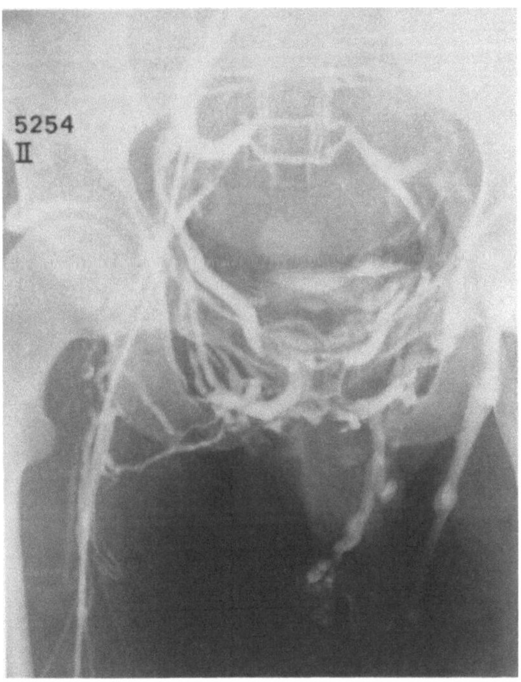

Fig. 5. Scrotal venography showing obstruction of the left common iliac with collateral circulation to the right common iliac vein.

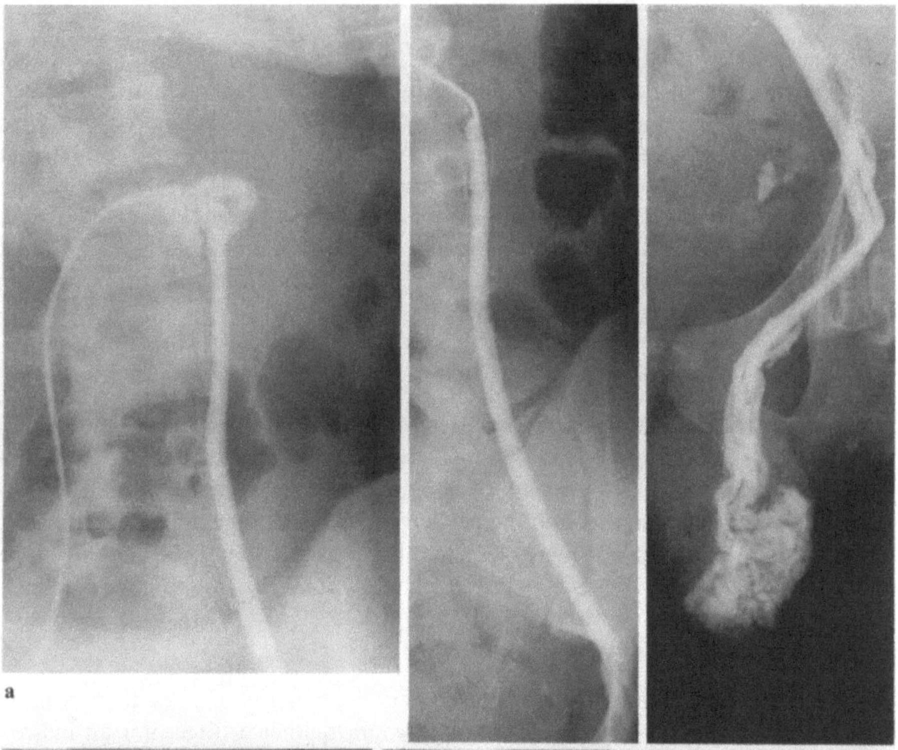

a

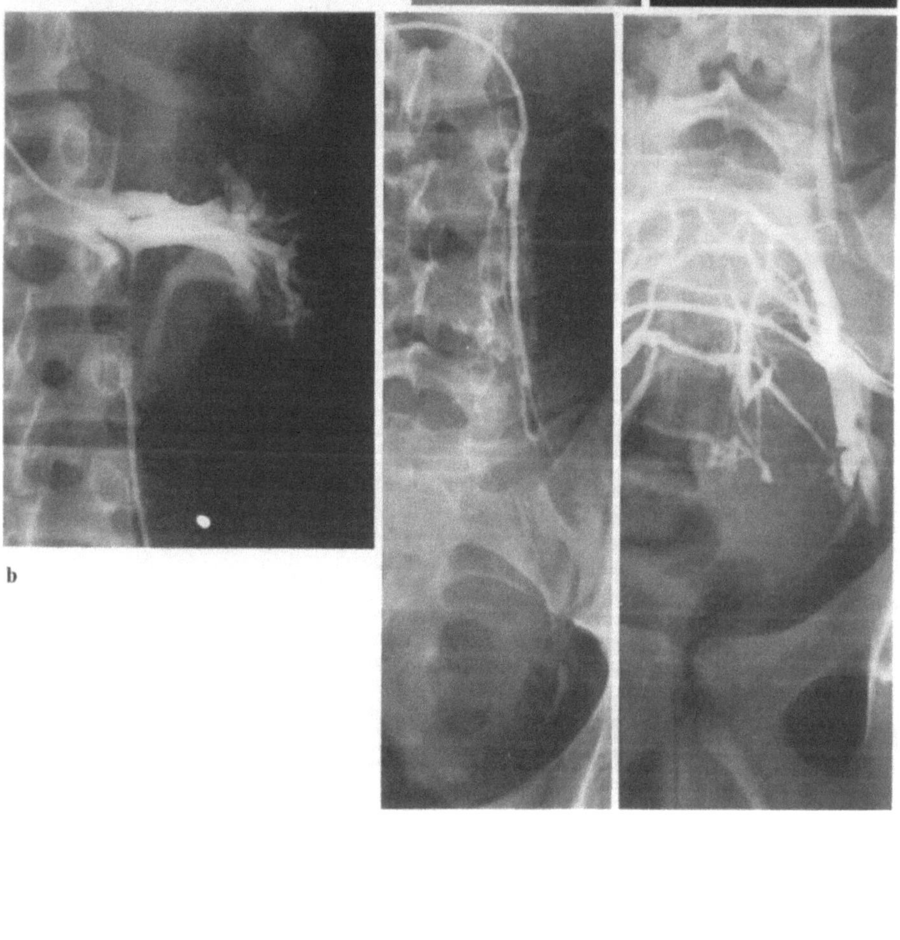

b

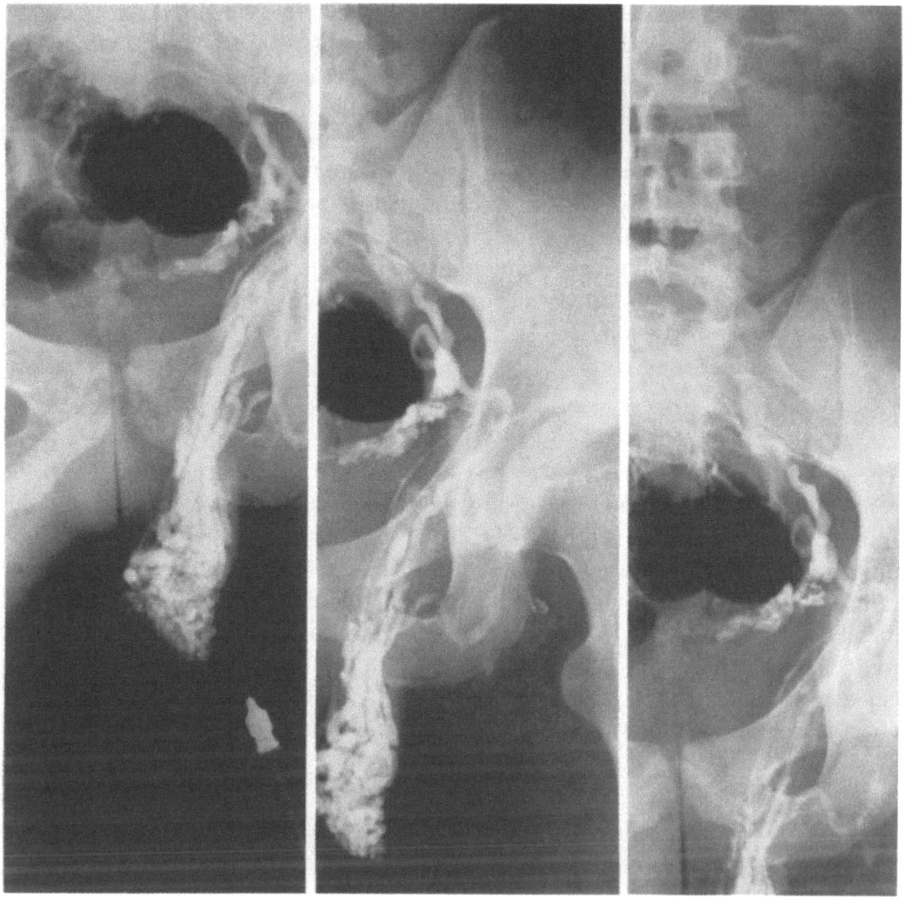

c

Fig. 6. a Standard venographic findings, i.e., passive reflux into a wide ISV, with a grade III varicocele. The ISV was ligated through a suprainguinal incision and partially resected but the varicocele persisted although to a lesser degree. **b** A further venography was performed together with that of the left common iliac vein. This showed an ISV of normal dimensions with a total block at the level of the ligation. The reduction in the size of the ISV is a common finding after such a procedure. The left common iliac vein was filled with contrast in search of a distal obstruction. This revealed an extensive collateral circulation which shunted the contrast material to the right side. This suggested a more distal obstruction and scrotal venography (**c**) clearly showed the drainage pathways of the varicocele. Once these vessels were ligated via a transinguinal incision the varicocele was cured. In this type of varicocele it is important to assess both the superficial and the deep drainage pathways, both of which have multiple anastomoses.

Hanley and Harrison (1962) reported 40 suprainguinal ligations including five cases in which the varicocele remained unchanged and three cases in which it even increased. These were cured by transinguinal ligation of the varicose veins.

Absence of a cause at what has been accepted as the classic site and the results of suprainguinal ligation as reported by Hanley and Harrison encouraged us to seek a more distal site. We carried out venographies of the left common iliac vein and an antegrade venography in some patients by injecting the varicocele.

Obstructions of the left common iliac vein were clearly evident in some patients, a phenomenon which we called the "distal Nutcracker." Flow from the common iliac vein into the vena cava is delayed and in some cases combined with an enormous pelvic venous collateral circulation, which shunts the blood from the left common iliac to the right (Fig. 5). Some of these cases had normal antegrade flow. There is no doubt whatever that this group can never be cured by a higher ligation, so that reports of 100% cures by such a procedure must be regarded with the utmost reserve. These cases require ligation of the varicose veins at the level of the internal ring of the inguinal canal with the patient in the anti-Trendelenburg position.

In many cases we found partial or total reflux into the ISV with signs of a secondary distal obstruction (Fig. 6).

Conclusions

The clinician and the research worker can both draw useful conclusions from the results of this investigation. The results of biochemical analysis of blood samples from the spermatic veins will be affected by the same hemodynamic factors which influence the development of the varicocele. The presence or otherwise of passive reflux in the ISV and of renal vein obstruction will affect the shunting of adrenal metabolites into the ISV. The results of varicocelectomy on seminal content and on frequency of pregnancy are contradictory and confusing. Before any definite conclusion can be drawn with regard to the influence of varicoceles on fertility the effect of treatment of the various groups of left-sided varicoceles on fertility must be investigated. A distinction must be made between the varicoceles:

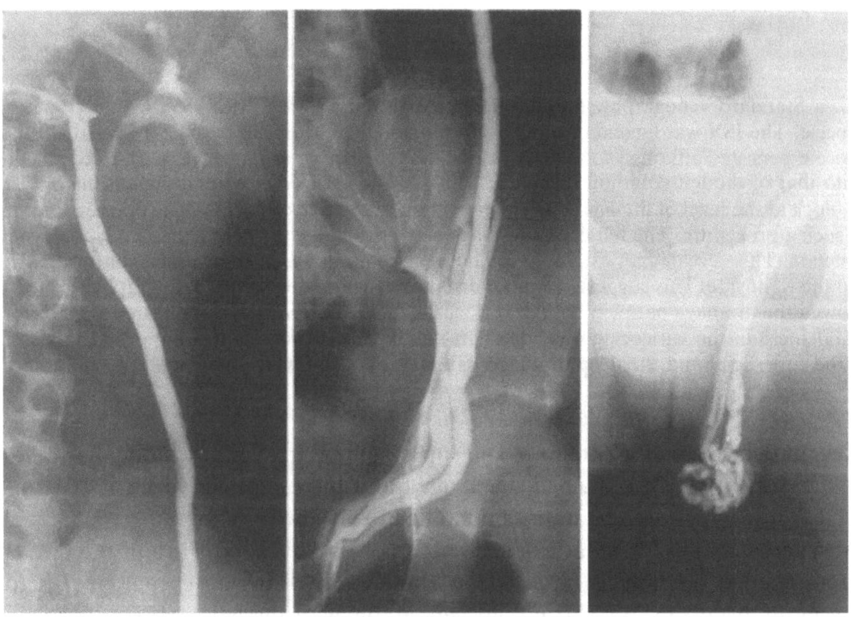

Fig. 7. ISV dividing in multiple veins at the suprainguinal level.

1) With and without passive reflux in the ISV;
2) with and without significant hemodynamic shunts;
3) with and without distal obstructions;
4) the various grades of varicoceles.

High ligation of the ISV is a safe and easy procedure but appears to have no effect on the venous outflow in 15% of cases. In some cases a high lumbar ligation is to be preferred to suprainguinal ligation, for example, in the presence of an extensive suprainguinal venous plexus (Fig. 7) and when the drainage vessels are closely situated to the refluxing ISV. The latter is difficult to determine through a suprainguinal incision. Another disadvantage of the suprainguinal approach is that it makes ligation of all the veins difficult when a complex network is present within the inguinal canal. When preoperative venography is not available, the method of choice is ligation of the various veins at the level of the internal ring with the patient lying in the anti-Trendelenburg position. Venography should be performed routinely in research centres to enable further differentiation of the varicocele syndrome to be made. This should allow a distinction to be made between those patients who will benefit from surgery and those who will not.

References

Brown JS (1976) Varicocelectomy in subfertile male: A ten-year experience with 295 cases. Fertil Steril 27:1046

Chait A, Matasar KW, Fabian CE, Mellinis HZ (1971) Vascular impressions on the ureters. AJR 111:729

Comhaire F, Vermeulen A (1975) Plasma testosterane in patients with varicocele and sexual inadequacy. J Clin Endocrinol Metab 40:824

Coolsaet BLRA (1978) Ureteric pathology in relation to right and left gonadal veins. J Urol 12:40

Coolsaet BLRA (1980) The varicocele syndrome: Venography determining the optimal level for surgical management. J Urol 124:833

De Schepper A (1972) Nutcracker fenomeen van de vena renalis en veneuze pathologie van de linker nier. J Belge Radiol 55:507

El-Safr AR, Mina E (1950) Anatomical and surgical aspects in operative management of varicocele. Urol Cutan Rev 54:257

Hanley HG, Harrison RG (1962) The nature and surgical treatment of varicocele. Br J Surg 56:64

Ivanessevich O (1960) Varicocele gauche dû à un reflux veineux. J Int Coll Surg 34:734

Lipshultz LI, Corriere JN (1977) Progressive testicular atrophy in the varicocele patient. J Urol 117:175

Macleod J (1969) Further observation in the role of varicocele in human male infertility. Fertil Steril 20:545

Nilsson S, Edvinsson A, Nilsson B (1979) Improvement of semen and pregnancy rate after ligation and division of the internal spermatic vein: fact or fiction? Br J Urol 51:591

Øster J (1971) Varicocele in children and adolescents. Scand J Urol Nephrol 5:27

Palomo A (1949) Radical cure of varicocele by a new technique. Preliminary report. J Urol 61:604

Seldinger SI (1953) Catheter replacement of needle in percutaneous arteriography: a new technique. Acta Radiol (Paris) 39:368

Steeno O, Knops J, Declerck L, Adimoelja A, Van de Voorde H (1976) Prevention of fertility disorders by detection and treatment of varicocele at school and college age. Andrologia 8:47

Verstoppen GR, Steeno OP (1977) Varicocele and the pathogenesis of the associated subfertility. I. Varicocelogenesis. Andrologia 9:133

Transfemoral Phlebography for Clarification of Persistent or Recurrent Varicocele

L. Weißbach and R. Janson

Introduction

It is necessary to be familiar with the normal anatomy of the venous drainage of the testis in order to be able to diagnose and treat persistent or recurrent varicocele. The pampiniform plexus consists of a network of 8–12 veins (Fig. 1), most of which are situated before the vas deferens (pars anterior). They drain the testis and surround the testicular artery. The smaller portion runs dorsally, mainly from the epididymus (pars posterior). In varicocele, the anterior group draining to the testicular vein undergoes varicose dilatation first and most intensely as a rule. The following drainage routes are possible for the two parts of the pampiniform plexus (Fig. 1):

1) Pars anterior, testicular vein (one or several main veins);
2) pars posterior, external spermatic vein, inferior epigastric vein, external iliac vein (Hanley and Harrison 1962).

Because of the great variations in venous anatomy, the frequency of persistence or of recurrence of idiopathic varicocele is understandable. It is reported as 0–25% in the literature (Weißbach 1978). In order to clarify the cause of the failed

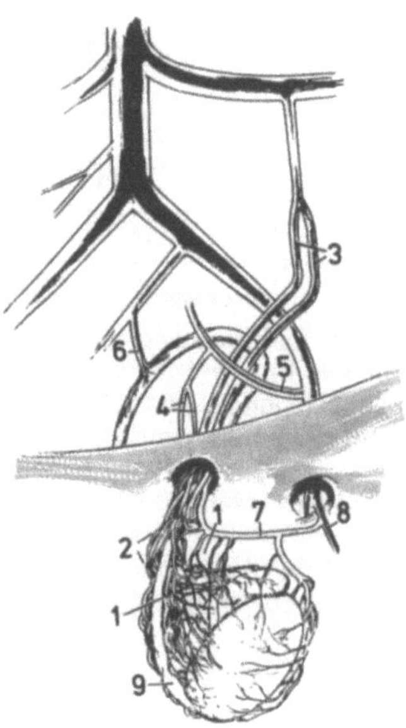

Fig. 1. The venous drainage of the testis. *1* Pars anterior of the pampiniform plexus; *2* pars posterior of the pampiniform plexus; *3* testicular vein; *4* external spermatic vein; *5* inferior epigastric vein; *6* vas deferens vein; *7* external pudendal vein; *8* greater saphenous vein; *9* vas deferens.

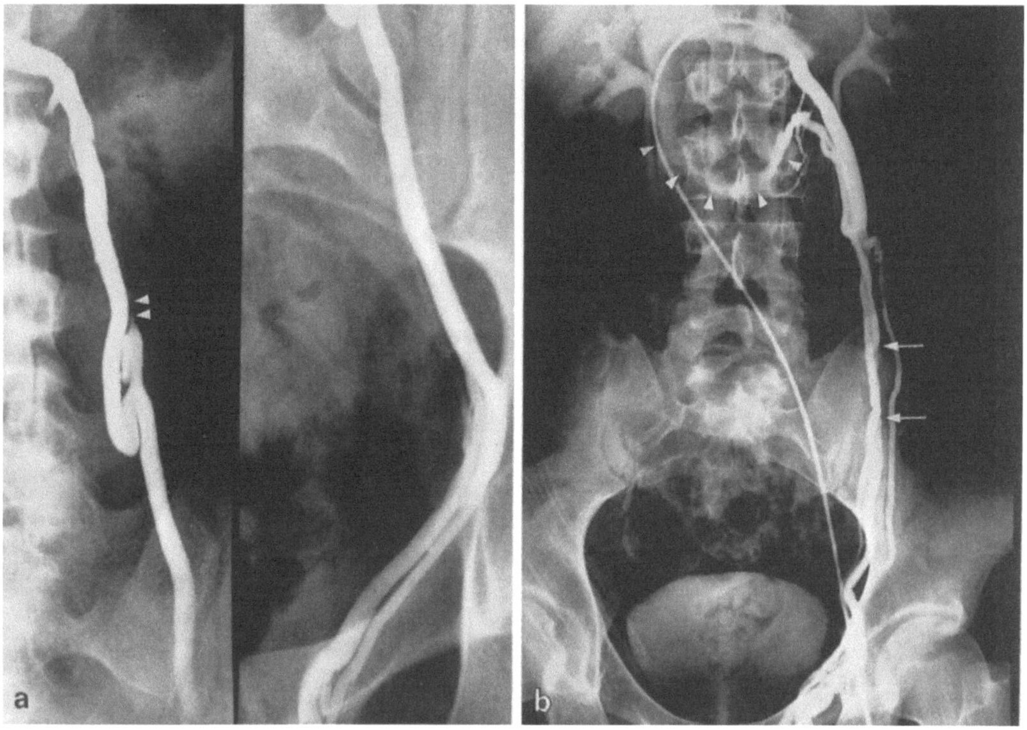

▲
Fig. 2 a, b. Selective injection into the testicular vein in persistent varicocele. **a** Vessel continuity maintained. Demonstration of the ligature site (◀) after first operation. **b** Continuity of several parallel branches of the testicular vein maintained. Demonstration of the ligature sites (→) after first operation. Collateral circulation (▶) via the paravertebral vein system to the inferior vena cava.

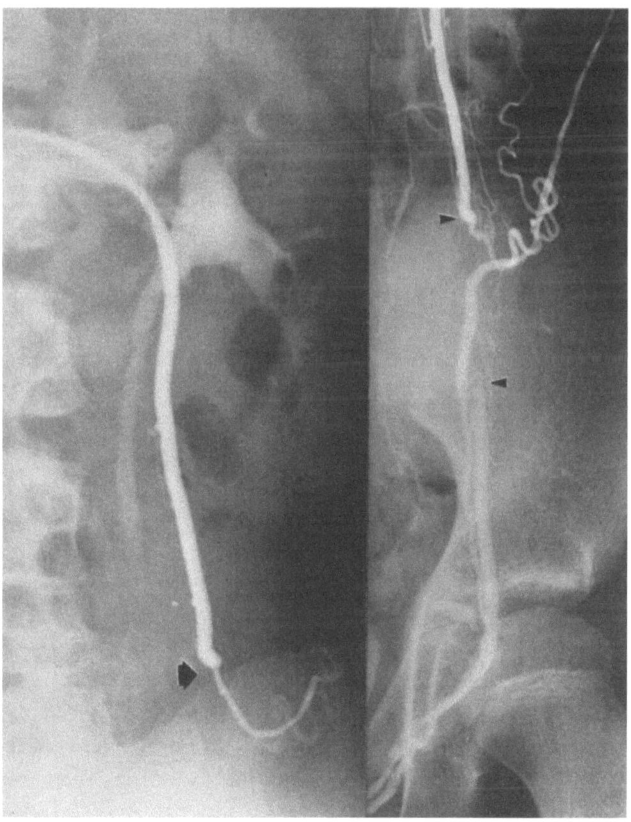

Fig. 3. Proximal resection site (➧) of the testicular vein after second operation. Filling of the proximal and distal vessel stumps (▶) via a collateral circulation deriving from the kidney capsule.

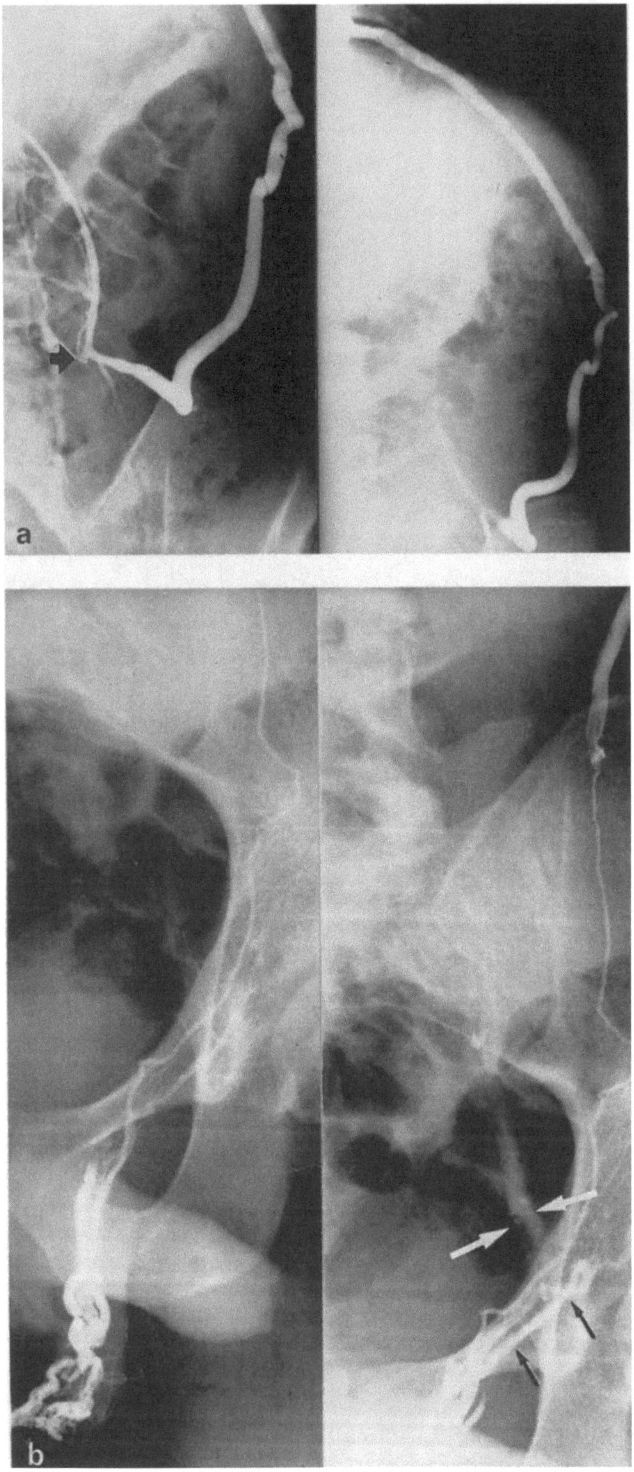

Fig. 4a, b

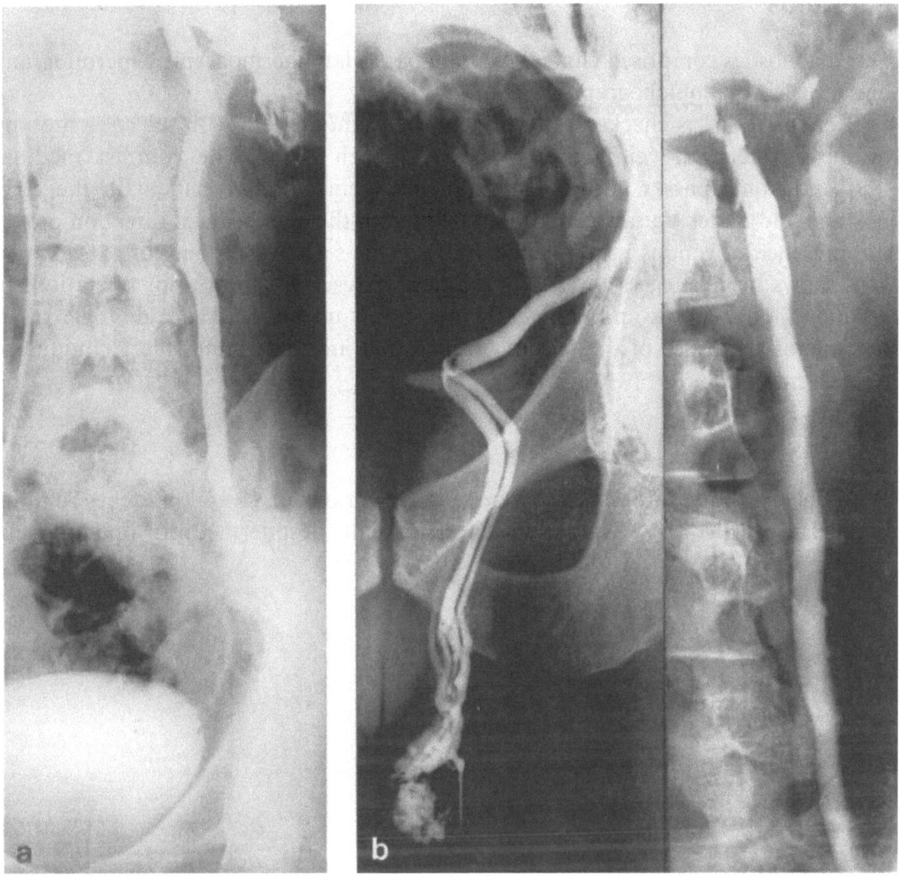

Fig. 5 a, b. Simulation of a sufficient ligature at the first operation. **a** Selective injection into the testicular vein with incomplete contrasting up to the lower sacral symphysis. **b** Injection into the pampiniform plexus with complete visualization of the testicular vein.

operation, 30 patients were investigated before a second-look operation. In most cases, there had been a prior high ligature of the left testicular vein. The nature of the prior operation in 30 patients with persistent or recurrent varicocele was a high ligature: $n=20$ (Bernardi, Palomo), $n=8$ (Ivanissevich), $n=2$ (Narath). Four of our patients had already been operated on unsuccessfully twice or three times. In a further case, embolization with the Gianturco coil had been performed 1 year previously.

Fig. 4 a, b. Transfemoral and scrotal phlebography in persistent varicocele. **a** Selective injection into the testicular vein with demonstration of the ligature site (➧). Hemodynamically ineffective collateral circulation via an atypical retroperitoneal vein to the azygos-hemiazygos venous system without filling of the pampiniform plexus. **b** Scrotal phlebography with demonstration of a relevant collateral circulation via the external spermatic vein (*black arrows*) into the external iliac vein (*white arrows*). Very thin connecting vein in the cranial direction.

Methods

Our diagnostics comprised clinical examination, plate thermography, spermiogram, and transfemoral phlebography.

Venous reflux is checked after puncture of femoral vein with selective probing of the left femoral vein (Janson and Weißbach 1978). The contrast medium frequently only passes into the left testicular vein with the patient in the erect position and under Valsalva conditions. Reflux in the craniocaudal direction proves the presence of venous insufficiency. Subsequent selective probing of the gonadal vein shows in most cases the site of ligation or resection from prior operation. In addition, anastomoses and collaterals are shown up better. The radiologic result determines the cause of the failure of operation and determines the technique of reintervention.

Results

With one exception, the testicular vein (Fig. 2a) or one or several branches running parallel to it (Fig. 2b) was open in all our patients despite the prior operation. In

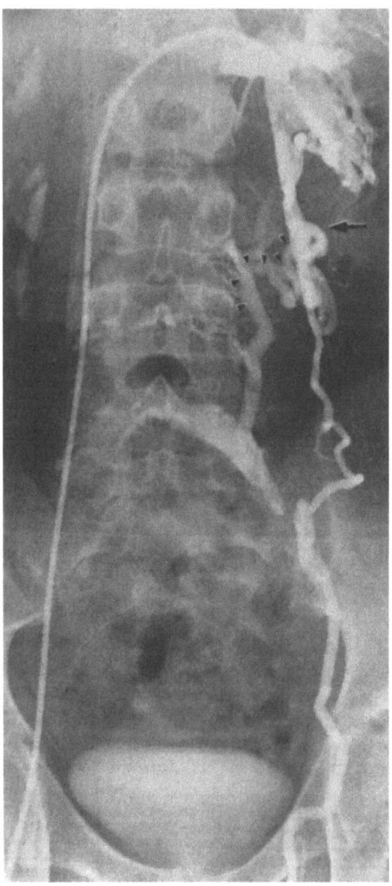

Fig. 6. Selective injection into the testicular vein with demonstration of a collateral circulation (▶) to the left ascending lumbar vein and contrasting of the common iliac vein (←) ligature site.

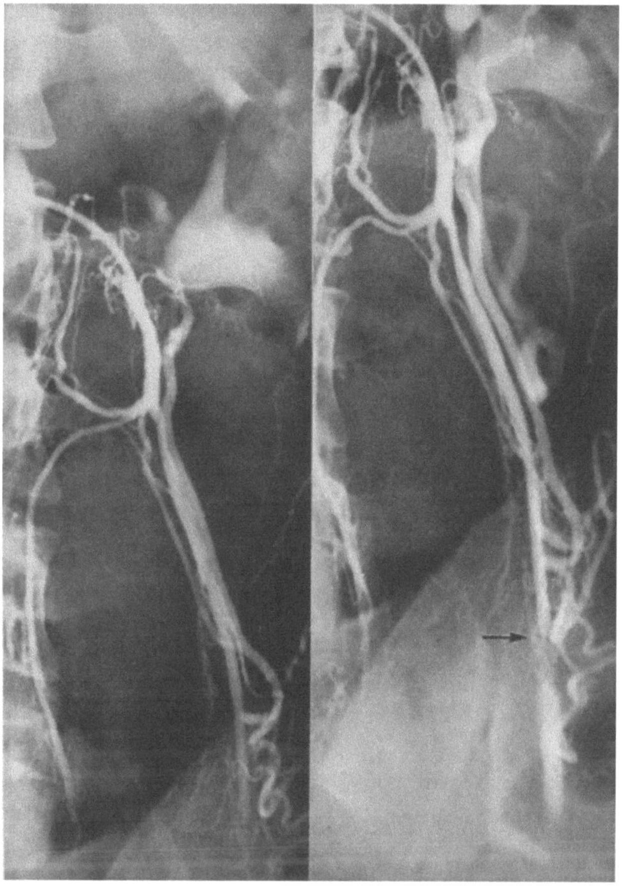

Fig. 7. Selective injection into the testicular vein with demonstration of the resection site (→) and representation of collaterals in the median direction to the lumbar venous plexus and in the lateral direction to the ureteric veins and the veins of the kidney capsule.

two cases, there was a blood supply via collaterals distal to the ligature (Fig. 3). In two further patients, the gonadal vein did not fill completely despite selective probing. Scrotal phlebography is indicated only in such cases. In one case, it shows the filling of the external iliac vein by the inferior epigastric vein and the external spermatic vein (Fig. 4a, b). In the other patient, we were able to demonstrate the maintained continuity of the testicular vein only by scrotal phlebography (Fig. 5a, b). An incomplete visualization of the testicular vein thus does not mean in every case that a proper ligature was performed. Hence the contrast medium drainage must always be checked with an oblique body position and during a press test in transfemoral phlebography.

We have found anastomoses to the veins of the kidney (renal parenchyma, renal pelvis, renal capsule) and ureter and to the lumbar venous plexus (Figs. 2b, 4b, 5, 6). In a few cases there were links to the azygos–hemiazygos system (Fig. 4a). In addition, we were able to demonstrate short circuits to the external iliac veins. More than half of our patients had one or several of the specified collaterals (Fig. 7). These must be carefully registered, since they are collapsed during the surgical intervention, so that they are readily overlooked. Later, these vessels can become a hemodynamically effective collateral circulation with connection to the distal vessel trunk of the testicular vein. Attention must thus be paid to an exact investigation technique.

Conclusions

A varicocele persists or recurs in about 10% of the cases after surgery. The causes are incomplete operation or variations of the retroperitoneal venous system (Riedl 1979). Radiologic clarification is hence always necessary before a second operation. Various methods are available for this:

1) Transfemoral phlebography (Ahlberg et al. 1965, 1966; Comhaire and Kunnen 1976; Janson and Weißbach 1978; Riedl 1979; Strecker and Sinagowitz 1979);
2) scrotal phlebography (Heising et al. 1979);
3) intraoperative visualization from the exposed gonadal vein.

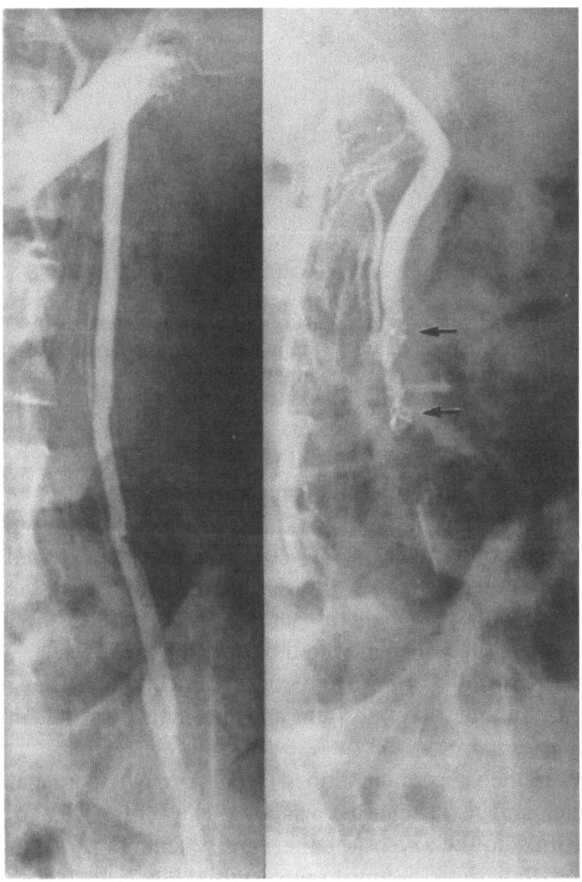

Fig. 8. Embolization of the testicular vein with two Gianturco coils (←) and subsequent thrombotic occlusion of the vessel.

We prefer the transfemoral retrograde technique, because it demonstrates the pathologic hemodynamics solely with preparation of optimal image documents. All variations are visualized best in this technique. In particular cases, embolization with the Gianturco coil (Fig. 8) can be performed immediately after phlebography for treatment or labeling (Thelen et al. 1979).

References

Ahlberg NE, Bartley O, Chidekel N (1965) Retrograde contrast filling of the left gonadal vein. A roentgenologic and anatomical study. Acta Radiol (Diagn) (Stockh) 3:385–392

Ahlberg NE, Bartley O, Chidekel N, Fritjofsson A (1966) Phlebography in varicocele scroti. Acta Radiol (Diagn) (Stockh) 4:517–528

Comhaire F, Kunnen M (1976) Selective retrograde venography of the internal spermatic vein: A conclusive approach to the diagnosis of varicocele. Andrologia 8:11–24

Heising J, Engelking R, Allhoff E, Geppert E, Hüls W (1979) Erfolglose Operation der Varikozele – Diagnostik und Reeingriff. Akt Urol 10:209–215

Janson R, Weißbach L (1978) Zur Phlebographie der Vena testicularis bei Varikozelen-persistenz bzw. -rezidiv. Fortschr Röntgenstr 129:485–490

Riedl P (1979) Selektive Phlebographie und Katheterthrombosierung der Vena testicularis bei primärer Varikozele. Eine angiographisch-anatomische und klinische Studie. Wien Klin Wochenschr [Suppl] 91:1–19

Strecker EP, Sinagowitz E (1979) Transfemorale Phlebographie der V. spermatica beim sogenannten Varikozelen-Rezidiv. Akt Urol 10:205–208

Thelen M, Weißbach L, Franken Th (1979) Die Behandlung der idiopathischen Varikozele durch transfemorale Spiralokklusion der Vena testicularis sinistra. Fortschr Röntgenstr 131:24–29

Weißbach L (1978) Die idiopathische Varikozele – Eine Übersicht. Extracta Urologica 1:255–268

Phallography
A New Technique of Nocturnal Tumescence Monitoring in Male Impotence

E. Wespes and C. C. Schulman

More men suffering from impotence are seeking treatment. The question of whether the condition is psychogenic or organic, or a combination of both, represents a difficult problem of differential diagnosis.

Phallography, or nocturnal tumescence monitoring (NPT), is a relatively simple procedure allowing differentiation of organic erection disability from psychogenic impotence. It gives the investigator a scientific basis for his differentiation between organic and psychogenic causes of impotence (Karacan 1970; Karacan et al. 1972 c). The concept is based on the regular cycle of nighttime erections in healthy adult males directly associated with rapid eye movement (REM) stages of sleep (Karacan et al. 1972 a, b). There ordinarily are three or four episodes of both REM and erections during the night, each lasting an average of 20–30 min (Fisher et al. 1965, 1975).

Description

The instrument is a recorder with two rings made of mercury-filled Silastic tubing (Karacan 1969). The appropriate strain gauges are selected in function of the size of the penis. Plastic cylinders of known diameters are used to calibrate the gauges and create a standardized baseline. One gauge is placed near the base of the penis and the other around the coronal sulcus. Changes in the circumference of the penis produce a change in electric gauge, which is amplified and recorded on the strip paper chart.

Recording

With normal erections the two lines go up and the baseline, which records the base of the penis, ordinarily expands more than the tip (Fig. 1). Poor expansion on the chart means that the penis is less rigid, making intercourse difficult. Several subjects show a gradual decline of the baseline during the first few hours of sleep since a drop in systemic arterial pressure during this period is well known (Richardson et al. 1969).

Interpretation

It is possible to see a normal nocturnal erection, a partial nocturnal erection, pulsations, fluctuation, short erection and poor expansion of the base of the penis, and no erection.

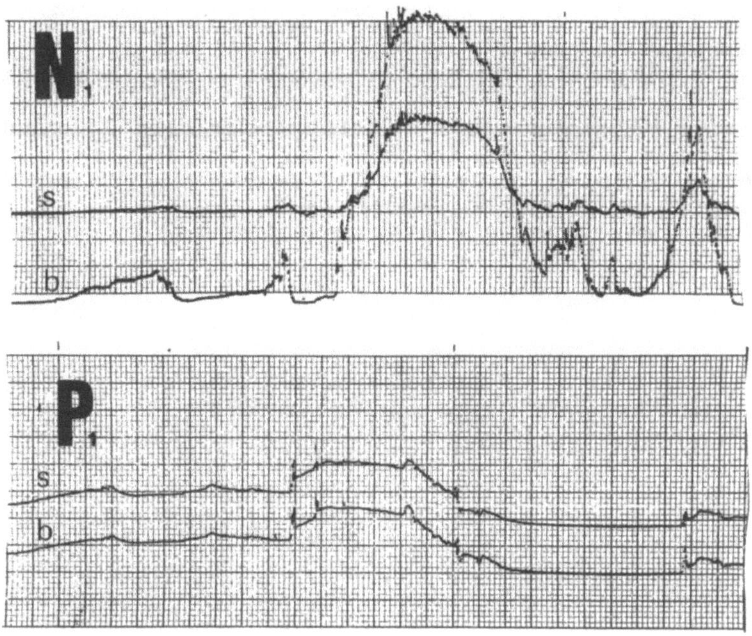

Fig. 1. Monitoring of nocturnal tumescence. *N 1,* Normal erection. *P 1,* Very partial erection. *s,* Top of the penis. *b,* Base of the penis.

After correlating NPT patterns from one patient with those from other patients, one may decide whether the patient NPT pattern is normal or pathologic. If it is normal, the neurophysiologic mechanism of erection is intact and the patient should be oriented to a psychological treatment. On the other hand, the absence of NPT in a patient complaining of impotence is strongly suggestive of some basic disturbance of the vascular or neurologic mechanism of erection.

Conclusion

Phallography is an excellent technique for screening patients complaining of erection failure. The test will separate organic from psychogenic impotence and can demonstrate different types of erection disability. This technique can provide objective evidence of erection failure and aids in the selection of patients for surgical or psychological treatment of erection difficulties.

References

Fisher C, Gross J, Zuch J (1965) Cycle of penile erection synchronous with dreaming (REM) sleep. Arch Gen Psychiatry 12:29

Fisher C et al. (1975) The assessment of nocturnal REM erection in the differential diagnosis of sexual impotence. J Sex Marital Ther 1:277

Karacan I (1969) A simple and inexpensive transducer for quantitative measurements of penile erection during sleep. Behav Res Meth Instr 1:251

Karacan I (1970) Clinical value of nocturnal erection in the prognosis and diagnosis of impotence. Med Asp Human Sexual 4:27
Karacan I, Hursch CJ, Williams RL (1972a) Some characteristics of nocturnal penile tumescence in elderly males. J Gerontol 27:39
Karacan I, Hursch CJ, Williams RL, Litell RC (1972b) Some characteristics of nocturnal penile tumescence during puberty. Pediatr Res 6:529
Karacan I, Hursch CJ, Williams RL, Thornby JI (1972c) Some characteristics of nocturnal penile tumescence in young adults. Arch Gen Psychiatry 26:351
Richardson DW et al. (1969) Variation in arterial pressure throughout the day and night. Clin Sci Mol Med 26:445

Angiography in Male Impotence

J. Struyven, G. Kuhn, and C. C. Schulman

Pudendal angiography is indicated in specific cases of male impotence after a thorough clinical, psychological, and plethysmographic evaluation provides a convincing probability of arterial lesion.

Anatomy

Erection is due to an increase of blood volume in the corpora cavernosa provoked by a venous occlusion mechanism under neurologic control. The blood supply of the corpora cavernosa is from the right and left cavernous arteries (a. profunda penis), which are terminal branches of the medial pudendal arteries. The internal pudendal artery, terminal branch of the hypogastric artery, after having given off the inferior hemorrhoidal artery, divides into a superficial branch (perineal artery) and a deeper branch giving off in succession the bulbar artery, the cavernous artery, and the dorsal artery of the penis (Figs. 1–3). Cavernous branches arise frequently from the dorsal artery of the penis, which courses between the bulb and the corpora cavernosa before reaching the dorsal face of the penis. In a small number of cases, an accessory internal pudendal artery arises from the pudendal artery, the hypogastric artery, or the obturator artery.

Examination Method

Pudendal arteriography requires general anesthesia to prevent pain induced by contrast media. A previous study, however, has demonstrated that examination could be performed under local anesthesia using well-tolerated nonionic contrast media. Both hypogastric arteries are usually catheterized by right femoral approach using a cobra catheter attached to a superselective wire guide. In 20% of cases this catheter is exchanged for a Sidewinder B Simmons catheter to obtain adequate catheterization.

If there is no evidence of proximal iliac stenosis, the catheter is drawn beyond the origin of the superior gluteal artery. Correct visualization of the cavernous artery and corporum cavernosum requires 30 ml contrast media injected at the rate of 3 ml/s. Usually 20 frames at the rate of 1/s are taken at the end of the injection. Initial examinations were recorded using 35-cm serial radiography. Pudendal arteriography is recorded on 105 mm spotfilms, which provide good resolution and decrease irradiation. The patient is positioned in a LAO projection for the investigation of the left cavernous artery and RAO for the right side.

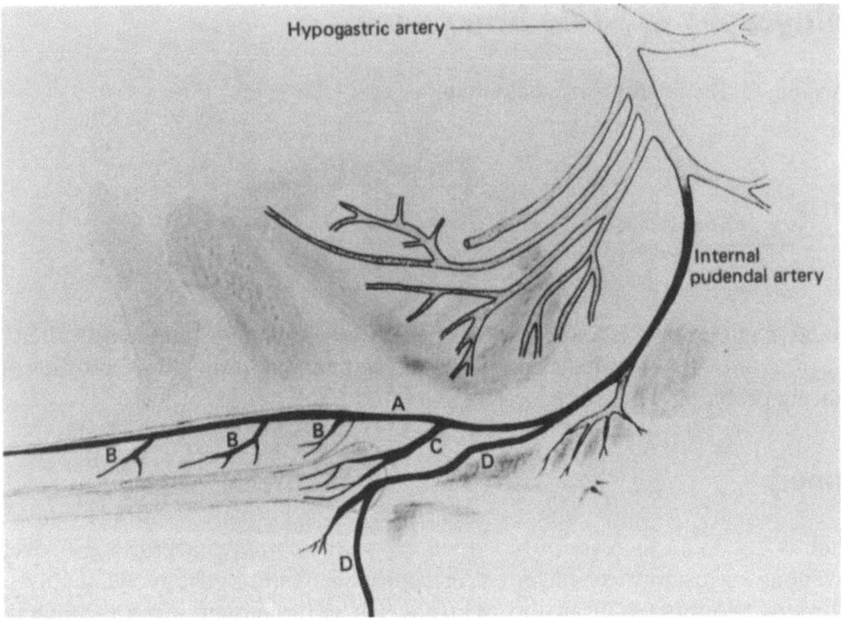

Fig. 1. Normal anatomy: *A,* Dorsal artery of penis. *B,* Cavernous artery. *C,* Bulbar artery. *D,* Superficial perineal artery.

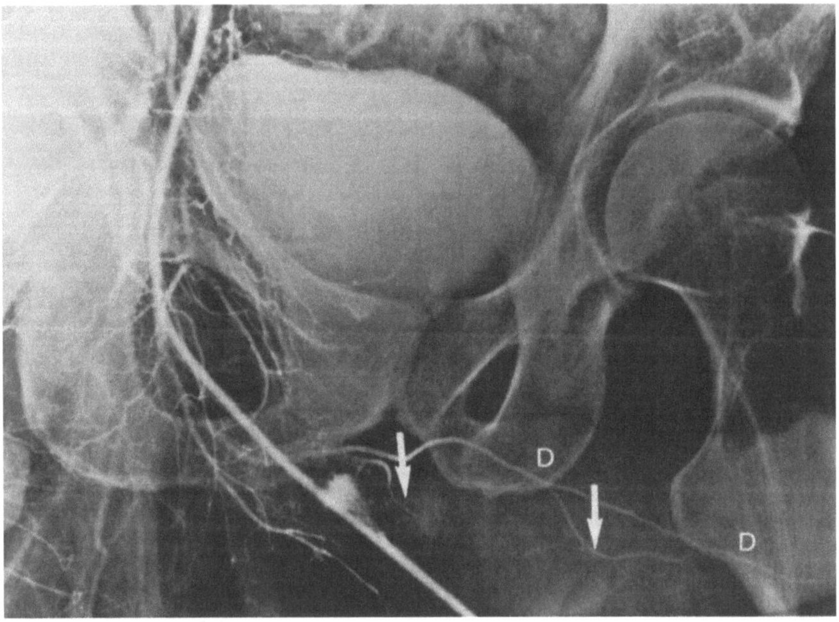

Fig. 2. Normal anatomy: *D,* Dorsal artery of penis. Two cavernous arteries (*arrows*) arise from the dorsal artery.

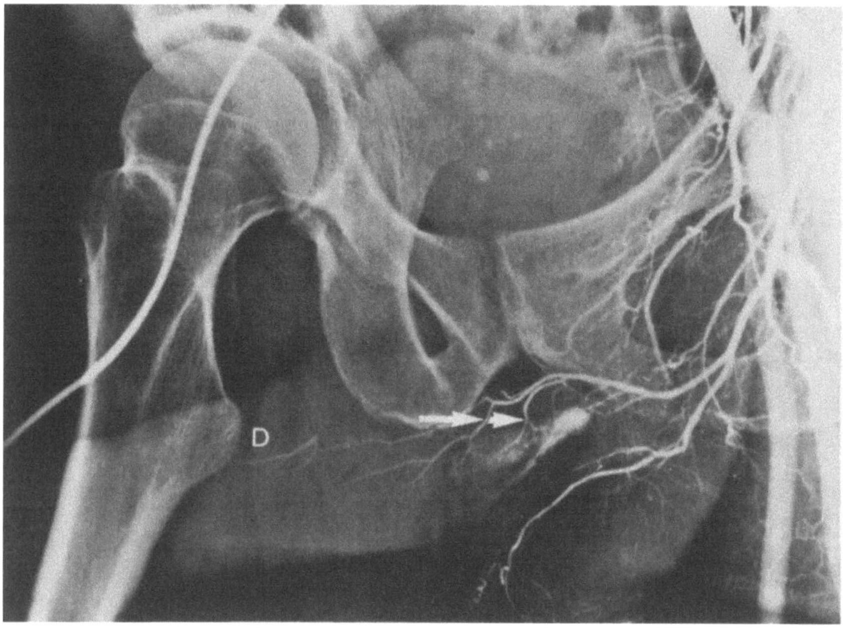

Fig. 3. Normal anatomy: *D,* Dorsal artery of penis. Multiple cavernous arteries (*arrows*). Reflux opacification of dorsal artery.

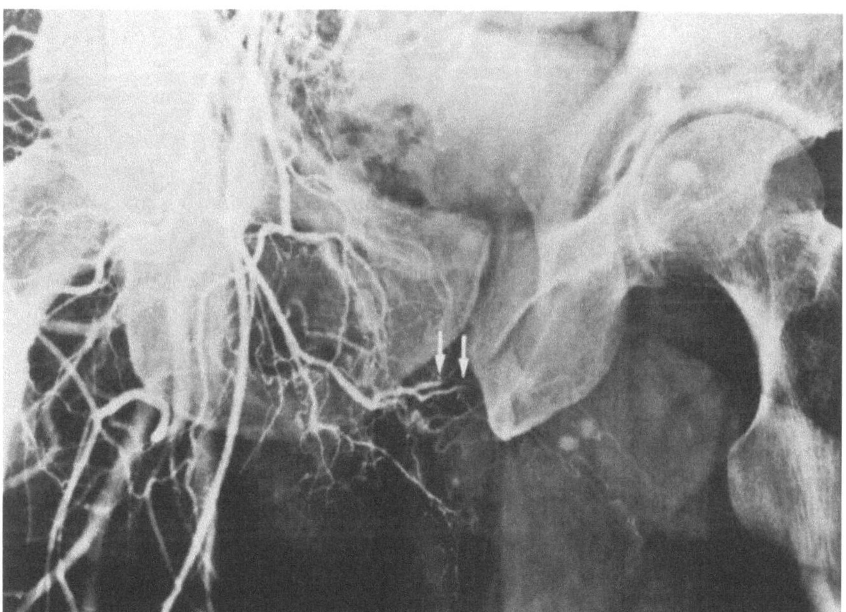

Fig. 4. Typical atheromatous lesion. Abrupt narrowing of dorsal artery of penis and cavernous artery (*arrows*).

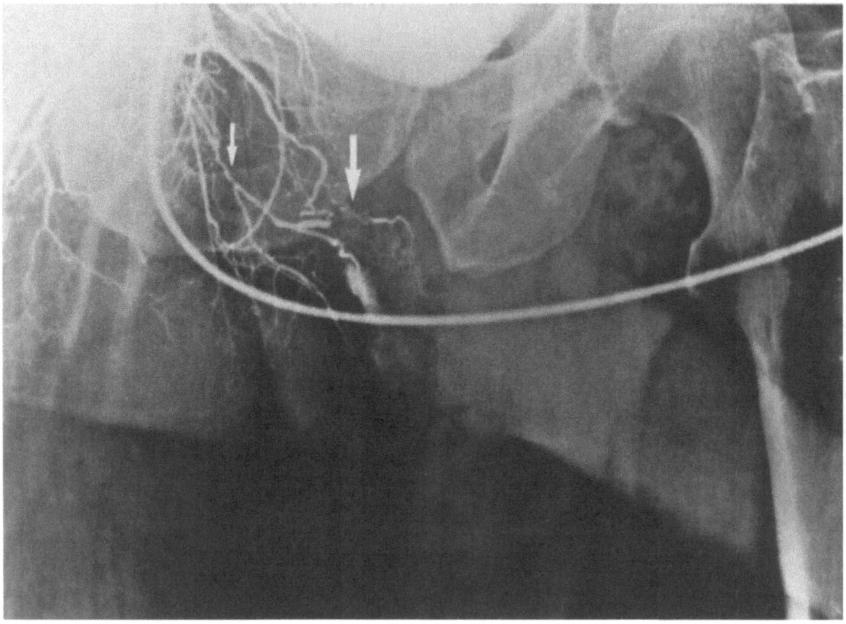

Fig. 5. Obstructive atheromatous lesion. Narrowing of the pudendal artery (*small arrow*). Narrowing on an accessory pudendal artery (*large arrow*).

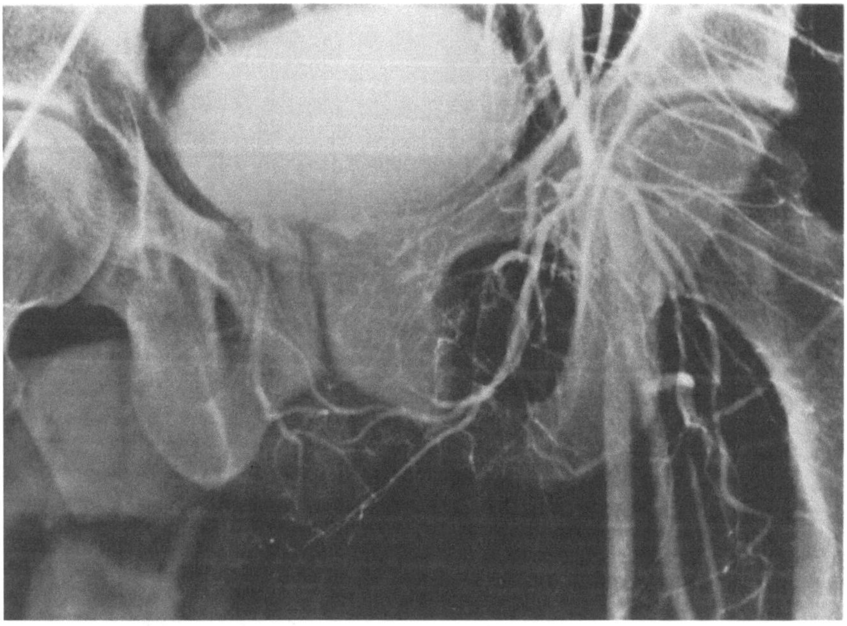

Fig. 6. Thromboangiitis in a 27-year-old man. Erection suddenly disappeared after severe septicemia following surgery of a pilonidal cyst. Complete obstruction of the cavernous artery and heterolateral shunting.

Indications

Pudendal arteriography is indicated in the detection of arterial lesions responsible for sexual impotence lasting at least 5 months. Psychological origin of impotence has to be excluded and convincing probability of arterial lesions can be demonstrated by a plethysmographic study.

Pathology

Thirty-six patients ranging between the ages of 19 and 61 with a unique complaint of impotence were investigated. Total impotence was from 6 months to 4 years with a mean of 1 year 4 months.

Classic lesions of pudendal arteries subdivide into three groups:

1) *Traumatic Lesions:* Deep trauma of the perineum, fracture of the pelvis, pelvis surgery.
2) *Obstructive Lesions:* Atheroma, thromboangiitis, diabetic arteritis.
3) *Dysplasia:* Absence of cavernous artery.

Of the 36 investigated ptients, 12 (39%) had a normal arteriogram. Obstructive atherosclerotic lesions were found in 16 (44%) patients (Figs. 4, 5). Diabetic arteritis was responsible for obstructive lesions in 4 (10%) patients. Dysplasia occurred in 2 (5%) patients with bilateral aplasia of cavernous arteries and in one with unilateral aplasia of the cavernous artery. Thromboangiitis was established in one patient (Fig. 6).

Lesions were bilateral in 85% of cases. A proximal hypogastric stenosis was found in 10% of cases, the pudendal artery was involved in 20% of cases, and 70% of lesions were documented on the dorsal or cavernous arteries.

Conclusion

In most cases, impotence is induced by distal lesions of the pudendal artery. Selective pudendal arteriography is essential in cases of sexual impotence in which peripheral vascular lesions are suspected. Angiography is essential before the planning of a revascularisation procedure.

Acknowledgment. Thanks to A. Degrelle and T. Perilleux for their valuable assistance.

References

Ginestié JF, Romieux A (1976) L'exploration radiologique de l'impuissance. Maloine, Paris
Struyven J, Gregoir W, Giannakopoulos X, Wauters E (1979a) Selective pudendal arteriography. Eur Urol 5:233–242
Struyven J, Jeanty P, Jeanmart J, Ghosen M, Schulman CC (1979b) Angiographic exploration of male impotence. J Belge Radiol 62:597–601

Peroperative Contact Radiography in Kidney Stone Surgery

J. Simon and C. C. Schulman

The aim of any surgery for renal stones is to remove fragments of calculus. Indeed, such residual concretion provides an opportunity for relapse since it is an ideal nucleus for crystallization so that when urine is supersaturated obstructive stones may rapidly occur, and there is a nidus of bacteria deeply trapped in the stone, which cannot be reached by antibacterial agents. Eradication of infection is then useless. The problem is not always to remove the small fragments but often to localize them. Contact radiography is the simpliest method and provides satisfactory control in kidney stone surgery.

Procedure

A double X-ray film included in a sterile sheath, the size of the kidney, is presented with a notch for the renal pedicle, and can be closely applied to the kidney (X-Omat KS film for kidney surgery from Kodak). It is exposed with a usual portable X-ray plant. X-rays are focalized with a metallic cone, which is sterilely held by the surgeon and placed against the kidney.

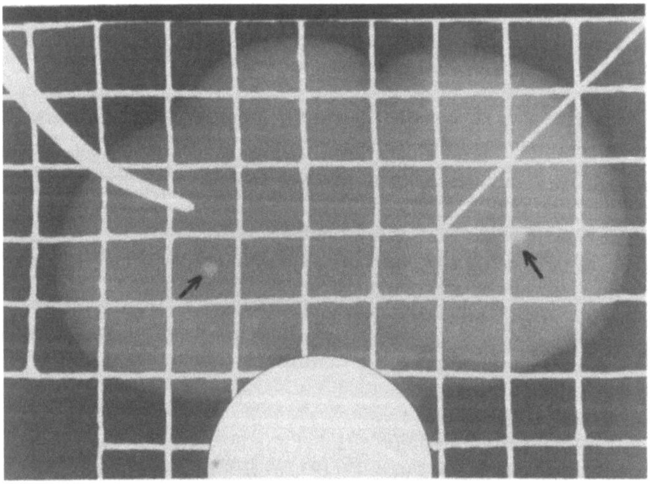

Fig. 1. Contact radiography showing two persisting little stones (*arrows*) at each pole of the kidney.

The sensitivity of the films (Kodak X-Omat KS) allows detection of very small concretions even when only slightly opaque. The use of two films in the same sheath provides exposures of different contrast.

Identical reference marks have to be available both on the kidney and film surfaces. This is achieved by a wire wetting against the kidney. Precise localization of the remaining fragments is then obtained and clips are placed directly on the renal capsule in front of the fragments. This allows work without a cumbersome device. Incidence can also be taken in profile to further improve localization.

The renal sinus area is sometimes difficult to visualize due to the notch in the film for the pedicle. It is then helpful to use perpendicularly orientated films to cover the whole area of the kidney. When developed, the plates are placed side by side to reconstitute the complete view (Fig. 1).

This procedure needs no costly device and is easy to perform. An increased sensitivity of X-ray films should still improve accuracy.

Radiographic Search for Renal Calculi During Nephrolithotomy by the Renodor Technique

K. F. Albrecht and J. Moncada

For the positive prevention of recurrent stone formation, even the tiniest fragments must be removed when staghorn calculi or multiple concretions are present in the kidney. If employed in good time, i.e. before intrarenal haemorrhage occurs, pyeloscopes, nowadays commercially available, can effectively assist in the removal of residual stones. However, this method does not guarantee that all fragments are removed. Therefore X-ray control will always be necessary at the end of the operation. After numerous comparative tests with mobile X-ray units with and without cones, with image converters and 6-valve generators featuring heavy-duty X-ray tubes and with stationary grids and stationary Bucky cabinets, we have to date relied on the radiographic method recommended by Leusch in 1970, based on the Status X installation from Siemes AG, Erlangen, and adapted for urological purposes. Since 1970 we have employed the unit carrying the tradename Renodor (Fig. 1) in about 600 nephrolithotomies.

The X-ray tube features a 9-cm-long and 1.2-cm-thick finger-shaped anode shaft and this is fitted to a rotary arm on a mobile stand. The anode shaft can be readily moved into the wound before, behind or below the kidney. A sterile mammography film (Kodak MR 1) packed in a flexible foil is cut in the darkroom to the size 9×12 cm and is placed on the other side, behind or on the kidney. The kidney must be mobilized, but not dislocated in front of the wound. Retractors or hooks can remain in the wound. Because of the large X-ray beam exit angle of 120°, the sterile applicator tip can be introduced into the wound for only one-half to two-thirds the kidney depth. The focus–kidney distance should be as large as possible, i.e. 3–5 cm. We obtain this distance by holding the kidney away from the anode shaft and close to the film by means of readily sterilizable, wooden and radiotranslucent fixation forceps. Owing to the relatively short focus–film distance, it is not possible to present the whole kidney on a single film. Thus, the caudal and cranial as well as the middle portion of large kidneys must be X-rayed separately. For orientation purposes and for better localization of the calculi, we always thrust two thin needles into the lower kidney pole and one needle into the upper kidney pole. Frequently, it is necessary to determine if a residual stone is lodged in the middle, in the anterior or in a dorsal calyx of the kidney.

By placing the film over the kidney pole and by applying the anode shaft below it by means of a curved metal holder, after Leusch (1970), the calculus can be verified as being in a dorsal, ventral or medial calyx.

The rating of the Renodor is 55 kV at 1 mA. Thus, the output is 20 times lower than that of the smallest X-ray unit (Heliosphere). As a result, the dose to the patient and surgeon is almost negligible. Measurements with the pen-type dose-

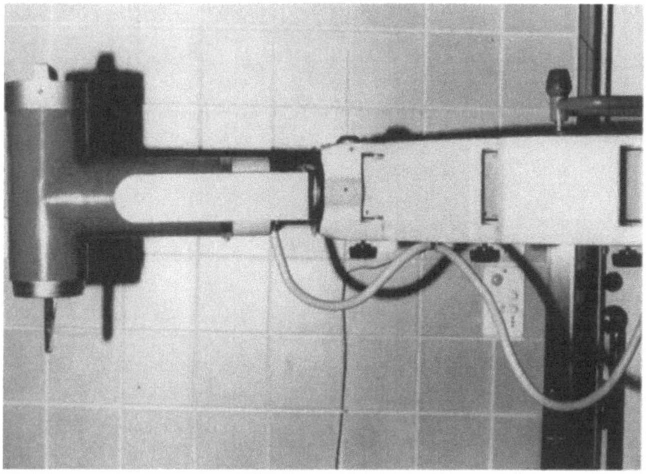

Fig. 1. Mobile X-ray unit Renodor (Siemens AG, Erlangen, West Germany) for intra-operative localization of renal calculi.

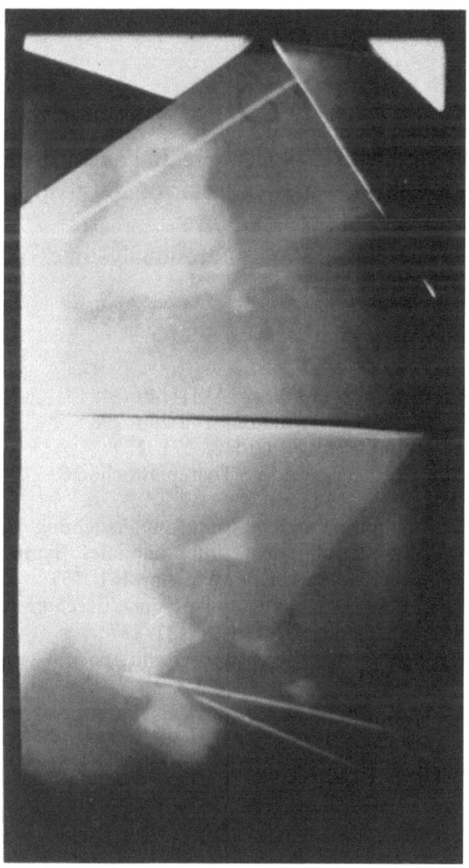

Fig. 2. Staghorn stone in the left kidney. Radiographic montage obtained by combining two intra-operative Renodor films before removal of the calculi. The upper pole (*above*) and the lower pole with two marking needles (*below*).

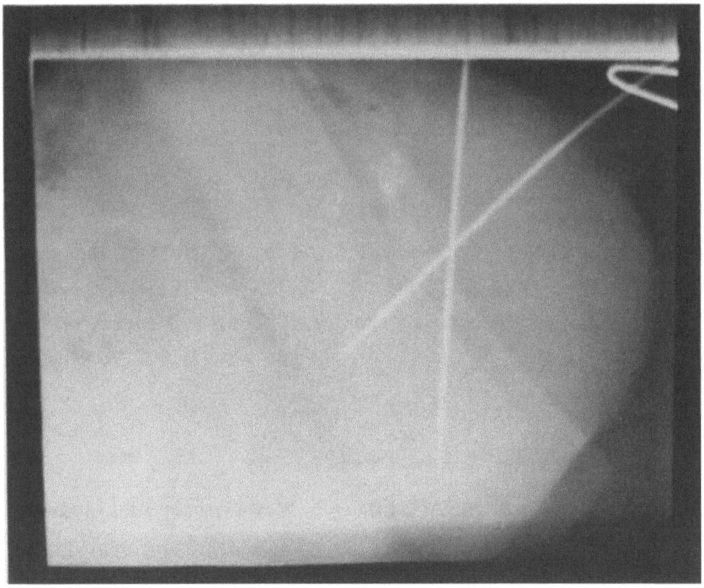

Fig. 3. Same patient as in Fig. 2. A small residual piece of concrement can be seen in the lower pole; it was successfully removed by directed nephrotomy.

meter in front of the lead apron and in front of the lead glove gave the following doses to the surgeon per exposure (0.8 s): hands 3–4 mR, breast bone 0.6 mR, gonads 0.3 mR. These values per exposure are lower by a factor of 200 than the permissible weekly dose in accordance with DIN 6811.

The use of the Renodor unit and the localization of residual stones are demonstrated in a clinical case (Figs. 2, 3).

References

Albrecht KF (1972a) Urologische Röntgenuntersuchungen. Urologe [A] 11:140–148
Albrecht KF (1972b) Urologische Röntgendiagnostik. Krankenhausarzt 45:290–298
Albrecht KF (1974) Operative Steinprophylaxe. Verh Dtsch Ges Urol 25:271–275
Albrecht KF (1976) Die operative Prophylaxe des Harnsteinrezidivs. Therapiewoche 26: 5860–5866
Albrecht KF, Moncada J (1979) Probleme der intraoperativen Röntgenuntersuchung bei Nierenausgußsteinen. In: Porpaczy P (ed) Kongreßbericht, Internationales Symposium zur Erforschung der Infektionen des Harntraktes. Egermann, Wien, pp 161–163
Albrecht KF, Hahn M, Brinkmann B (1971) Die Entfernung von Korallensteinen durch große longitudinale Nephrotomie (sogenannter Sektionsschnitt). Urol Int 26:122–137
Baur HH (1972) Intraoperative Röntgenuntersuchung bei Nierensteinoperationen mit dem Röntgengerät "Status-X". Urologe [A] 11:190–195
Baur HH (1973) Der Renodor – ein neuartiges Röntgengerät für den intraoperativen Nachweis von Nierensteinen. Electromedica (Siemens AG) 80–84
Leusch G (1970) Ein neues Röntgenverfahren in der Nierensteinchirurgie. Urologe [A] 9:182–188

Bidimensional Radioscopy
A Rapid Method for Peroperative Localization of Residual Calculi

W. A. De Sy and W. Oosterlinck

Safe, easy running, and reliable radiologic equipment is one of the most important requirements in staghorn calculus surgery. Indeed, it is essential that all stone fragments should be removed to avoid stone recurrence and to sterilize urine. Looking out for the last residual stone fragment may be a tedious and time-consuming task.

After removal of the bulk of the stone we use contact films to carry out peroperative forward-backward and oblique radiography with metal markers on the kidney surface. This is usually sufficient for localization of the remaining stones. If, however, after this procedure one or more stone fragments remain "unfindable", we prefer bidimensional radioscopy over a series of time-consuming radiographies to localize the stone and to guide a small nephrotomy.

Method

Easy running, small-sized radiologic equipment for peroperative radioscopy with an image intensifier and a television screen must be used. We personally use the Siremobil II (Siemens). It is equipped with an automatic dose rate control, which facilitates considerably peroperative working. Its image intensifier and television screen with 1225 lines give a very high definition of the images. A very efficient small field collimator reduces the radiation exposure outside the beam to a minimum and also contributes to the image quality.

The kidney must be completely mobilized and lifted up from the wound. A broad lumbotomy from the dorsal paravertebral muscles to the rectus sheet is necessary, but this is always so when complicated staghorn calculi must be removed.

The procedure is illustrated in Fig. 1. A forward-backward exposure quickly shows whether the stone is localized in the upper, middle, or lower pole. Under television screen control the stone is localized by means of two perpendicularly placed fine needles or clips (Fig. 1 A). The kidney is then turned over 90° with the help of a spoon, specially designed for this purpose (Fig. 2). In this way, either the hilus or the back of the kidney is exposed to the X-ray beam. The stone can again be localized by a needle cross in the ventral or dorsal part of the kidney (Fig. 1 B). Then the kidney is brought into its previous foreward-backward position and if the stone is in the dorsal part of the kidney, a new marker is placed under radioscopic control on the dorsal kidney surface on the stone. Then a fine intradermal needle

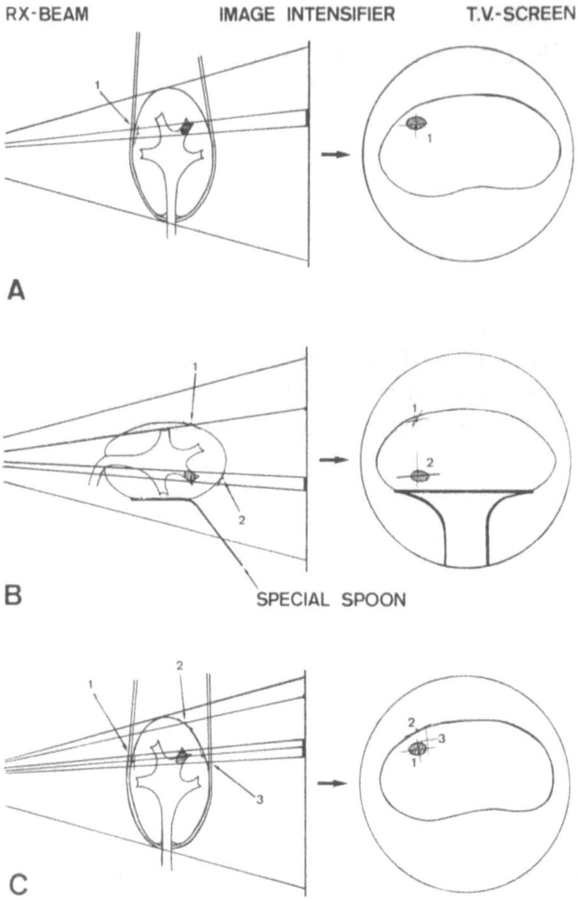

Fig. 1. A Kidney is brought out of the wound in the forward-backward position in front of the image intensifier. The stone is located by a needle cross or marker on the ventral kidney surface (*1*). **B** The kidney is turned over 90° with the help of a special spoon. Now the stone can be localized in the ventral or dorsal part of the kidney by another needle cross or marker (*2*). **C** If the stone is in the dorsal part of the kidney, a new marker is placed at the dorsal kidney surface (*3*).

is introduced obliquely at the kidney surface right on the stone and a small nephrotomy, which allows extraction of the stone, can be easily performed. The entire procedure takes about 5 min.

Radiation Exposure

The Siremobil has a very efficient small-field collimator, reducing radiation exposure outside the beam to a minimum. It consist merely of slight secondary irradiation from the exposed kidney and the surrounding tissues. In the middle of the beam a dose of 1500 mrem/h was measured (Fig. 3). At 15 cm from the middle of the beam it was 126 mrm/h while at 45 cm it was reduced to 1.1 mrem/h. If the

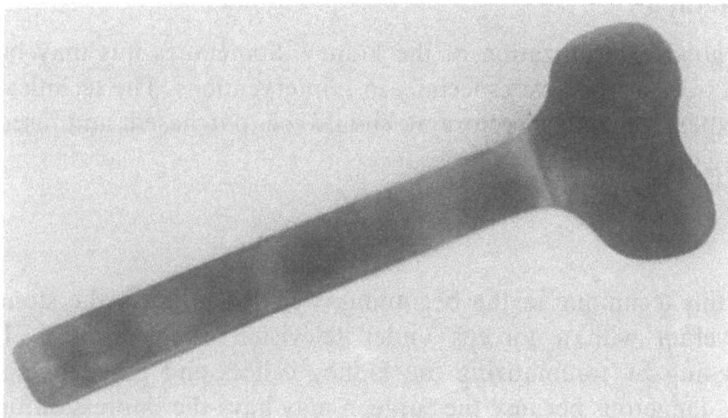

Fig. 2. A special homemade kidney spoon for easy presentation of the kidney in oblique position.

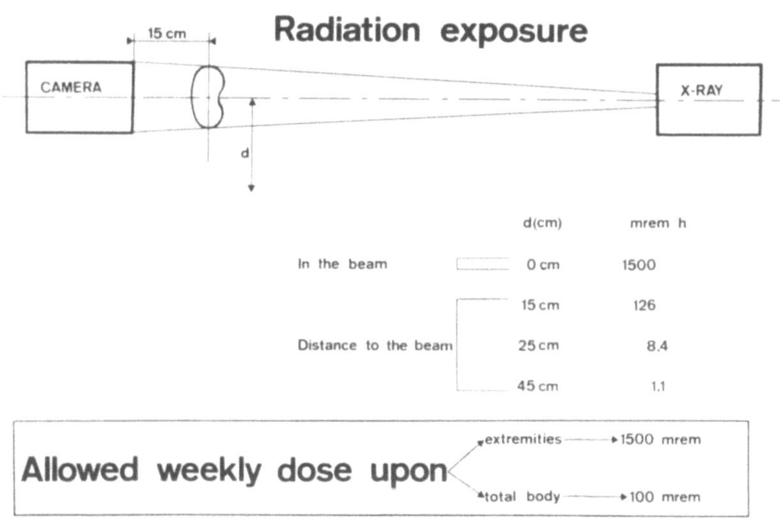

Fig. 3. Radiation dose in and outside the RX-beam of the Siremobil II during peroperative radioscopy.

surgeon remains for 1 h with his hands in the beam he will have received the weekly allowed radiation dose. With a certain experience and practice one does not come into the beam at all, the markers or needles being placed with a long clamp.

Results

In a series of 65 staghorn calculi only three little stone fragments were left. We thought that a further search for the stones would have been more disastrous to the kidney than a small residual stone itself.

Limitations of the Method

The method needs a good exteriorization of the kidney. Sometimes this may be impossible with a fibrotic short pedicle especially in reinterventions. The technical equipment is very expensive and therefore it should be purchased and used together with other surgical disciplines.

Danger

Once, when we used this technique in the beginning, we tried to grasp the stone through the open pyelum with a forceps under television screen control. It provoked serious bleeding by traumatizing the kidney calices and parenchyma. This maneuver is very dangerous because the surgeon may have the impression on the television screen that he is nearly at the stone and will be able to grasp it. In his overenthusiasm he may force through the renal parenchyma. Indeed, the last unfindable stone is nearly always at a place where it cannot be reached with forceps from the pyelum.

Conclusion

We consider this easy-running and safe radiologic equipment a valuable and time-saving aid for staghorn calculus surgery.

Three-dimensional Radiography of the Kidney

J. M. Gil-Vernet

The methods and materials used at present for the intra-operative radiographic exploration of the kidney are somehow very deficient. This is reflected in the great number of recurrences which, in most cases, are due to residual calculi not detected at the time of surgery because of the poor quality of the radiographic material, or because it was not possible to find them, not having an adequate technique to localize the small fragments with exactitude in the renal space. The surgery and the radiographic exploration of renal lithiasis have up to now been carried out in a very simplistic manner.

The surgeon is usually satisfied with a plain radiograph which indicates the presence of the calculus and some intravenous pyelogram (IVP) films which show the repercussions on the intrarenal excretory system. He extracts the stone as he would a tooth, and scarcely uses any radiological control during the operation, or this control is ineffective. Furthermore, he does not make a radiographic examination of the patient on discharge from the clinic, and thus in the future, if faced with a renal calculus, does not know whether it is a real or false recurrence, or whether the kidney has been damaged in the course of the operation. This attitude is correct in the case of a simple pyelic stone, but cannot be accepted in multiple pyelocalyceal lithiasis and particularly in staghorn calculi. The latter presents a problem which must be tackled in depth. It means that the surgeon cannot be satisfied with routine pre-operative radiographic examination, nor can he accept as valid the old-fashioned and ineffective radiological techniques for intra-operative control or surgical removal of renal calculi.

Present day surgery for staghorn or multiple renal calculi should be carried out under certain important postulates (Truc and Grasset 1960) and guidelines (Gil-Vernet 1965). The postulates are three: (1) it should be conservative, (2) it should be complete and (3) it should be atraumatic.

Conservative Surgery. For renal calculi it is quite important to avoid total nephrectomy, and even partial resection of the renal parenchyma, which has been frequently abused under the pretext of removing the so-called lithogenic focus.

Complete Removal of Renal Calculi. It means that the extraction of the stone must be total. Otherwise the operation lacks sense since a recidive is certain, particularly if there is infection. If the surgeon is not able or equipped to extract all the calculi, regardless of the cause or the reasons, it is preferable not to operate because the next operation will be worse or more difficult.

Atraumatic Surgery. Whenever possible an effort should be made to avoid nephrotomy removing all renal calculi through an intrasinus pyelotomy. If an incision through the renal parenchyma is needed or unavoidable, it should be minimal, radially placed and well controlled from the haemostasia standpoint and straight towards where the calculus is located.

In our opinion, the following *radiological guidelines* should be followed in pyelocalyceal and staghorn calculi:

1) Meticulous or exhaustive radiological exploration prior to renal surgery.
2) Perfect radiological control during the operation, which will make it possible to detect and/or locate even the smallest calyceal calculi in a precise manner.

The following guidelines will make easier the *complete removal* of the calculi since they provide us with precise information:

1) The shape and size of the primary calculus and the number and localization of the secondary calculi.
2) The shape and size of the cavities in which the calculus is lodged and, particularly, the morphological characteristics of the calices and their infundibula.

The pre-operative radiological study of the staghorn calculus includes a series of simple radiographic plates covering the following: anteroposterior position; internal profile; obliques from different angles; and tomographies.

This set of plates will make possible a visualization of the number and orientation on different planes of all branches of the staghorn calculus, as well as its possible articular surfaces, and also the number and location of the accessory calculi. This is very important not only to avoid leaving behind a fragment or a free calculus, but also for studying the force lines of the calculus, its branches and the axis and direction in which the traction is to be applied, in order to follow the suitable rules for the removal of staghorn calculi (Gil-Vernet 1970). An IVP taken according to the direction of the beams and planes described will make it possible to see the morphology of the cavities where the calculi are lodged and the route through which they will eventually be removed.

Renal Contact Radiography

For control during surgical removal of renal calculi different radiological techniques have been used: radioscopy with an image intensifier, television, simple radiography and intra-operative contact renal radiography. We consider the last mentioned to be the very best of all and it also offers the following advantages:

1) Better structural detail, as the plate is situaed in close contact with the kidney surface.
2) Less enlargement of the image for the same reason.
3) An important reduction in all of the radiological characteristics (kilovolts, exposure time and milliamperes), because half the body thickness has been eliminated by the intra-abdominal position of the plate and, thus, there is no need for antidiffusors.

Materials and Techniques

At present, there are special radiographic plates on the market prepared for this technique. However, a serious drawback is their fragility. They bend easily during handling for proper placement in the lumbar space, distorting thereby the renal image and causing alterations in the radiographic emulsion with the subsequent appearance of photographic spots. However, the greatest and most serious defect and/or hazard of these plates is the fact that they neither have intensifying screens, which means that an increase in the exposure time is necessary, nor lead protection for preventing subsequent secondary radiation, with resulting loss of contrast. In short, the renal contact radiographic plates in existence on the market, provide images of a very low quality and lack definition, since calculi of small size and low density go unnoticed.

With these plates, and to improve the radiographic quality, the surgeon releases the kidney from its surrounding attachments and brings it outwards in order to prevent any interference from the tissues between the kidney and the X-ray tube. Undoubtedly, this is a potential traumatic manoeuvre and even though a better contact radiograph will be obtained than the one performed with the kidney "in situ", the traction or stretching on the renal pedicule is dangerous since it can cause irreversible anatomical lesions in the division branches of the renal artery, especially when they emerge prematurely, and in the polar arteries. At times, it causes a truncal vasospasm in spite of the anaesthetic infiltration and, as a result, the kidney develops an ischaemic tubulopathy. Clinically and experimentally we have verified that forceful exteriorization or stretching of the kidney causes important haemodynamic and biochemical changes with repercussions on renal function.

The quality of the radiographic image obtained with our method, as it is described below, is much better and also much less traumatic on the kidney as it is radiographed in situ, without any pulling or bringing it outwards.

Renal Contact Chassis

In 1968, we solved the aforementioned drawbacks by making a small chassis (Paitre et al. 1941), composed of a metal sheet and two intensifying screens with the radiographic film between them. This is all contained within an opaque cover which can be sterilized by ethylene oxide or by immersion in iodine or other antiseptic solutions (Fig. 1).

In this way, the equivalent, although much reduced in size, of a normal radiographic chassis is obtained, but with the advantages of X-ray intensification produced by the reinforcement screen (V. Müller Surgical Instruments, Chicago, IL), plus the absorption of secondary radiation by the metal sheet and the addition of a certain rigidity of the unit, which gives greater security to the film. The above improvements result in images of great radiographic quality.

With a portable X-ray machine and this minichassis, perfect radiographic studies can be obtained since, in general, an output of 50–55 kV, 12 mA suffices, at a focus plate distance of 70 cm.

Calculation of Direct and Indirect Radiation

Exposure at 1 m: 0.048 R (100 cm^2 field);
Dose on surface: 0.052 rad;
Dose at a depth of 1.5 cm: 0.021 rad.

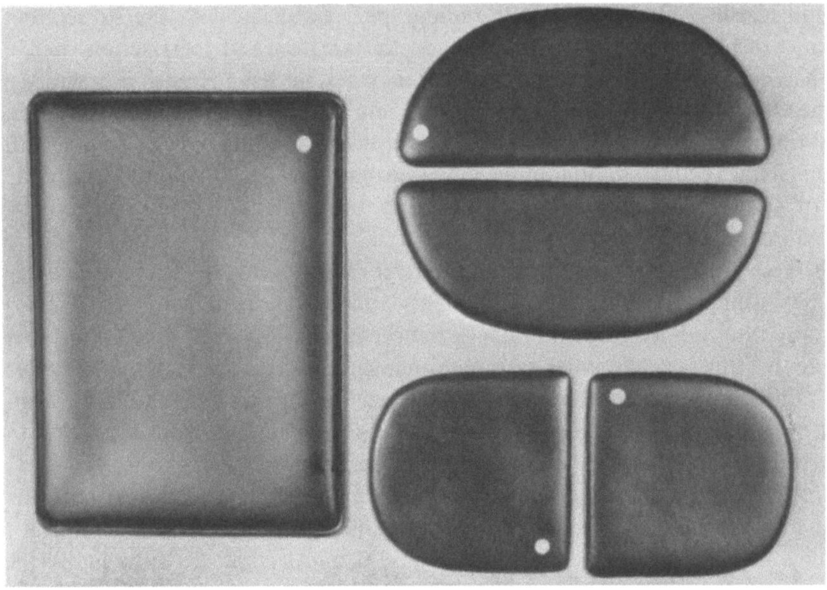

Fig. 1. Set of minichassis for three-dimensional radiographic exploration of the kidney.

This calculation of the radiation dose demonstrates that X-rays made with our contact minichassis have no dangerous effects, not even when considering the accumulative factor, since 0.021 rad allow a far greater number of radiographic shots than those normally necessary.

Before obtaining the radiography we should be certain that the kidney surface is well placed against the minichassis and that the central X-ray beam is perpendicular to the kidney chassis as a whole.

Sequential Arrangements of the Plates. In the course of intra-operative radiographic exploration our normal practice has been to take first the contact plate of the posterior surface of the kidney. In this manner we obtain an anteroposterior (AP) radiographic view of the kidney, that is, from front to back.

However, we have found that by placing the plate in contact with the anterior surface of the kidney and obtaining a postero-anterior (PA) X-ray, that is, from back to front, the superimposition of calcified costal cartilages and ribs, which could lead to error, is avoided.

It is important that the first contact X-rays be made after the kidney has been released and immediately prior to the removal of the calculi. Thus, it can aid us to adjust the radiological characteristics to the density of the calculus, which will also ensure the good quality of the X-rays later on in order to localize the small calculi or residual concretions. Actually the important thing is to localize them, that is, to know in which calyx they are located. For this purpose, it is absolutely necessary to use metal clips which, when placed just under the fibrous renal capsule, will serve in the radiological control as points of reference for the localization of the residual calculi. Four to six clips are placed longitudinally on the posterior surface of the kidney, except one of them, which is placed across so as to facilitate identification of one of the poles. The position of these clips can eventually be modified during the operation so that they can be superimposed on, or brought near to the remaining calculus or calculi and this radiographic finding will allow their removal.

Three-dimensional Radiography

To know exactly where the residual calyceal calculus is located is indeed the great question which often faces the surgeon during the removal of a staghorn calculus. A fact, which at times can be very distressing, can be now learned by means of a new technique which we call *"three-dimensional radiographic exploration of the kidney"*. Up to now, the conventional intra-operative contact X-rays have provided us with two dimensions of the kidney and calculus: their length and width, whereby we know only the height of the renal zone in which it is projected. However, we still need to know the third dimension of the kidney, that is, its thickness or depth. Obtaining the radiographic third dimension of the calculus means that its exact position within the kidney can be pin pointed.

The excretory ducts begin in the small or second order calyces, which, joined together, form the major calyces.

The number of second order calyces, except when there are morphological variants, averages from six to eight. These are arranged according to their height in

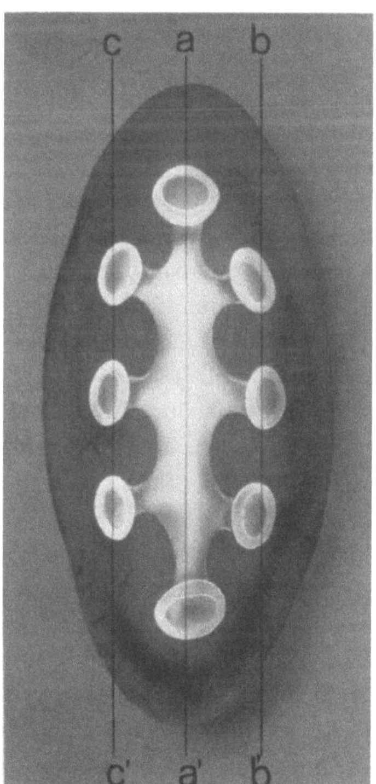

Fig. 2. Profile of the kidney, showing the three rows of calyces in the renal space. *a–a'*, Calyces of the superior and inferior groups in the mid-frontal plane. *b–b'*, Ventral calyces in the anterior plane. *c–c'*, Dorsal calyces in the posterior plane.

two main groups: a primary superior group and a secondary inferior one. According to the *thickness* of the kidney, the calyces are placed in three rows (Fig. 2), one on the mid-frontal plane, a–a′, the other two in front, b–b′, and behind this plane, c–c′. Thus, a single nephrotomy on one plane cannot open all calyces at the same time. Only the large calyces which are located on the frontal plane itself (Paitre et al., 1941) can be opened by one single incision of nephrotomy.

There are usually three large or first order calyces: superior, middle and inferior. The large superior calyx is long and vertical and the large inferior calyx is shorter and also vertical, but the large middle calyx is horizontal and perpendicular to the superior one. The small calyces which empty into the large middle calyx are grouped in two longitudinal rows; one of them is made up of the anterior or ventral calyces of the kidney and is situated in the anterior renal hemisphere. The other row is made up of the posterior or dorsal calyces and is located in the posterior renal hemisphere. Since a nephrotomy on the median line of the renal convexity or on its posterior aspect on the so-called Hyrtl avascular line (which is neither real nor entirely avascular) (Hyrtl 1870) does not permit a simultaneous approach to the two rows of the middle calyces, and when complete removal through an extended intrasinusal pyelotomy is not possible, it is preferable to approach the calyces by means of small selective radial nephrotomies, which should fall on the peripheral zone of the calyx. However, an exact knowledge of the location of the calculus is an indispensable prior condition.

Material

To obtain the third dimension of the calculus, that is, to discover its depth and subsequently its situation in the renal space, it is necessary to take external profile X-rays, that is, at a 90° angle. For this purpose we use a set of minichassis and two articulated clamps with two flat surfaces which can be taken apart like forceps; these plate holders come in two different models. Each one has the shape of a half ellipse, in transverse (Fig. 3) or in longitudinal section (Fig. 4), and is made of metal. The radiographic plates are arranged on these surfaces in a similar manner. The two halves of the radiographic film are placed on both metal plates of the clamp, thus avoiding secondary radiation from behind.

The half-elliptical shape, either in transverse or longitudinal section, which we have selected for the radiographic film is the most appropriate one. In this way each renal hemisphere, whether it be the anterior or posterior one, or the superior or inferior renal half, can be projected onto it, and on joining both we have the complete kidney in a profile view.

First, a conventional AP X-ray is made followed by another from a PA direction (Fig. 5). Then the two external profile X-rays are obtained. If the type I plate holder is used disassembled, one of its branches is placed in front of and the other behind the pedicule (Fig. 6), and when type II is used afterwards, one of its branches is placed above and the other below the pedicule (Fig. 7). The plate holder is closed at the moment the X-ray is taken. This closing – which is not complete – does not involve even the slightest trauma to the vessels of the kidney. The ischaemia time, very relative and 2–4 s, needs no comment.

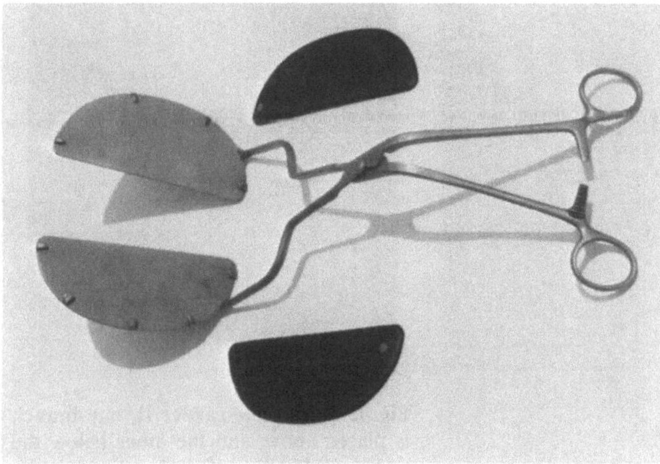

Fig. 3. Plate carrier type I for X-raying the anterior and posterior renal hemispheres.

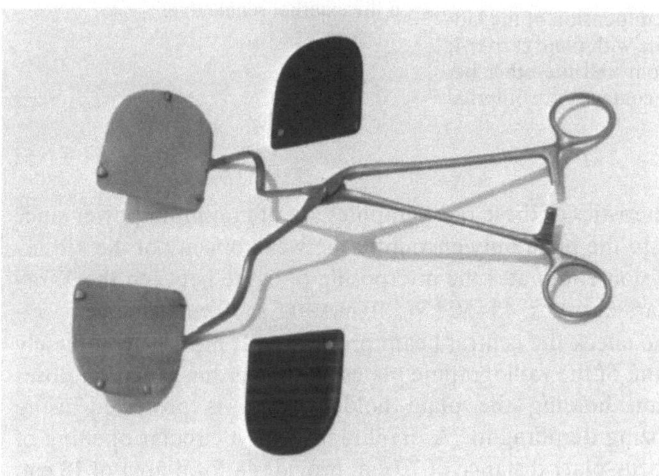

Fig. 4. Plate carrier type II for X-raying the superior and inferior renal halves.

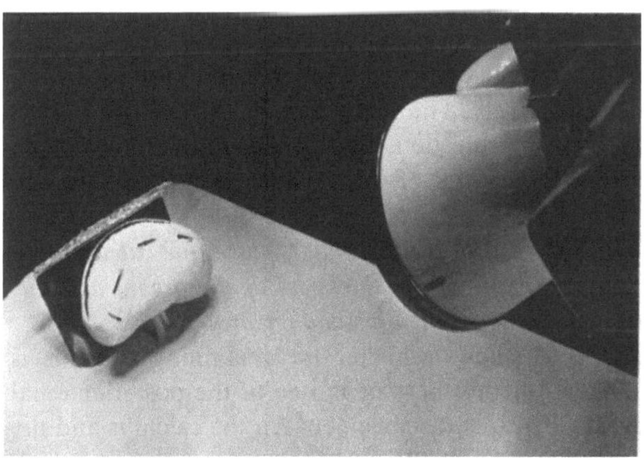

Fig. 5. X-ray, in AP or PA, to obtain the two dimensions of the kidney and its contents.

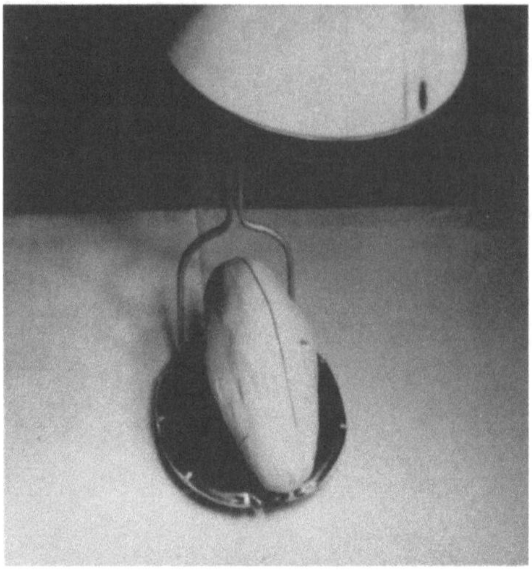

Fig. 6. Obtaining the third dimension of the kidney. X-ray in external profile with plate carrier I; one branch is placed in front and the other behind the pedicle, both in contact with internal edge of the kidney.

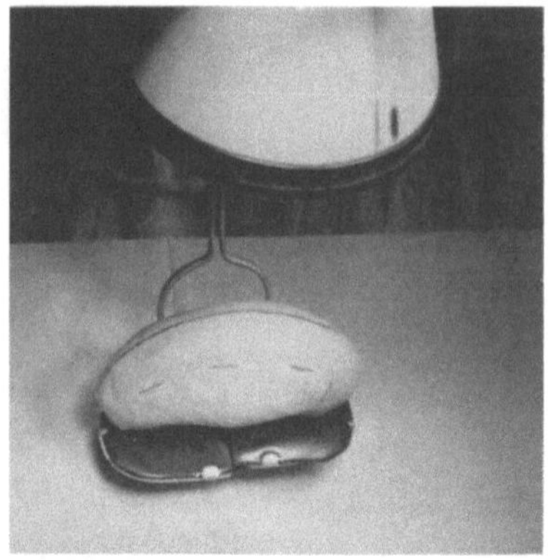

Fig. 7. With plate carrier II, one branch is placed above and the other below the pedicle. Metallic reference clips on the posterior surface and an opaque thread on the external renal edge.

The technical characteristics of these radiographies are of minimum power since the X-rays on their way to the plate only encounter the weak opacity of the kidney because the surgical incision eliminates the interposing of tissue between the X-ray tube and the kidney. Characteristics: 45–50 kW; 10 mA; 0.5 s; 70 cm distance.

It is very important to check the central beam previously. It must be completely perpendicular to the plane of the radiographic plates. Although the radiation doses are minimal, the person holding the plate holder clamp is protected using radiological beam-focalizing diaphragms. A diaphragm with a circular opening of 1 cm in diameter, at a focus-plate distance of 70 cm, provides a focal area of 18 cm, sufficient in size to cover the entire kidney, thus avoiding direct radiation around it.

Results

Figures 8–10 show a plain pre-operative X-ray, a pre-operative IVP and a bidimensional pre-operative X-ray, respectively. The X-ray at a 90° angle with respect to the chassis properly placed on AP projection, that is, the radiography of an external profile, provides the *third dimension* of the calculus in the renal space (Figs. 11–14).

The importance of this radiography rests in the fact that it places the calculus in a front to back direction, that is, in the plane of the thickness of the organ, and this constitutes a valuable and decisive aid for its localization and removal.

An external profile contact X-ray shows whether the remaining calculus is found in a calyx of the anterior renal hemisphere or in one of the posterior renal hemispheres; in addition, it reveals the exact distance between the calculus and the surface of the organ, that is, the thickness of the parenchyma covering it, which

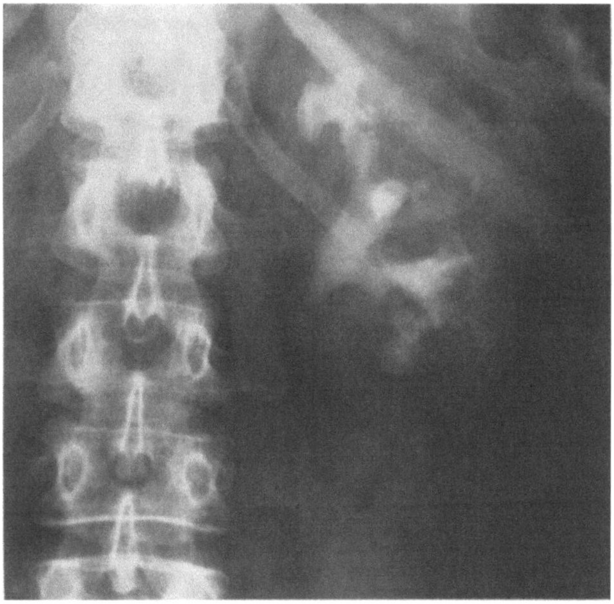

Fig. 8. (Ob. I). Plain pre-operative X-ray. Staghorn and low-mineralized soft calyceal stones.

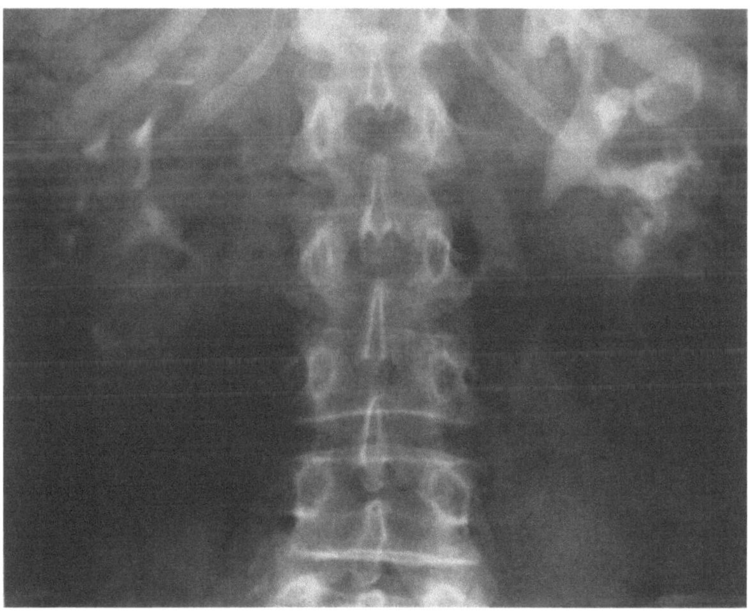

Fig. 9. (Ob. I). Pre-operative IVP.

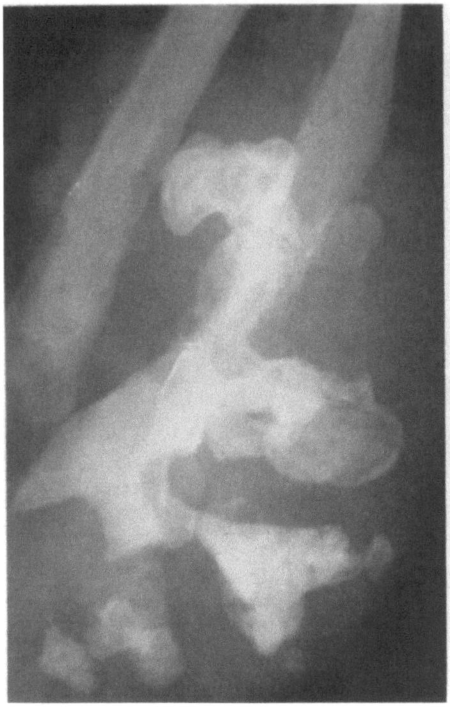

Fig. 10. (Ob. I). Bidimensional pre-operative X-ray with the kidney in situ in AP.

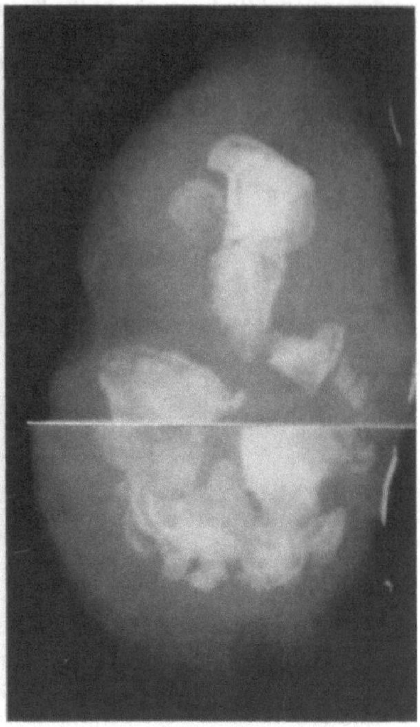

Fig. 11. (Ob. I). X-ray in external profile with plate carrier II, obtaining the third dimension of the kidney. Certified mucoprotein images appear neatly.

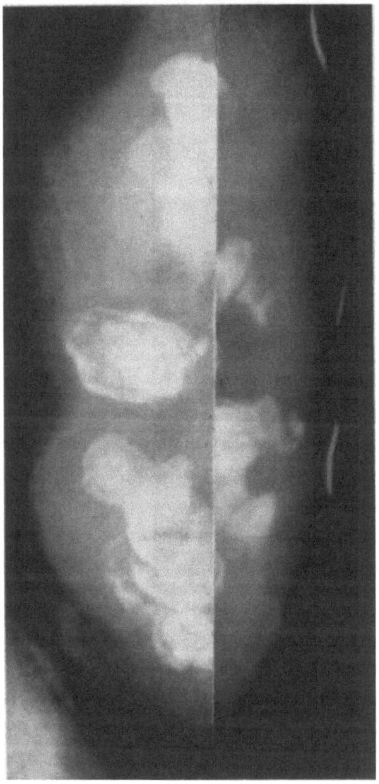

Fig. 12. (Ob. I). X-ray with plate carrier I, obtaining the third dimension of the kidney. Parenchyma thickness covering stones and their exact localization in the renal space can be seen.

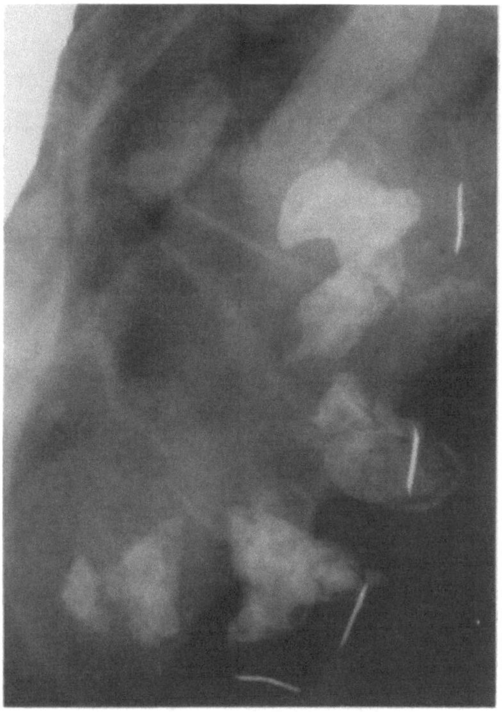

Fig. 13. (Ob. I). In external profile X-ray, low-mineralized stones appear neatly.

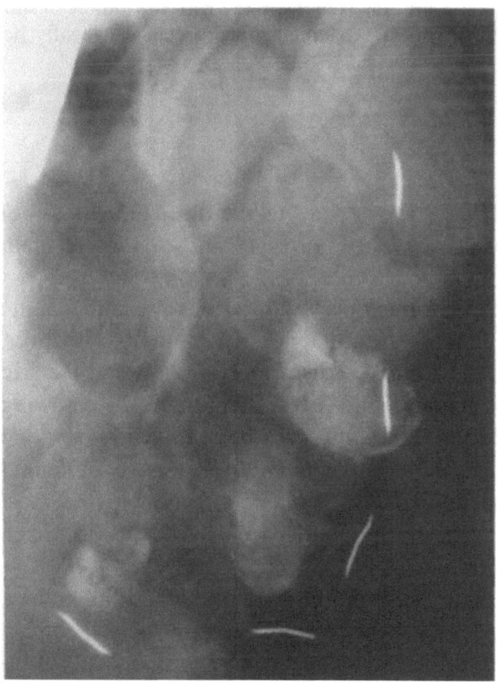

Fig. 14. (Ob. I). External profile X-ray with plate carrier II.

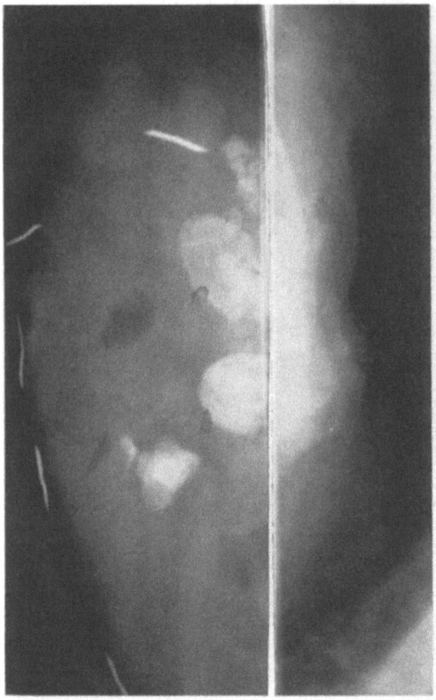

Fig. 15. (Ob. I). Renal contact X-ray with the kidney in situ in AP.

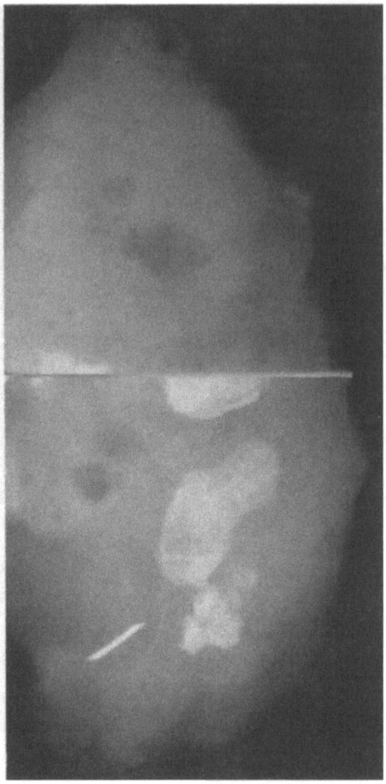

Fig. 16. (Ob. I). X-ray with the kidney in situ in AP. Calcified mucoprotein can neatly be seen.

when combined with the AP X-rays (Figs. 15, 16), gives us the three dimensions of the calculus, whereby we learn its *exact location.* Figures 17 and 18 show a plain postoperative X-ray and a postoperative IVP.

This is a great help in the localization of calculi within any calyx, and for the complete removal of its contents by means of an extended pyelotomy. However, when this is not possible because there is a marked disproportion between the size of the calculus and that of the infundibulum of the calyx, then, thanks to knowing exactly in which calyx the calculus is found, the latter can be removed by a radial and small nephrotomy incision which should be *minimal,* that is, of a length equivalent to the thickness of the calculus and in a *radial* direction in the most *peripheral* zone of the calyx, which is the shortest transparenchymatous approach and the one with the least vascular risk.

As there is no superimposition of tissue between the X-ray tube and the kidney, radiographies with greater clarity than even those carried out with the AP contact chassis are obtained, and this is very important when concretions or little mineralized calculi are to be detected. It must be emphasized that in 16% of cases we

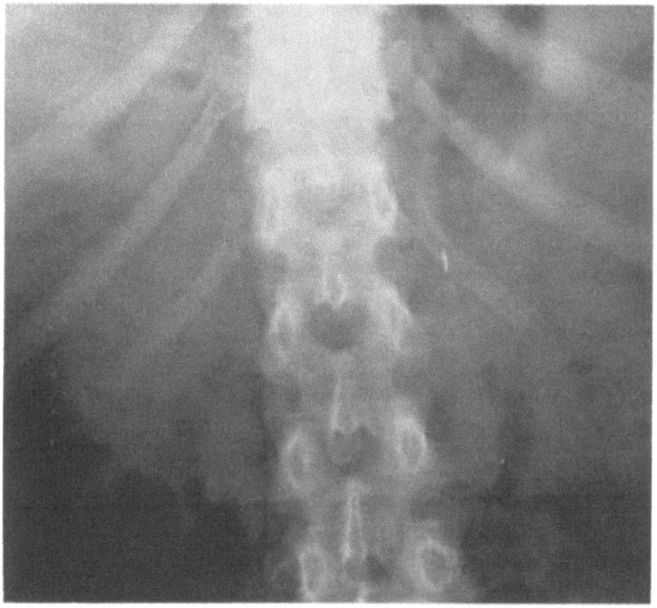

Fig. 17. (Ob. I). Postoperative plain X-ray. Complete removal.

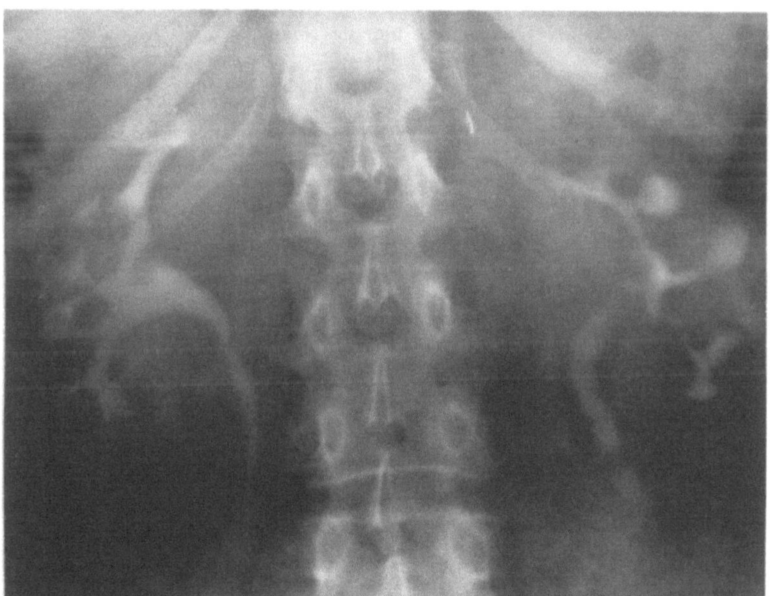

Fig. 18. (Ob. I). Postoperative IVP.

have been able to discover calculi or calcifications which had not been revealed either in the pre-operative radiographic explorations or in the anteroposterior contact intra-operative X-ray.

Summary

A practical renal contact chassis which we have designed and used for radiological control during surgical removal of difficult renal calculi is described in this report. It allows discovery of the smallest calculi due to the purity or quality of their images, which are far superior to those obtained from plates available on the market, and with less radiation exposure to the patient and staff in the operating room. We have established the bases for intra-operative, three-dimensional radiographic exploration of the kidney, which up to the present time has not been achieved and is, indeed, of great importance during surgical removal of renal lithiasis. In short, it represents a decisive aid for the intra-operative localization of residual calculi of any size and, therefore, allows us to remove these completely with a minimum of trauma to the renal parenchyma.

References

Gil-Vernet JM (1965) New surgical concepts in removing renal calculi. Urol Int 20:255

Gil-Vernet JM (1970) La cirurgia intrasinusal de los cálculos coraliformes. Rapport XVe Congr Soc Inter Urol Tokyo 1:11

Hyrtl J (1870) Das Nierenbecken der Säugetiere und des Menschen. Wiener Sitzungsberichte, B, LIV

Paitre F, Giraud D, Dupret S (1941) Prac. Anatomoquirúrgica ilustrada. In: Salvat (ed) Los elementos del pedículo, en fasc. 3. Barcelona, p 255

Truc E, Grasset D (1960) Lithiase rénale. Encyclop Med Chir 9:5

Three-dimensional Intra-operative Stone Localization

H. Melchior and G. Lang

In 1978, Matouschek recommended a new method of intra-operative stone localization by X-ray control. Stereoscopic X-ray photographs of intrarenal stones and of reference markers on the kidney surface were taken by two X-ray tubes, which were coupled in a defined angle. The vertical position of the concrements was calculated from the projection distances between the double images of the stones and the markers. The idea of a mathematical determination of the stone localization within the three-dimensional space of the pyelocaliceal system appeared logical while the use of the relatively unwieldy X-ray unit with light beam localizer seemed less favorable because of the resulting technical problems.

To utilize the advantages of stereoscopic stone localization and to improve the intra-operative handling of the X-ray unit, two small X-ray tubes, which are generally employed in dental diagnostics, were coupled and furnished in 1979 with a special joint collimator to guarantee constant X-ray exposure data (Fig. 1).

In order to further facilitate the intra-operative handling of the X-ray unit, only one Oralix tube with a collimator was attached to a tripod with weight balance, enabling an adequate movability of the tube as well as its stable locking in the required position (Fig. 2).

Method

The technique of three-dimensional intra-operative stone localization is based on the geometrical laws of stereoscopic photography: While the horizontal stone position is determined conventionally from the situation of the stone images in relation to the X ray markers, the vertical stone position can be calculated from the diameter of the kidney, the projection distance between the double images of the concrements, and the projection distance between the double images of the markers (Fig. 3):

$$\frac{h_s}{d_s} = \frac{f - h_s}{a} \qquad (1)$$

$$\frac{h_m}{d_m} = \frac{f - h_m}{a}\,. \qquad (2)$$

The elimination of "a" leaves the equation:

$$h_s = \frac{d_s \cdot h_m}{\frac{h_m}{f}(d_m - d_s) + d_m}\,. \qquad (3)$$

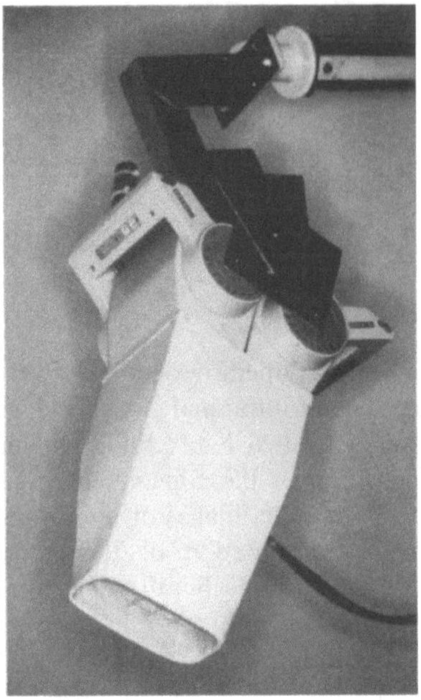

Fig. 1. Two X-ray tubes (Oralix) coupled with a special collimator; a type of reticle is attached within the collimator.

Fig. 2. An X-ray tube (Oralix) on a tripod with load balance which enables free movability and stable locking.
▼

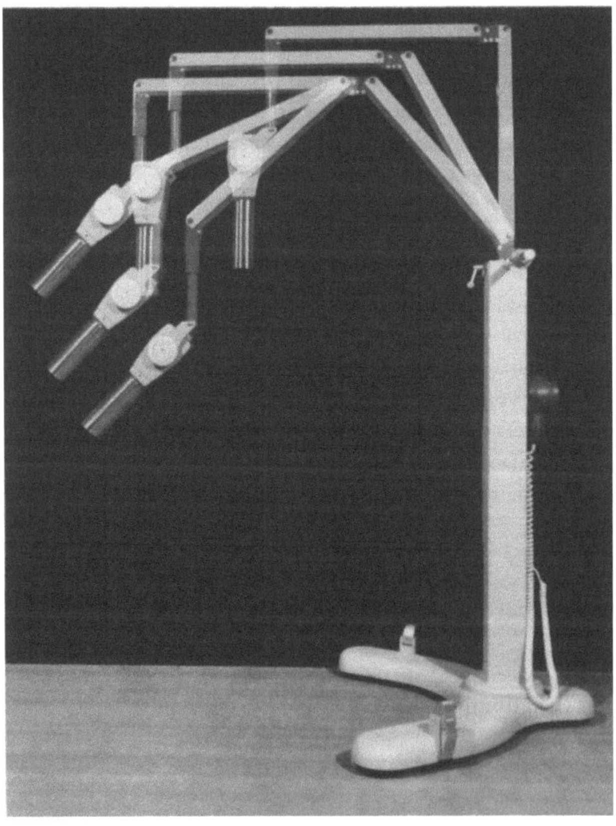

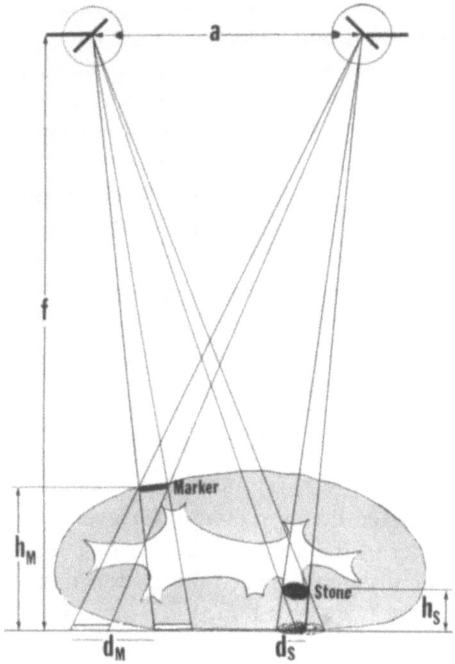

Fig. 3. Vertical stone localization based on the geometric laws of stereoscopic photography. *a*, Shifting angle of the X-ray tube. *f*, Film-focus distance. *h*, Distance to the level of the X-ray film. *d*, Projection distance between the double images. *M*, Marker. *S*, Stone.

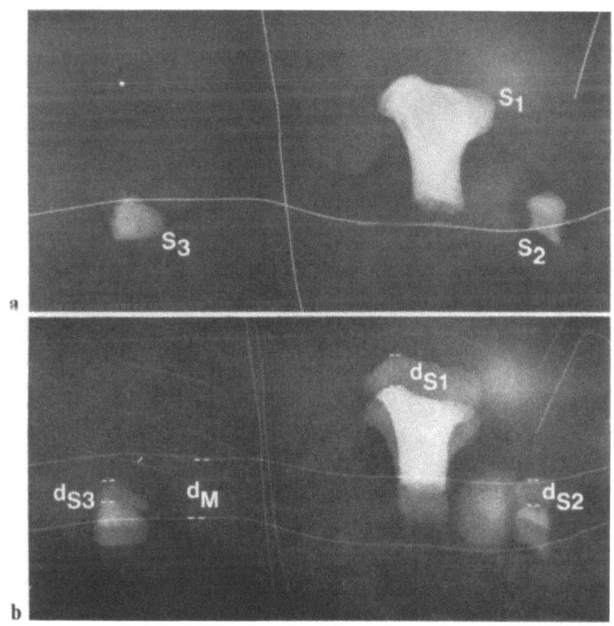

Fig. 4a, b. Vertical stone localization (example). **a** Standard exposure. S_1, Stone 1; S_2, stone 2; S_3, stone 3. **b** Double exposure. d_M, Distance between marker images. d_{S1}, d_{S2}, d_{S3}, Distances between the images of stones 1, 2, and 3, respectively.

Because $\frac{h_m}{f}(d_m - d_s) \ll d_m$, Eq. (3) results in the approximation:

$$h_s \approx \frac{d_s \cdot d_m}{d_m}, \tag{4}$$

where s = stone, m = marker, h = distance to the level of the X-ray film, d = projection distance between the double images, a = shifting angle of the X-ray tube, and f = film–focus distance.

In this calculation, the curvature of the X-ray film and the displacement of the X-ray images caused by oblique irradiation are not taken into consideration, but the inaccuracy caused by this neglect is irrelevant in clinical practice. The discrepancy ranges between 3% with stones situated far from the X-ray film and 25% with concrements near the film level.

Figure 4 shows examples of X-ray photographs obtained with this method. Three concrements are visible in the kidney and the X-ray marker is situated on the kidney surface (Fig. 4a). The distance between the marker and the level of the X-ray film (h_m) is determined by the diameter of the kidney, which is 40 mm. In the double-exposed photograph (Fig. 4b), the distance between the marker images (d_m) is 10 mm, the distance between the images of stone 1 (d_{s1}) is 6 mm, that of stone 2 (d_{s2}) is 3 mm, and that of stone 3 (d_{s3}) is 5 mm. According to the equation:

$$h_{stone} \approx \frac{d_{stone} \cdot h_{marker}}{d_{marker}}$$

the distances between the concrements and the film level are: $h_{s1} = 24$ mm; $h_{s2} = 12$ mm; and $h_{s3} = 20$ mm.

Discussion

Three-dimensional intra-operative stone localization by stereoscopic X-ray photography is a very simple technique. The small Oralix tube with a collimator attached to a tripod with a weight balance guarantees optimal intra-operative handling as well as constant X-ray exposure data and easy focusing. The horizontal stone position is determined conventionally from the situation of the stone images in relation to the X-ray marker while the vertical stone position is calculated according to the geometrical laws of stereoscopic photography. Equation (4)

$$h_{stone} \approx \frac{d_{stone} \cdot h_{marker}}{d_{marker}}$$

only requires the intraoperative determination of the diameter of the kidney equaling the distance between the markers on the kidney surface and the level of the X-ray film, and the determination of the projection distances between the double images of the markers and the concrements.

If the mathematical problems of a rule of three are too difficult, the procedure can be further simplified, with a loss of exactness, however.

a 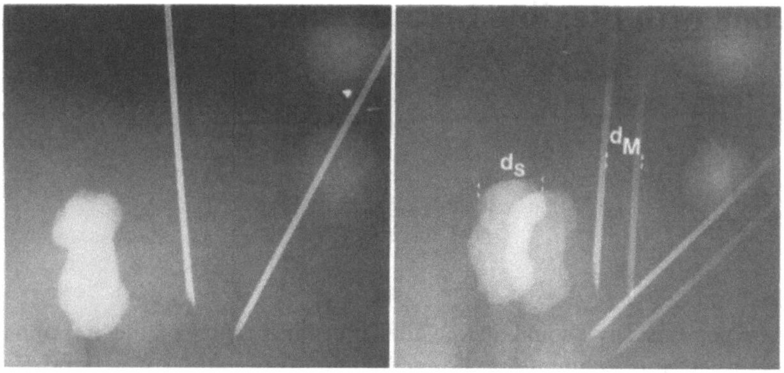 b

Fig. 5 a, b. Vertical stone localization approximation (example). **a** Standard exposure. **b** Double exposure. d_S, Distance between the images of the stone. d_M, Distance between the images of the marker needle.

Another example of this technique can be seen in Fig. 5, which shows two needles and one concrement in a kidney. The distance between the stone images is nearly the same as the distance between the double images of each needle. Therefore, the concrement must be situated at the same level as the marker pins.

This method of intraoperative stereoscopic stone localization allows a fairly exact estimation of the postion of concrements within the three-dimensional space of the kidney:

1) If the distance between the stone images is smaller than that between the double images of the marker pins, the concrement is situated behind the pins, near the film.
2) If the distance between the stone images and the distance between the double images of the needles are the same, the concrement is situated at the same level as the needles.
3) If the distance between the stone images is greater than that between the double images of the marker pins, the concrement is situated before the pins, in front of the surgeon.

Generally, the technique of approximative stereoscopic stone localization will be preferable; in certain cases, however, the exact calculation of the vertical position of residual stones may be the method of choice.

Reference

Matouschek E (1978) Über eine Methode zur intraoperativen Lokalisation schattengebender Nierensteine in drei Ebenen. Urologe [A] 17:236–237

Pyeloscopy with Flexible Instruments

L. V. Wagenknecht

Pyeloscopy or nephroscopy should define the direct inspection of the intrarenal system. If perfected, this technique would facilitate in a spectacular way intrarenal surgery for complete stone removal.

In 1941 Rupel and Brown described the first extraction of a stone via a nephrostomy canal by the use of a cystoscope. The same was done 33 years later by Bissada and co-workers, and termed nephrostoscopy.

The first pyeloscope was developed by Trattner in 1948. This was a conventional warm-light instrument with an angle of 90°.

Pyeloscopy should be restricted to intraoperative inspection of the intra-renal system. Radiologic preoperative "pyeloscopy," however perfected, should be termed selective pyelography.

Pyeloscopes now commercially available are still angulated instruments, which have the advantage of cold light and better optics. These instruments are as invalid as their construction. In our hands it was never possible to inspect completely the intrarenal system. Nevertheless, Hertel and Vatz and co-workers reported stone extractions with these inflexible instruments. Some years ago we abandoned angulated pyeloscopes for lack of flexibility and vision at the expense of traumatic introduction.

A flexible choledochoscope, first used by Stuart in 1974 for nephroscopy, was modified later to our requirements. It is 77 cm long. The anterior end has a diameter of 16 Charrière and can be moved foreward and backward through an arc of 60°. The smallest detectable distance between the object and the pyeloscope is 5 mm. The instrument has one canal with two different connections: one for water irrigation and another one with a valve mechanism for introduction of biopsy forceps or stone retrievers.

As part of some modifications of this instrument, it may be disinfected entirely (with the exclusion of the optical part). Disinfection is done for 10 min in a glutaraldehyde bath. The flexibility of this instrument allows its introduction into practically all calices under direct vision even when the kidney cannot be entirely mobilized. For intrarenal use, high-pressure irrigation of the pyeloscope is necessary. This is done by adjusting a pressure cuff around a flexible water bag which is connected to the scope. Good visibility within the intrarenal system is only ensured when the latter is sufficiently filled with water. We recommend a small pyelotomy for introduction of the instrument and digital compression of this insertion while guiding the instrument at the same time.

As for all endoscopic techniques, special adaptation and experience is required for this method. By systematic inspection of the intrarenal system with this flexible pyeloscope we are able to control if a kidney is free of stones. So far we have used this instrument in 42 patients. Following radiologic control, we demonstrated by direct pyeloscope inspection small remaining papillary calcifications in four of these patients, although the kidney was believed to be free of stones.

In three patients small intrarenal tumors were inspected and clearly identified. Direct vision on dubious-lesions may differentiate tumors from vascular impressions or inflammatory areas. In another patient with suspected upper ureteral tumor, no tumor was found by direct surgical inspection through ureterotomy. With this 16-Charrière fibroscope the upper third of the ureter was inspected and a tumor safely excluded.

In cooperation with the industry, this instrument will be modified in some details:

1) The length of 77 cm is excessive and will be reduced to about 50 cm.
2) Biopsy forceps and stone retrievers have to be manageable through the instrument at maximal flexion of the distal end.
3) Complete sterilization.
4) Smaller diameter of the scope.

There are the following indications for the pyeloscope:

1) *Renal lithiasis* is the prime indication. Direct inspection of the intrarenal system makes traumatizing and time-consuming search with various other instruments dispensable. Radiologic controls during surgery are complimentary to this technique.
2) *Dubious intrarenal lesions* are a further indication for pyeloscopy. We expect that renal hematuria of uncertain origin – in combination with suspicious cytology and/or radiologic filling defect – might be cleared up by pyeloscopy.
3) The direct inspection of renal papillae for calcifications or inflammation may be of value for postoperative prophylaxis of patients with chronic stone formation and nephrocalcinosis.

We now use a bronchoscope of 4.3 mm diameter, which allows a foreward movement of 60° and a backward movement of 20° at the distal end, continuous irrigation, introduction of biopsy forceps for stone removal, and perfect vision.

Lymph Node Evaluation by Combined Methods of Investigation

G. Pizzocaro, F. Zanoni, B. Damascelli and R. Musumeci

Lymph node evaluation is essential in planing an adequate therapy in urologic tumors. No single method of investigation, however, is usually adequate in giving as much information as is necessary.

The clinical examination may evidence enlarged inguinal or supraclavicular nodes and an abdominal mass may be palpable, but these are signs of advanced disease.

Lymphangiography (LAG) has tremendously improved lymph node evaluation, particularly in the retroperitoneal area. We reviewed the records of 152 patients with nonseminomatous germ cell tumors who had no previous therapy after orchidectomy. All these patients were clinically staged as categories N0 and N1–2 and underwent surgery for retroperitoneal lymph node dissection (Table 1). The false negative rate was relatively high (22.3%), while false positive examinations were very few (8.5%). In 12 patients (8%) the examination met technical difficulties and it was inconclusive (NX). These data support that LAG is a relatively easy examination, with a high specificity and a relatively low sensitivity. The lack of sensitivity is due to the fact that LAG is unable to visualize nodes completely replaced by tumor and, furthermore, bipedal LAG alone usually misses the lymph nodes of first drainage in urologic tumors.

Ancillary procedures are necessary in patients with negative LAG. Funicular lymphangiography (Chiappa et al. 1966) visualizes the testicular lymph node center (Fig. 1) and also penile LAG was described (Riveros et al. 1967).

Urography may disclose metastases displacing the ureter even if missed by LAG (Fig. 2).

Phlebograms are more useful in evaluating the extent and resectability of large retroperitoneal nodes than in diagnosing small retroperitoneal deposits. Left renal and spermatic phlebography (Fig. 3) is useful in the case of large paraaortic nodes

Table 1. Lymphangiography and pathology correlation in nonseminomatous tumors.

LAG	No. cases	Pathology		
		N0 (%)	N1–2 (%)	N3 (%)
N0	81	63 (77.7)	17 (21.1)	1 (1.2)
N1–2	59	5 (8.5)	49 (83.0)	5 (8.5)
NX	12	6 (50.0)	6 (50.0)	
Total	152	74 (48.7)	72 (47.4)	6 (3.9)

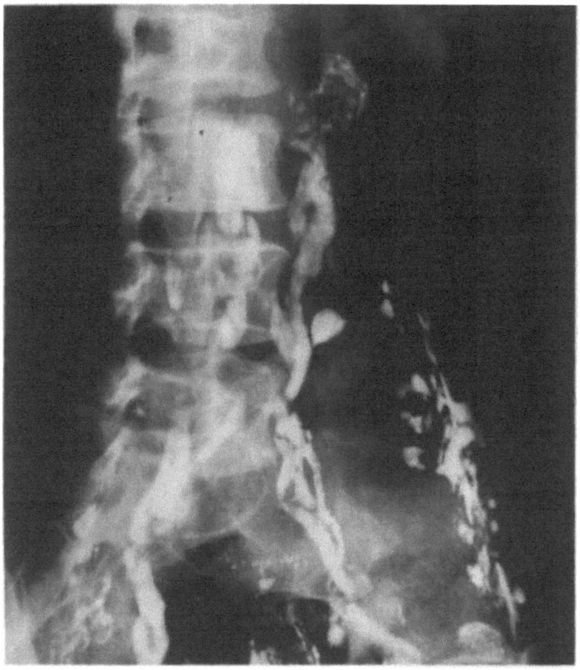

Fig. 1. Combined funicular and pedal lymphangiography: Metastases to the testicular lymph node center.

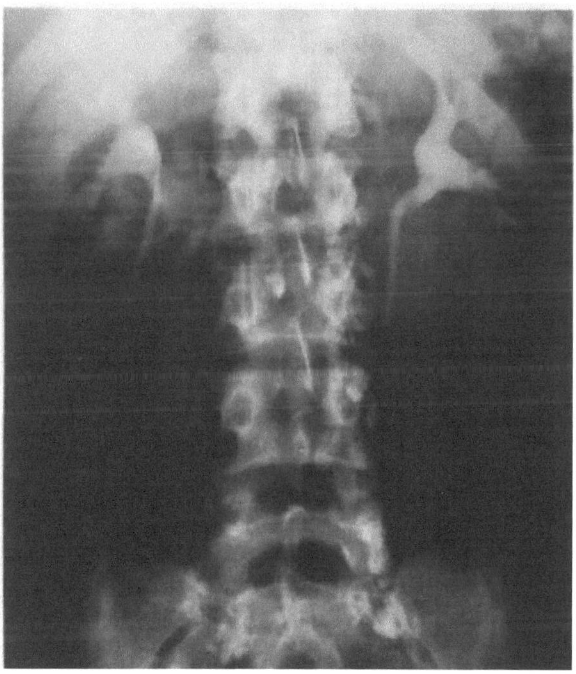

Fig. 2. The displacement of the right ureter discloses large retroperitoneal involvement missed by bipedal lymphangiography.

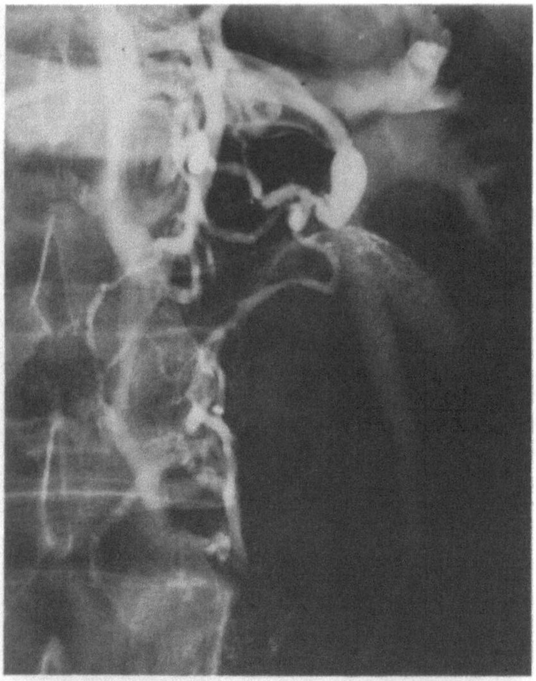

Fig. 3. Left renal phlebography evidencing a large hilar metastasis draining into the left spermatic vein.

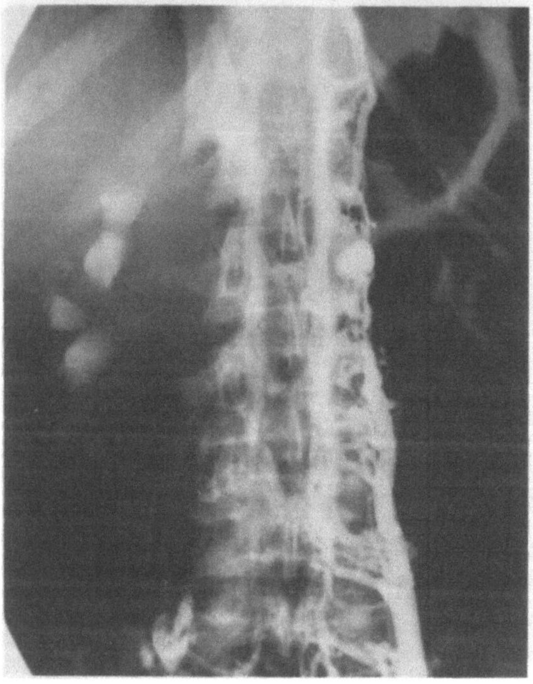

Fig. 4. Occlusion of inferior vena cava by large retroperitoneal adenopathies and collateral venous drainage.

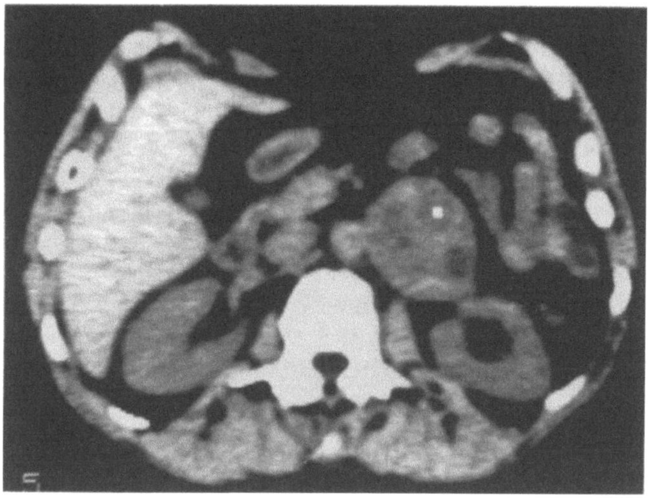

Fig. 5. A large retroperitoneal metastasis on CT-scan. Relationships with aorta and renal hilum are evident.

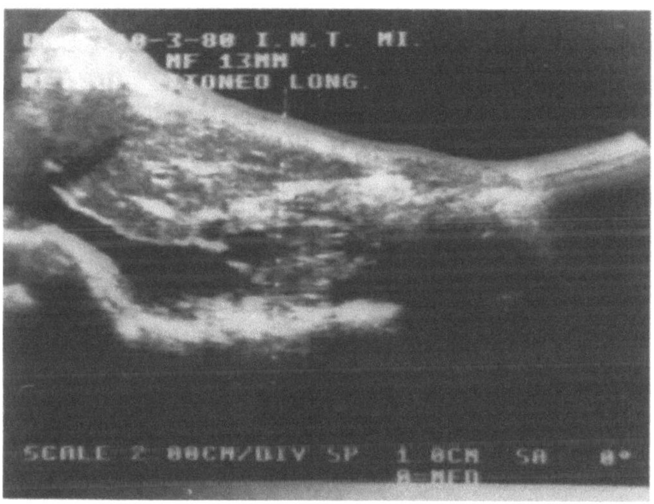

Fig. 6. Retropancreatic metastasis on echotomography in a patient with testicular teratoma.

on the left side, while an inferior venocavogram (Fig. 4) is indicated when the retroperitoneal involvement is on the right side of the aorta.

Serum markers (HCG and AFP) are reported to improve LAG staging accuracy in testicular cancer from 59% to 86% (Barzell and Whitmore 1979). In our experience, however, 33 out of 91 patients with negative markers after orchidectomy had proven retroperitoneal metastases (36.2%). The false positive rate was very low (7.2%) and these findings may be due to residual circulating markers after the removal of the primary tumor.

CT scan is a relatively new diagnostic method. According to several authors it could replace LAG in evaluating retroperitoneal nodes. It is able to detect paraaortic nodes larger than 1.5 cm and the relationship with neighboring organs is also easily assessed (Fig. 5). However, the false positive rate is relatively high (Pizzocaro et al. 1981) because the examination is unable to differentiate between metastases and other conditions of lymph node enlargement. Besides it has serious limitations in detecting pelvic nodes, as well as in very thin patients because of the lack of retroperitoneal fat.

Echotomography has severe limitations in fat patients and in patients with bowel gas distension because of ultrasound reflection interferences. After a good bowel preparation (oral charcoal) and in thin patients, it is as good or even superior to CT scan and it can detect retroperitoneal nodes missed by lymphangiography (Fig. 6).

In conclusion, LAG or CT scan are nowadays the major methods of investigation of retroperitoneal nodes. They are complementary because LAG is very specific and CT scan is very sensitive. Furthermore, CT scan is superior to LAG in paraaortic node evaluation and vice versa in pelvic nodes. Usually LAG needs ancillary procedures, so CT scan should be done first and LAG should follow in doubtful positive cases. In very thin patients echotomography should substitute for CT scan.

References

Barzell WE, Whitmore WF Jr (1979) Clinical significance of biologic markers: Memorial Hospital experience. Semin Oncol 6:48–52

Chiappa S, Uslenghi C, Bonadonna G, Marano P, Ravasi GL (1966) Combined testicular and foot lymphangiography in testicular carcinoma. Surg Gynecol Obstet 123:10–14

Pizzocaro G, Durand JC, Fuchs WA, Merrin CE, Musumeci R, Schmucki O, Vahlensieck W, Whitmore WF Jr, Zvara VL (1981) Staging and surgery in testicular cancer. Eur Urol 7:1–10

Riveros M, Garcia R, Cabanas R (1967) Lymphadenography of the dorsal lymphatics of the penis: technique and results. Cancer 20:2026–2030

Transabdominal Fine Needle Biopsy of Lymph Nodes for Urologic Cancer Staging

K. Rothenberger, A. Hofstetter, N. Rupp, and K.-J. Pfeifer

Accurate staging of malignant urologic tumors related to the tumor node metastasis (TNM) system has become general. It is particularly this procedure that allows best treatment planning. Clinicians often underrate the frequency of lymphogenous dissemination. Patients affected by carcinoma of the prostate show metastasis in a lymph node with 20% in stage B and 64% in stage C (Spellmann et al. 1977), i.e., these patients are to be classified as stage D. For this reason a staging operation should be performed prior to radical operation for both tumor of the bladder and carcinoma of the prostate. These surgical interventions mean discomfort to the patient and call for preoperative diagnosis with the greatest possible accuracy. Lymphography, however, represents a high percentage of false negatives and false positives (Fuchs 1965). In this case, sonography and computed tomography were not sufficient to furnish improvement of major importance. Both methods do not allow detection of metastasis in a lymph node at an early stage of growth, as it is exclusively the increase in tumor masses that can be determined (Feuerbach et al. 1979; Rothenberger et al. 1979).

Material and Method

Lymphography is followed by puncture utilizing a 23-gauge needle. (Göthlin 1976; Rothenberger et al. 1978; Rupp et al. 1979; Zornoza et al. 1977). Under fluroscopic guidance we transperitoneally punctured five to ten lymph nodes along the lymphogenous pathway of metastasis (Fig. 1). Puncture is performed only in general sedation (Diazepam). Contraindications include bleeding, ileus, and inflammable processes of the abdominal skin. This method excludes discomfort to the patient, and complication was not encountered. In the meantime, after lymphography, 126 patients from our hospital have undergone a fine needle biopsy of retroperitoneal lymph nodes. Using this method cytologic specimens could be obtained from 545 lymph nodes.

Results and Discussion

The rate of impact was 75%. Table 1 shows the number of patients considered, the diagnoses, and the number of patients with positive cytology. Out of 126 patients, 28 (22%) were proved to have metastasis in lymph nodes by cytologic diagnosis (Fig. 2).

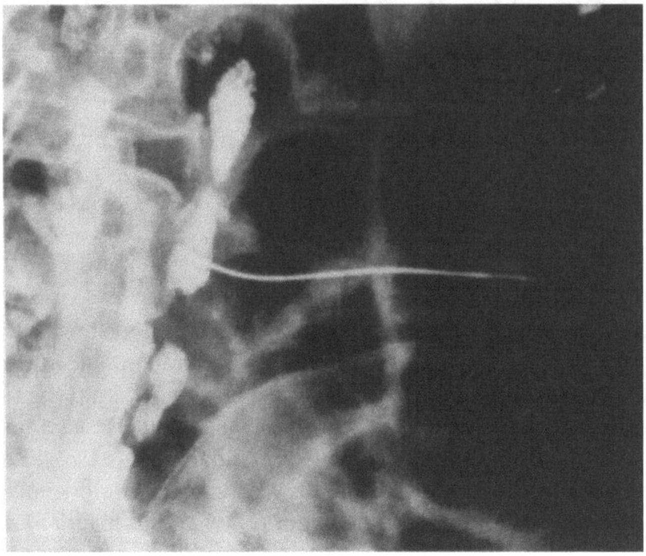

Fig. 1. Fluoroscopically guided fine needle biopsy of lumbar lymph node. Oblique position.

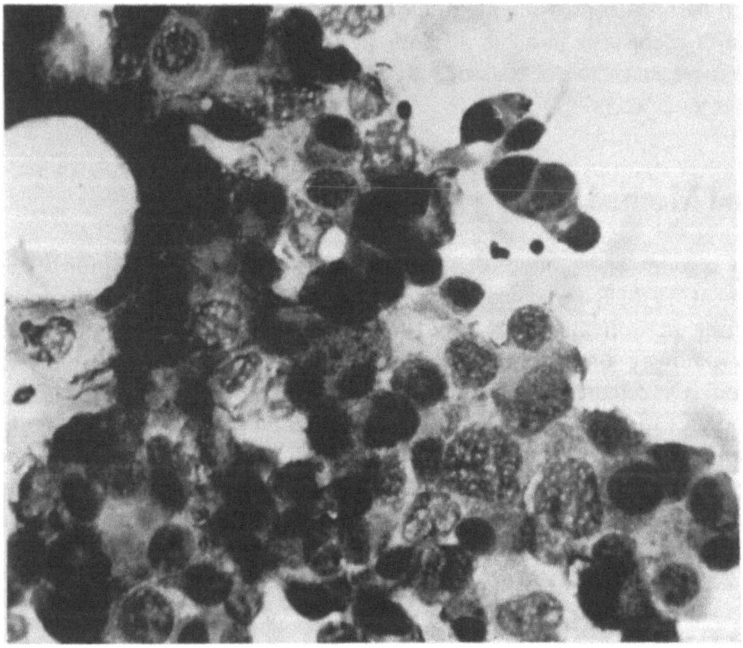

Fig. 2. Aspiration biopsy smear of a lymph node. A cluster of carcinoma celles (adenocarcinoma of the prostrate). May-Grünwald-Giemsa, ×400.

Table 1. Transabdominal fine needle biopsy of retroperitoneal lymph nodes; 730 punctures, 545 lymph nodes (rate of impact 75%).

Diagnosis	Number of patients $n = 126$	Positive cystology $n = 28$
Carcinoma of the urinary bladder	45	10
Carcinoma of the prostate	33	7
Testis teratoma	7	0
Testis seminoma	13	3
Kidney carcinoma	7	1
Penis carcinoma	6	2
Melanoma	4	3
Other tumors	11	2

Table 2. Comparison of cytologic findings with results of lymphography. Fine needle punctures in 545 lymph nodes.

Diagnosis	Cytology	Lymphography		
		Corresponding	False positive	False negative
Metastasis	73 (10)	35 (4)		38 (6)
Lymph node without pathological findings	468 (85)	417 (81)	51 (4)	
Doubtful	4 (0)	4 (0)		

The results shown in Table 2 are based on comparison of cytologic results with results obtained by lymphography of these 545 punctured retroperitoneal lymph nodes; using cytology we were able to determine tumor cells in 73 lymph nodes. Lymphography findings were correspondingly positive in 35 lymph nodes and false negative in 38. The figures in parentheses indicate histologically controlled lymph nodes. Cytology did not reveal 468 lymph nodes, and in 417 cases lymphography was correspondingly negative. Fifty-one lymphographic positive nodes did not show metastasis by way of cytology, the results of which were confirmed four times by histology. As it is particularly the positive cytologic findings that provide sufficient proof, a staging operation seems to be necessary to be on the safe side. The negative cytologic findings do not reliably exclude tumor affection since not all lymph nodes can be punctured, and some afftected lymph nodes store no contrast medium and are thus not accessible. But even with the most careful staging operations, some lymph nodes are left in situ and thus will not be available for fine tissue examination either. In addition, tumor cell nests in lymph nodes without pathologic findings by means of macroscopy may be easily overlooked during histologic control since expenditure and employment do not allow series sections of all lymph nodes.

The effectiveness of the fine needle biopsy, which is employed for retroperitoneal lymph nodes, should be assessed by histologic control (Table 3). In all cases cytology corresponded to histology. In 27 patients who underwent an operation we were able to prove that in 21 cases without and in two cases with metastasis in a lymph node, lymphography findings corresponded to cytology and histology. Three patients had metastasis and represented negative lymphography, one patient had no metastasis and represented positive lymphography. In 28 patients we were able to determine metastases. Fifteen of these patients showed positive lymphography and thus lymphography was in agreement with cytology.

Table 3. Cytologic results of puncture confirmed by histology in 27 patients.

Lymphography	Cytology	Patients
Negative	Negative	21
Negative	Positive	3
Positive	Positive	2
Positive	Negative	1

It should be emphasized that 13 patients showing lymphography without pathologic findings were proved to have metastasis in a lymph node by means of cytology – a result of high significance. A staging operation was not necessary due to cytologic demonstration of tumor in retroperitoneal lymph nodes.

Considering both the complexities of the staging operation and the method of transperitoneal fine needle puncture for retroperitoneal lymph nodes, neither of which involves any discomfort to the patient from complications of the procedure, the method presented may be recommended for widespread application.

Summary

Lymphography for staging lymphogenous metastasis represents a high percentage of false negative and false positive respones. In 28 patients, after puncture of lymph nodes along the pathway of metastasis, we were able to determine metastases by means of cytology. Thirteen of these patients showed negative lymphography. In all these cases a staging operation was not necessary due to cytologic demonstration of metastases. Of our patients with malignant disease, 22% showed metastasis in a lymph node. By means of fine needle puncture the rate of impact reached 75%. The method presented eliminates discomfort to the patient and may be recommended for widespread application.

References

Feuerbach St, Rupp N, Rossmann W, Heller HJ, Rothenberger K, Tauber R, Schmidt G (1979) Lymphknotenmetastasen-Diagnose durch Lymphographie und CT. Fortschr Röntgenstr 130:3

Fuchs WA (1965) Lymphographie und Tumordiagnostik. Springer, Berlin Heidelberg New York

Göthlin JH (1976) Post-lymphographic percutaneous fine needle biopsy of lymph nodes guided by fluroscopy. Radiology 120:105

Rothenberger K, Rupp N, Feuerbach St, Bayer-Peitsch E (1979) Lymphknoten-Metastasennachweis durch transabdominelle Feinnadelbiopsie. In: Verhandlungsbericht der Deutschen Gesellschaft für Urologie 1978. Springer, Berlin Heidelberg New York, p 65
Rothenberger K, Hofstetter A, Pfeifer K-J, Rupp N (1979) Transperitoneale Feinnadel-Biopsie retroperitonealer Lymphknoten in der Karzinomdiagnostik. Fortschr Med 97:2218–2222
Rupp N, Rothenberger K, Bayer-Pietsch E, Feuerbach St, Esch U (1979) Die perkutane Feinnadelbiopsie von Lymphknoten. Fortschr Röntgenstr 130:3, 328
Spellmann MC, Castellino RA, Ray GR, Pistenma DA, Bagshaw MA (1977) An evaluation of lymphography in localized carcinoma of the prostate. Radiology 125:637
Zornoza J, Wallace S, Goldstein HM, Lukeman M, Jing B-S (1977) Transperitoneal percutaneous retroperitoneal lymph node aspiration biopsy. Radiology 122:111

Lymphography, Computed Tomography, and Sonography

A Comparison in Evaluations of the Metastatic Spread in Malignant Tumors of the Urogenital Tract

H. Schmoller, R. Köhle, and J. Frick

Lymphography, computed tomography, and sonography are the methods of evaluating metastatic spread in malignant tumor of the urogenital tract. A comparison concerning their diagnostic value is limited, because every method has its own independent value, with a strong indication for application.

Computed tomography can be done in principle in every patient, except in pregnancy. Computed tomography is superior to sonography in adipose patients and if there is abundant gas. Also in the minor pelvis, computed tomography yields more evidence than sonography. A metastatic lymph node is visible if it is more than 1.5–2 cm thick. The length of the lymph node is less important and not pathognomonic for metastatic involvement.

Sonography should be done in slender patients. Abundant gas can considerably disturb the examination and make it impossible. It is of interes, that there is no radiation, no complications can occur and the examination can be done with more flexibility. The examination is fast, provided that a real-time-scanner is used.

It is possible to make cross, longitudinal, and also oblique sections. Enlarged lymphonodi may be seen if they are more than 1.5–2 cm thick (Schmoller et al. 1979).

Computed tomography and sonography also allow us to evaluate, in contrast to lymphography, these lymph node stations, which cannot be seen in lower-limb lymphography. It is also possible to evaluate the abdominal parenchymal organs for metastatic spread in the same examination (Lackner et al. 1979).

Lower-limb lymphography shows only a limited number of lymph nodes. But there is the advantage that also small lesions in the filling state of a lymph node are visible, even before enlargement is evident.

Lymphography is a time-consuming examination and is indicated only in special problems (equivocal or negative computed tomogram and sonogram with urgent clinical suspicion for metastatic spread). Today we have less lymphographies, but the number of positive findings is higher.

Clinical Results

Last year we performed sonography, computed tomography, and lymphography in an unselected group of 14 patients with cancer of the urogenital tract. In nine cases (three definitely positive and six definitely negative) all three methods agreed. In

Table 1. Comparison of three methods of evaluating cancer in the urinogenital tract. *CT,* Computed tomography; *US,* sonography; *LY,* lymphography.

	$N=14$ Correlation positive	False positive	Correlation negative	False negative
CT	3	3 ?	6	0
US	3	2 ?	6	0
LY	3	3 ?	6	0

the remaining five cases, which had been truly correctly negative because of their clinical course and in one also because of surgical staging, computed tomography was questionably positive three times, lymphography also three times but sonography only twice (Table 1).

This small advantage of sonography compared with computed tomography and lymphography agrees with the reports of Burney and Klatte (1979), which give both imaging methods about the same value. Whalen (1979) is of the opinion that computed tomography is superior to sonography in this problem because the pictures show more details and therefore better anatomic relations, and adiposity and gas do not disturb the examination.

Conclusions

In large metastases (over 2 cm), in slender patients with not much bowel gas and no pathologic findings, all three methods agreed in our series. The most difficult decision in this problem arises in questionable findings in one or several of these methods. If one starts with sonography, the best way to confirm or exclude a metastatic spread into lymph nodes is to complete the investigation with computed tomography. If the result is still questionable, lymphography should be carried out. We start in thin patients with sonography because sonography is cheaper, faster,

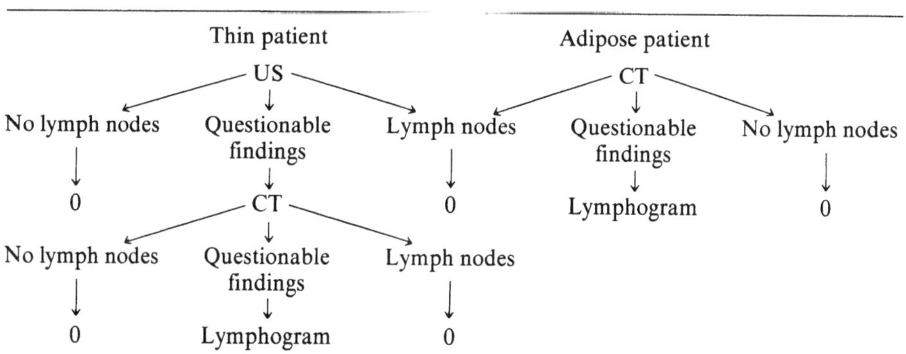

Fig. 1. Diagnostic approach to retroperitoneal adenopathy.

there is no radiation, and computed tomography should be dismissed. Based on our findings, we prefer the diagnostic approach for metastatic lymph nodes which is shown in Fig. 1.

References

Burney BT, Klatte EC (1979) Ultrasound and computed tomography of the abdomen in the staging and management of testicular carcinoma. Radiology 132:415–419

Lackner K, Weiszbach L, Boldt KI, Scherholz K, Brecht G (1979) Computertomographischer Nachweis von Lymphknotenmetastasen bei malignen Hodentumoren. Fortschr Röntgenstr 130/6:636–643

Schmoller H, Kunit G, Frick J (1979) Ultrasonic diagnosis of the retroperitoneal space. Eur Urol 5:113–116

Whalen JP (1979) Radiology of the abdomen: Impact of new imaging methods. Am J Roentgenol 133:585–618

The Value of Echotomography in Diagnostic Urology

W. Fiegler and R. Felix

Ultrasound was first employed in detection and differentiation of mass lesions of the kidney and is now of great value in other diagnostic problems of urology.

Kidney

Indications of Ultrasound in Urologic Kidney Disease

1) Detection and differentiation of space-occupying lesions;
2) nonfunctioning kidney;
3) obstruction of the collecting system;
4) filling defects of the renal pelvis;
5) pregnant and allergic patients;
6) puncture of cysts and percutaneous nephrostomy.

Renal Scanning Technique

The right kidney is best evaluated with scans through the liver with the patient supine. The left kidney can be imaged in the prone position because in the supine position the left kidney is often hidden behind overlying intestinal gas. A complete sonogram of kidneys includes longitudinal as well as transverse sections at 1 cm intervals.

Anatomy of the Normal Kidney

In longitudinal sections the kidney shows an ovoid shape. Gray scale technique and high-frequency transducers produce an accurate anatomic demonstration of the kidney; the cortex and medulla can be seen (Scheible et al. 1979). The vessels, calices, and other hilar structures produce the dense central echoes.

Renal Space-Occupying Lesions

It is useful to distinguish between *signs of a space-occupying lesion, signs of a cyst, and signs of a tumor.* The signs of a *space-occupying lesion* are:

1) Deformation of the typical kidney shape;
2) displacement or disappearance of the central echoes.

The *renal cyst* presents a characteristic image (Fig. 1):

1) Echo-free, even when high sensitivity adjustment is used;

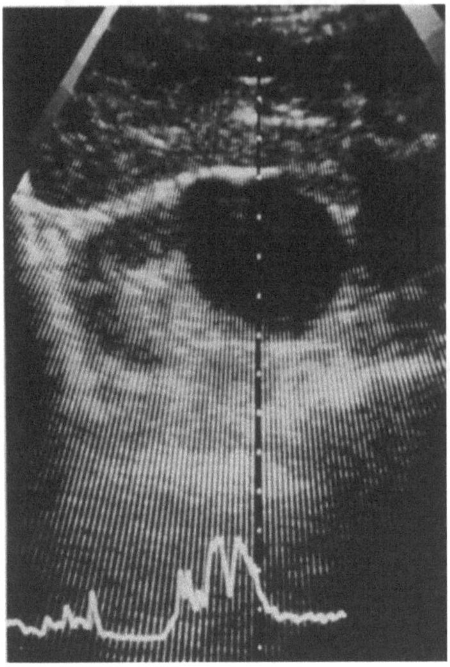

Fig. 1. Longitudinal scan of a renal cyst (real time). Mass in the lower pole of the right kidney with deformation of the kidney shape, absence of internal echoes (also in the A scan), and smooth wall. Transmission through the cyst is significantly greater than through a space-occupying lesion or a tumor.

2) sharply outlined;
3) usually circular in configuration;
4) transmission through the cyst is significantly greater than through space-occupying lesions or tumors.

The lower limit of resolution of a cyst depends on the frequency of the transducer and is about 1–1.5 cm.

There are certain limitations, however, to be considered:

1) In cysts, repetition echoes from ribs can appear as artifacts.
2) Intrararenal vascular deformations are difficult to distinguish from cysts. Doppler ultrasound can facilitate the differentiation. By means of real-time technique the pulsation in large aneurysms can be sometimes observed (Pollack et al. 1979).
3) Necrotic tumors and lymphomas may show only weak echoes and could therefore be misinterpreted as cysts.
4) Infected and hemorrhagic cysts may show echoes in the space-occupying lesion if cell detritus or blood clots are present.
5) Ultrasound cannot determine whether or not a malignant degeneration of the cyst is present. For this reason puncture of the cyst should be performed for further differentiation (Heckemann 1979).

Renal tumors are characterized by:

1) Echoes in the space-occupying lesion;
2) irregularity in the wall contours;

3) transmission through the tumor is not greater than through space-occupying lesions or cysts.

At the present state of technology tumors can, due to their similar structure to that of normal renal parenchymas, only be determined as such by means of secondary symptoms of a space-occupying lesion (Triller et al. 1978; Frommhold et al. 1976). That is why tumors can, depending on their localization, only be recognized at a size of 2–3 cm (Triller et al. 1978).

Renal cell carcinomas grow into the renal vein and vena cava inferior. Renal tumors therefore require sonographic visualization of the vena cava. Ultrasound can detect filling defects in the vena cava.

Rare Renal Tumors

Angiomyolipoma has a typical sonographic appearance: very high echogenicity, even at low gain settings and a very good sound transmission (Scheible et al. 1979).

Diagnostic Accuracy

Many investigators have performed quantitative studies. They have achieved the following accuracy: King (1972) 90%, Pitts et al. (1975) 92%, Fiegler et al. (1975) 93%, Koischwitz et al. (1976) 93%, Voegeli et al. (1980) 95%.

Nonfunctioning Kidney

Ultrasound is indicated in azotemic patients and in unilateral, nonvisualized kidneys and should be used first as a simple, noninvasive procedure. Sonography is independent of the remaining renal function and indicates the size of the organ and can differentiate between solid and cystic lesions. Ultrasound has an accuracy of 77%–92% [Marangola et al. (1976) 77%, Fiegler et al. (1979) 88%, Behan et al. (1979) 92%] in evaluation of non-functioning kidneys.

Hydronephrosis

Ultrasound is very sensitive in detecting a dilated collecting system and can be employed as a screening procedure when obstruction is the clinical question (Ellenbogen et al. 1978). The dilated collecting system causes a splitting of the central echoes. In cases of middle-grade hydronephrosis, the central echoes are set up in a circular arrangement (ring sign) or in a C-shaped arrangement (Fig. 2). However, not all dilated collecting systems are obstructed: reflux, congenital megacalyces, papilary necrosis, and renal tuberculosis show similar findings.

Renal calculi with an acoustic shadow can obscure the dilatation of the related caliceal system. If a hydronephrosis has been recognized, further examinations are necessary in order to document the postrenal stop (retrograde pyelography, anterograde pyelography). The pelvis also has to be examined sonographically in order to exclude a pelvic tumor. Pyonephrosis is characterized by fine echoes from debris within the dilated collecting system.

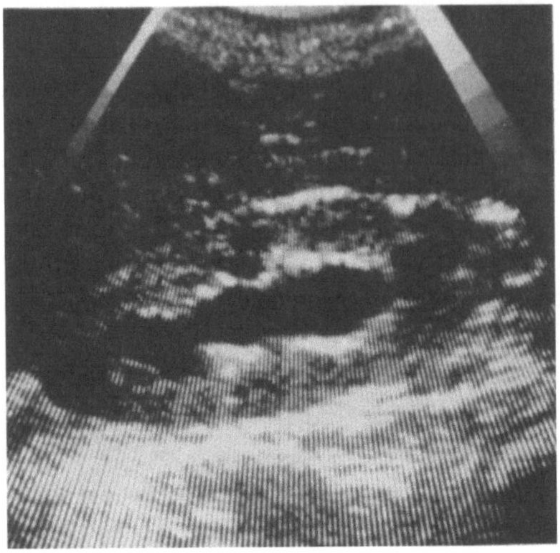

Fig. 2. Longitudinal scan of a hydronephrosis (real time). Separation of the collecting system echoes with a central sonolucency.

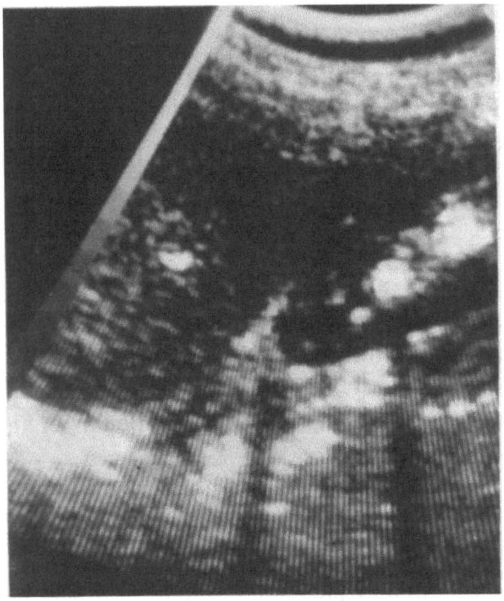

Fig. 3. Longitudinal scan of a kidney with renal calculi (real time). Within the renal pelvis is a very strong echo with shadowing. Another calcification is in the renal capsula with shadowing.

In filling defects of renal pelvis, noted during intravenous urography, ultrasound can differentiate between nonopaque stones (Fig. 3) – strong echo and shadow (Roters et al. 1979) – and other causes of filling defects, i.e., blood clots and papillary tumors – no strong echo, no shadow (Scheible et al. 1979; Pollack et al. 1978).

Ultrasonic Guidance of Puncture

Ultrasound is indicated in percutaneous nephrostomy and in percutaneous puncture of renal cysts.

Retroperitoneum and Perirenal Space

Fluid collections (urinoma) are characterized by an echo-free space. The kidney may appear displaced, rotated, or compressed. Organizing hematomas can be sonographically indistinguishable from an abscess or necrotic tumor. Retroperitoneal lymph node metastases greater than 3 cm can be diagnosed with an accuracy of about 85% (Asher et al. 1979).

Renal Transplant

The superficially placed renal transplant achieves ideal conditions required for ultrasound. Ultrasound examination can exclude obstruction, lymphoceles, and hematomas, which can mimic the rejection. *Obstruction* of the transplanted kidney causes dilatation of the collecting system. However, a distended urinary bladder may cause temporary hydronephrosis (Scheible et al. 1979). *Fluid collection* (urinoma, lymphocele, abscess, hematoma) can be detected very accurately. Puncture of the fluid accumulation allows exact determination. The *rejection* of the allograft is characterized by enlargement, compression of the renal sinus and patchy areas of sonolucency in the renal parenchyma due to edema, hemorrhage, or infarction (Scheible et al. 1979).

Bladder, Prostate, and Scrotum

The *prostate* can be demonstrated by "standard contact scanning" – using a suprapubic approach through the vesical ultrasonic window – and transrectal ultrasound – using an intrarectal transducer. Prostatic enlargement is easily noted and Japanese authors achieved an accuracy of 80%–89% in evaluation of prostatic disease (Watanabe et al. 1975; Harada et al. 1979).

Ultrasound is used for detection and staging of *bladder tumors* and determination of residual volume of the bladder. The urinary bladder is usually examined by direct contact scanning through the abdominal wall. Some authors use transurethral intravesical scanning (Niijima 1979; Holm et al. 1974).

Moreley, in a comparative study of suprapubic surgery and autopsy, achieved an accuracy for staging of bladder tumors of 48% in Jewett O and A (IUCC T1); 78% in Jewett B1 and B2 (IUCC T2 and T3A); and 91% in Jewett C and D1 (IUCC T3B and T4) (Morley 1978). It is difficult to differentiate between stages B1 and B2 (Russel et al. 1979) and a deep B2 is sonographically similar to an early stage C (Morley 1978). Fluid-filled lesions and solid masses of the *scrotum* can be detected excellently with an Octoson machine (the scrotum is immersed in a water bath).

A negative sonogram is highly reliable. Ultrasound is highly accurate in screening the scrotum for abnormalities and a clear differentiation of the origin of an abnormality was possible in 80% of cases (Sample et al. 1978).

References

Asher W, Freimanis AK (1969) Echographic diagnosis of retroperitoneal lymph node enlargement. Am J Roentgenol 105, 2:438

Behan M, Wixson D, Kazam E (1979) Sonographic evaluation of the nonfunctioning kidney. J Clin Ultrasound 7:449–458

Ellenbogen PH, Scheible FW, Leopold GR (1978) Sensitivity of gray scale ultrasound in detecting urinary tract obstruction. Am J Roentgenol 130:731–733

Fiegler W, Friedrich M, Sörensen R (1975) Der Wert der Sonographie in der Diagnostik renaler raumfordernder Prozesse. Fortschr Röntgenstr 125:452–457

Fiegler W, Friedrich M, Sörensen R (1979) Der Wert der Sonographie bei der Abklärung der einseitig urographisch stummen Niere. Roentgenblaetter 32:355–361

Frommhold H, Koischwitz D, Brühl P (1976) Einsatzmöglichkeiten der Sonographie zur Differentialdiagnostik raumfordernder renaler Prozesse. Fortschr Röntgenstr 125: 452–457

Harada K, Igari D, Tanahahi Y (1979) Evaluation of internal echo pattern of the prostate. 4th World Congress of Ultrasonics in Medicine. Miyazaki (Japan)

Heckemann R (1979) Ultrasound diagnosis of renal and pararenal tumors. In: Löhr E (ed) Renal and adrenal tumors. Springer, Berlin Heidelberg New York, pp 170–187

Holm HH, Northeved A (1974) A transurethral ultrasonic scanner. J Urol 3:238

King DL (1972) Renal ultrasonography. Radiology 10:633–640

Koischwitz D, Frommhold H, Brühl P (1977) Die Treffsicherheit der Sonographie in der Diagnostik von Nierenerkrankungen. Fortschr Röntgenstr 127, 2:97–106

Marangola J, Broyon P, Azimi F (1976) Ultrasonic evaluation of the unilateral nonvisualized kidney. Am J Roentgenol 126:853–862

Morley P (1978) Clinical staging of epithelial bladder tumours by echotomography. In: Hill CR, McCready VR, Cosgrove DO (eds) Ultrasound in tumour diagnosis. Pitman, London, pp 145–161

Niijima T (1979) Ultrasonic diagnosis of bladder cancer staging. 4th World Congress on Ultrasonics in Medicine. Miyazaki (Japan)

Pitts WR, Kazam E, Gershowitz M, Muecke Ec (1975) Review of one hundred renal and perinephric sonograms with anatomic diagnosis. J Urol 114:21–26

Pollack HM, Arger PH, Goldberg BB, Mulholland SR (1978) Ultrasonic detection of nonopaque renal calculi. Radiology 127:233–237

Pollack HM, Banner MP, Arger PH, Goldberg BB, Mulhern CB (1979) Comparison of computed tomography and ultrasound in the diagnosis of renal masses. In: Rosenfield AT (ed) Genitourinary ultrasonography. Churchill Livingstone, New York, pp 25–72

Roters HM, Scherer K (1979) Ultraschalldiagnostik von Nierensteinen. Fortschr Röntgenstr 131, 4:379–385

Russell JM, Resnick M (1979) Ultrasound in urology. Urol Clin North Am 6, 2:445–468

Sample WF, Gottesman JE, Skinner, DG, Ehrlich RM (1978) Gray scale ultrasound of the scrotum. Radiology 127:225–228

Scheible W, Talner LB (1979) Gray scale ultrasound and the genitourinary tract. Radiol Clin North Am 18, 2:281–300

Triller J (1978) Stellenwert der Sonographie in der radiologischen Nierendiagnostik. In: Fuchs WA, Triller J (eds) Aktuelle Probleme der Röntgendiagnostik Bd. 4, Ultraschall-Computertomographie. Huber, Bern

Voegeli E, Kwasny R, Hofer B (1980) Möglichkeiten und Grenzen der Sonographie und Angiographie bei renalen Raumforderungen. Fortschr Röntgenstr 132, 1:55–62

Watanabe H, Igari D, Tanahashi Y, Harada K, Saitoh M (1975) Transrectal ultrasonotomography of the prostate. J Urol 114:734–739

Prenatal Diagnosis of Foetal Urological Abnormalities by Ultrasonography

N. Elkhazen, C. Picard, and C. C. Schulman

Performance of maternal abdominal ultrasonography during pregnancy is rapidly increasing. It is usually used to determine foetal growth, gestational age, location of the placenta and foetal position and in the search for certain congenital malformations in high-risk pregnancies.

When maternal echography is performed after the foetus has started to produce urine, the foetal kidneys and the bladder can be identified. The foetal kidneys can usually be visualised by echography during the second trimester of intra-uterine life. Antenatal diagnosis of congenital malformation of the urinary tract may thus be made, particularly since the genito-urinary tract is the most common site of congenital malformation. Hence, one can anticipate finding about two foetal urological abnormalities in every 1000 pregnancies.

Normal Foetal Kidney

During the mean of the second trimester of intra-uterine life, the kidney can be visualised in the paravertebral subdiaphragmatic location. The capsular limit is well delineated since it is echogenic. The identification is characterised by the mobility associated with the diaphragmatic movement during foetal respiration in the uterus.

On longitudinal section, the kidney already has the form of a bean measuring 40–60 mm × 25–45 mm at the time of delivery in normal pregnancies (Fig. 1). The walls of the renal cavities (renal pelvis and calices) show a clear echogenic limit but the renal pelvis appears as a simple cavity, which is distinctly different in hydronephrosis. On transverse section, the kidney has an oval-shaped cavity (Fig. 2). When the ureters are visualised in normal foetuses, they can only be observed in the upper portion at the level of the renal pelvis.

Bladder

The bladder, with its liquid contents, is visualised earlier than the kidneys. Its volume is variable and its maximal diameter can reach 50–55 mm. Above this size, increased diamter can correspond to indirect signs of malformations such as urethral valves or neurogenic bladder associated with neurological disorders (myelomeningocele, etc.).

Urethra

The female urethra is well outlined. When looking for the sex of the foetus, its diameter is very small but the lumen is well visualised if ultrasonography is performed during micturition.

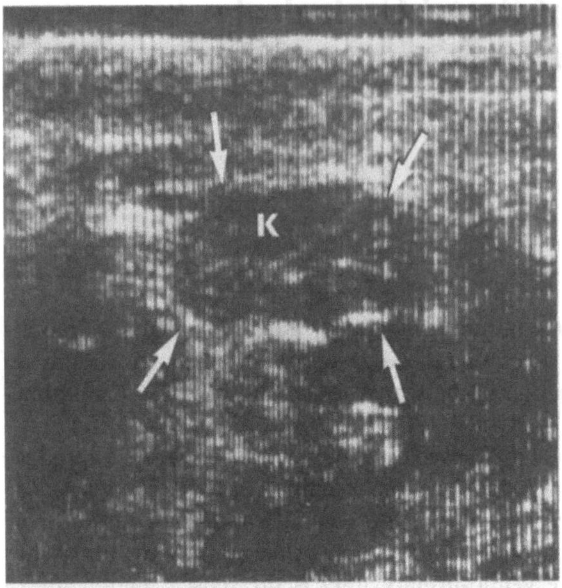

Fig. 1. Longitudinal section in the abdomen of a 36-week-old foetus – the kidney (*K*) (*arrows*) is well outlined with the diffuse and variable echogenicity of the renal cavities.

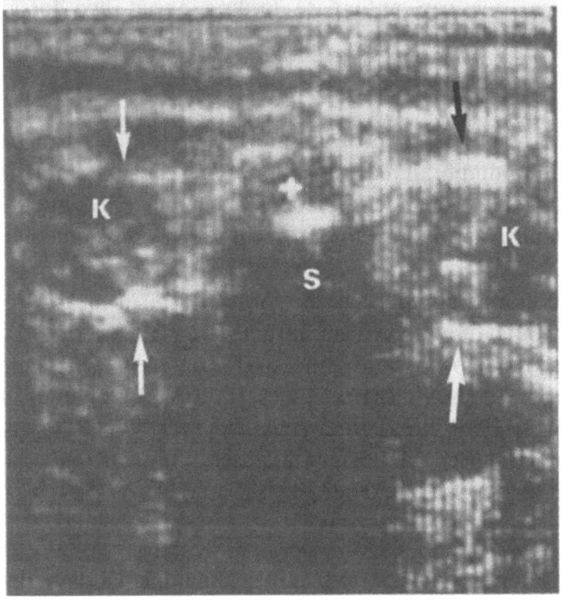

Fig. 2. Transverse section in the abdomen of a 36-week-old foetus: both kidneys (*K*) are well delineated (*arrows*) on each side of the spine (*S*).

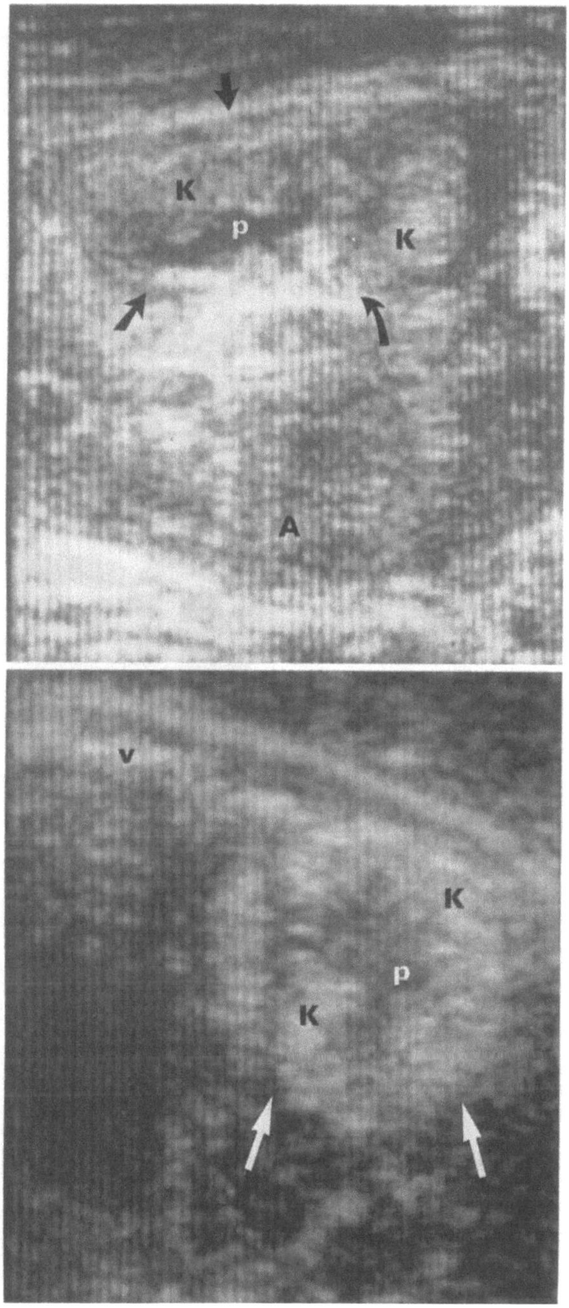

a

b

Fig. 3 a, b. Polycystic kidney disease. **a** Longitudinal section in a polycystic kidney (*K*) of a foetus. The longitudinal axis of the kidney is enlarged (76 mm), the general shape is well conserved (*arrows*), the renal pelvis (*p*) is normal, but the general echogenicity of the kidney parenchyma is diffusely enhanced. *A*, Abdominal cavity. **b** Transverse section of a foetal polycystic kidney (*K*). The general shape of the kidney is maintained (*arrows*), the renal pelvis (*p*) appears normal, but the general echogenicity and density of the parenchyma is much more important. *v*, Vertebrae.

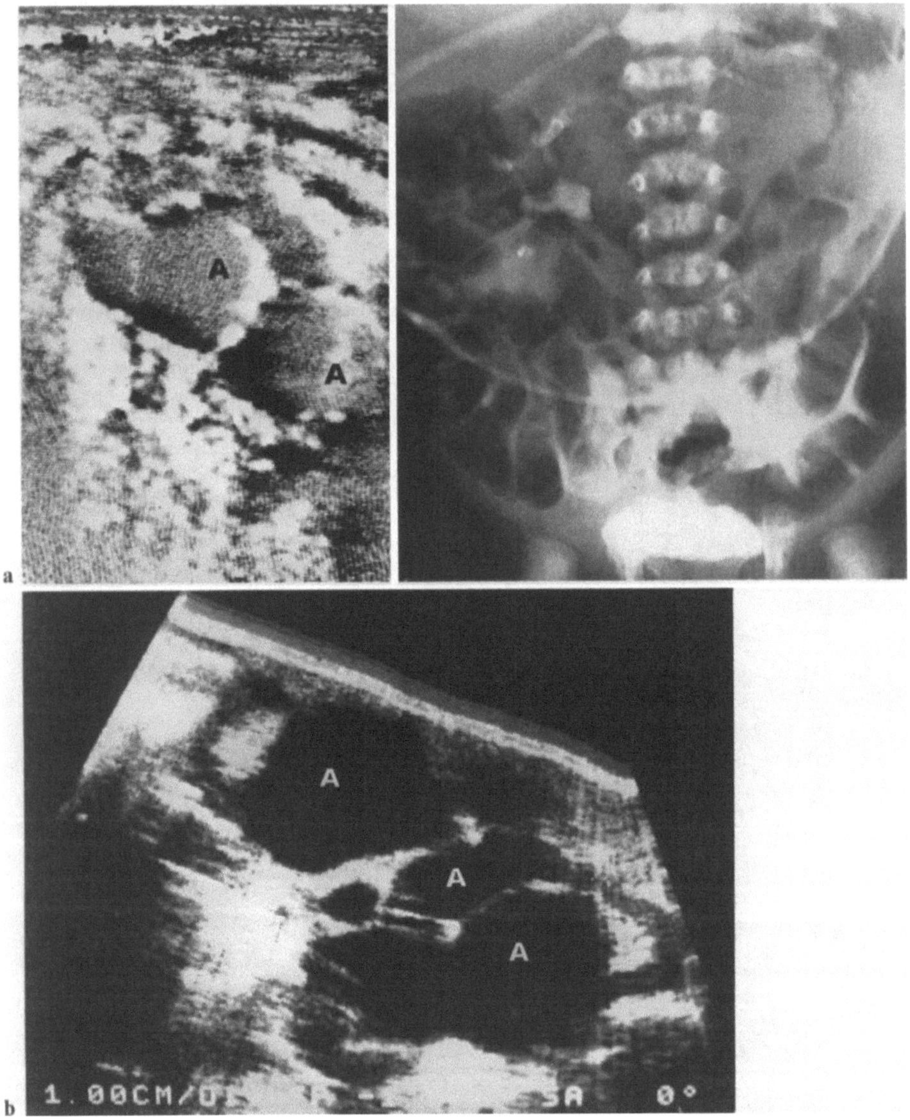

a

b

Fig. 4a–c. Multicystic kidney. **a** Foetal ultrasonography revealing hugely dilated cavities (*A*) without visible renal parenchyma. **b** Postnatal echotomography confirming the presence of huge cystic formation (*A*) on the left side without visible renal cortex. **c** Urogram: non-functioning left kidney. Surgical exploration at 1 month confirmed the existence of a left multicystic kidney.

The Male Urethra

The male urethra is not easy to visualize or outline in its entire length and this depends on the incidence of the echographic section.

Sex

The sex of the foetus can easily be recognised when the perineal region is observed, which is the case in about 75% of the examinations. During the scanning of the genital area the presence of testicles, penis and appearance of the urethra are the main features allowing sex determination.

Malformations of the Foetal Urinary Tract

Polycystic Kidneys

The general shape of the kidney is conserved but its size is increased on both sides (Fig. 3). Its longitudinal dimension varies between 60 and 80 mm. The renal parenchyma is more echogenic than in a normal kidney since the microcystic formations are particularly rich in echoes. The renal capsule is less refringent to ultrasounds and it appears with a less regular outline.

However, the limit of resolution does not allow distinguishing of the microcystic cavities, which are of very small size. The diagnosis thus mainly relies on the increase in size and the increased echogenicity of the kidneys on both sides.

Multicystic Kidneys

The general shape of the kidney is not conserved (Fig. 4). The liquid formations in the renal area are free from echo and round shaped, with a size varying from a few millimeters to 15–20 mm in diameter. This multicystic mass may compress other abdominal structures. As a rule, most multicystic kidneys are unilateral.

Upper Urinary Tract Dilatation

The description of the lesions depends on the level of the obstruction. The shape of the kidney is normal and the cortex is more or less normal in thickness but may be severely reduced in case of massive hydronephrosis. The diagnosis is mainly based on the problems of a dilated renal pelvis with hydronephrotic cavities, which may eventually be accompanied by a massively dilated ureter, which can be easily visualised at the lumbar or even lower level in cases of mega-ureter (Fig. 5).

Discussion

Echotomography performed during the last third of pregnancy is able to demonstrate congenital malformations of the urinary tract in the foetus. The definite antenatal diagnosis is not always possible but the suspicion of abnormalities in the foetus urinary tract should call the attention of the clinician and lead to the

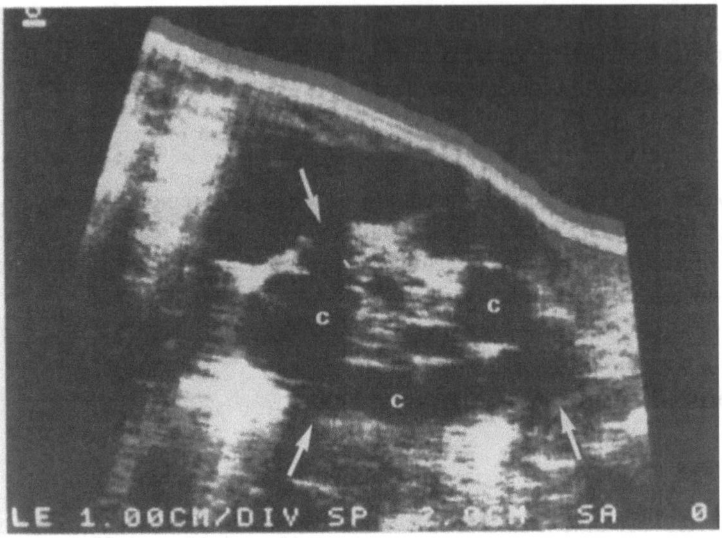

a

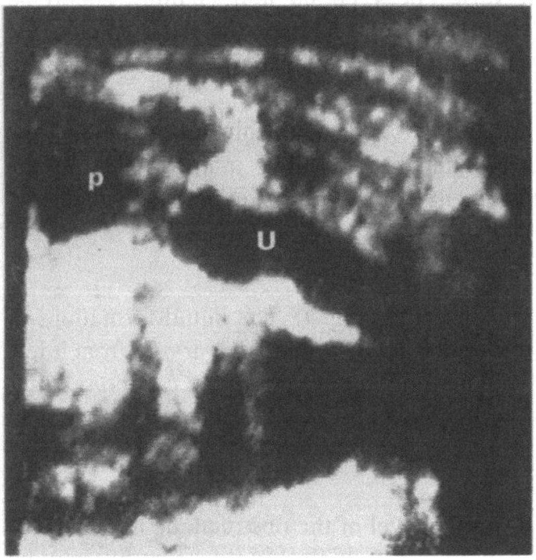

b

Fig. 5 a–d. Bilateral mega-ureters with ureterohydronephrosis. **a** Foetal echotomography reveals the presence of dilated renal cavities (*c*) with the presence of renal parenchyma (*arrows*). **b** Echotomographic section at the lower pole of the left kidney reveals a dilated renal pelvis (*p*) with a massively dilated ureter (*U*).

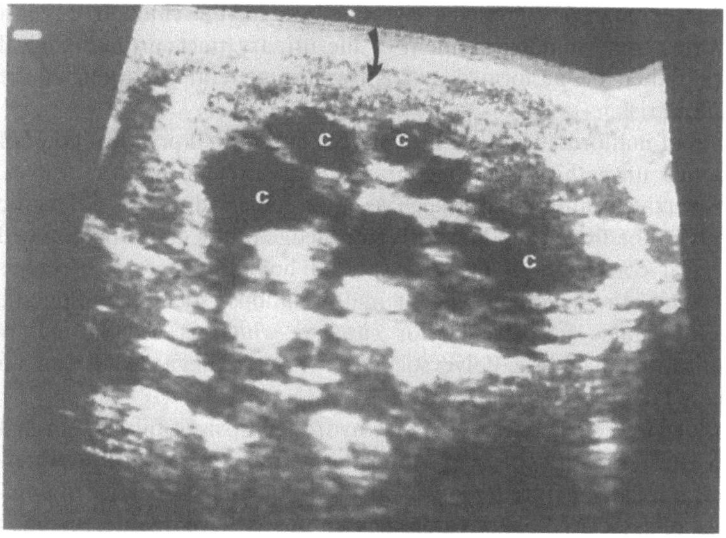

c

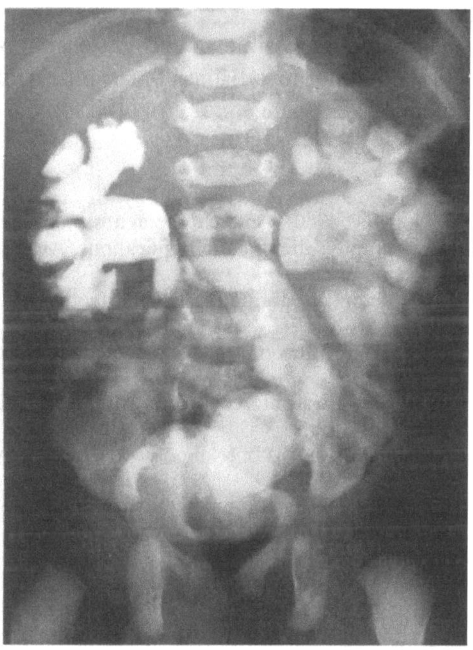

d

Fig. 5 c, d

c Postnatal echotomography: A longitudinal section of the left kidney confirms the existence of massively dilated renal cavities (*c*) with the persistence of a sick renal cortex (*arrow*). **d** Urogram: Bilateral mega-ureter with ureterohydronephrosis, more important on the left side. A bilateral reimplantation was performed at the age of 2 weeks without complications.

performance of echotomography immediately after birth of the child. If this last examination confirms some maldevelopment of the urinary tract, uroradiological investigation should then be performed as soon as the general condition of the child allows it without risk.

Two main types of malformations can be distinguished from a practical point of view: the obstructive uropathies (hydronephrosis, mega-ureters, urethral valves, etc.) and non-obstructive malformations such as multicystic kidneys or polycystic disease. It is mainly in the first group that early knowledge of the malformation will allow earlier surgical correction of the disease, and hopefully before infectious complications develop. In the other type of malformations, such as multicystic kidney, there is of course no urgency for surgery, which is usually mainly performed to confirm the diagnosis. Polycystic kidney disease diagnosed at such an early stage is usually fatal.

One may consider in the presence of massive hydronephrosis, if bilateral or in a solitary kidney, performing a percutaneous transuterine puncture with decompression to preserve the renal function and prevent the frequently associated pulmonary complications of associated oligohydramnios. In this last eventuality, one may also consider earlier delivery of the child.

Echotomography during pregnancy has made it possible to recognize abnormalities of the urinary tract in the foetus and thus to advance the frontiers of diagnoses and make possible earlier treatment of some congenital uropathies.

References

Colodny AH, Bauer SB, Retik AB, Birnholz J (May 1980) Antenatal diagnosis of fetal urologic abnormalities by intrauterine ultrasonography: therapeutic implications. Annual Meeting, American Urological Association, San Francisco

De Vore GR, Hobbins JC (1979) Diagnosis of structural abnormalities in the foetus. Clin Perinatol 6:293–319

Friedberg JE, Mitnick JS, Davis DA (1979) Antepartum ultrasonic detection of multicystic kidney. Radiology 131:198

Garret WJ, Kosoff G (1976) Selection of patients by ultrasonic echography for fetal and immediate neonatal surgery. Aust Paediatr J 12:313–318

Garret WJ, Grunwald G, Robinson DE (1966) Prenatal diagnosis of fetal polycystic kidney by ultrasound. Obstet Gynecol 28:164

Morrisson-Lacombe G, Monfort G Cristofari J (1980) Diagnostic anténatal des malformations congénitales par l'échotomographie. Chir Pediatr 21:249–252

Slovis TL, Perlmutter AD (1980) Recent advances in pediatric urological ultrasound. Urol 123:613–620

Sonographically Guided Percutaneous Puncture of Renal Cysts

E. Schindler, M. Preßler, H. Zöckler, P. Kolle, and N. Papandreou

Aspiration of renal masses dates back to 1861, when Thompson "repeatedly emptied by tapping an enormous sac connected with the kidney" (Buttarazzi et al. 1968). Fish (1939) probably was the first to recommend exploration of a suspected cyst with the aspirating needle. In 1939, he presented an air-filled cystogram and published two cases that were successfully treated by aspiration and instillation of 50% dextrose as a sclerosing agent. Dean (1939) advocated puncture as the treatment for renal cysts, based on 15 cases of his own. He was supported by Wheeler (1941), who, at a meeting of the New England Section of the AUA, drew attention to "hypernephric cysts." In the following discussion, Deming, to our knowledge, was the first to suggest the injection of contrast material into the cyst. Lindblom (1946) reported a series of five cystograms performed by the instillation of 2–7 cc 35% diodrast. Ever since, an increasing number of authors have favored aspiration in the diagnostic workup of renal cysts (Phillips 1963; Witherington and Rinker 1966; Pearman 1966; Klosterhalfen 1963; Lang 1966). The danger of seeding a malignant tumor in the site of needle puncture has been conjectured but never been proven (Devine et al. 1968). Lang (1966) stressed, above all, the diagnostic value of cyst puncture. He inaugurated the double-contrast technique with introduction of air and contrast material into the cyst; additionally, he recommends qualitative and quantitative assessment of the aspirated fluid for fat together with a Papanicolaou smear. Beginning at the end of the 1960 s, ultrasound has increasingly been instituted as a means of differential diagnosis of renal masses (Goldberg et al. 1971; Pollack et al. 1974; Sanders 1975). Cyst puncture under fluoroscopic guidance after sonographic evaluation seems to be the most widely practiced method, but aspiration under ultrasound guidance has been favored with the introduction of enhanced technical equipment (Lang 1977). In a survey of 5674 cases, Lang (1977) reported an incidence of major complications of cyst aspiration of 0.75%–1.4% (perirenal hematoma, pneumothorax, arteriovenous fistulae, traumatic urinomas). Flexible puncture equipment and the extensive experience of the investigator lessened the risk of complications.

Probably due to insufficient investigative methods, renal cysts once were considered a rare and uncommon lesion. But Branch (1929) noted that solitary serous cysts of the kidney are observed in approximately 3%–5% of all routine autopsies. A similar rate was reported by Lang (1971). Excluding all urologic cases, we encountered 30 liquid renal masses in 1000 routine sonograms. The mean age was 69 years for men and 67 years for women, the youngest patient being 49 years old (the incidence rate in the urologic patients was 14.8%). In a series of 2000 CT scans, we found renal cysts in approximately 10% of patients. Donker and

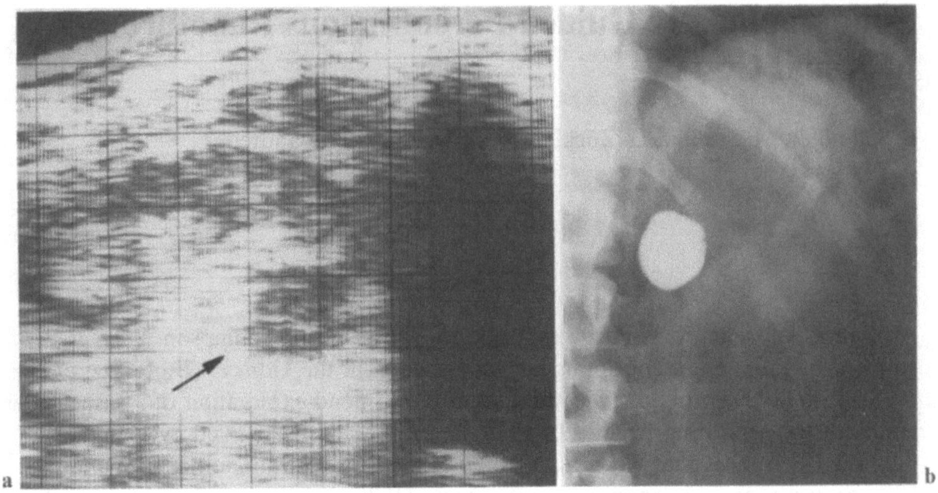

Fig. 1. a Sonography of left kidney (longitudinal section): liquid mass (*arrow*) in central upper portion with some acoustic reverberations within the cyst, but sizable posterior echo. **b** Cystogram: Smooth, well-defined circular wall.

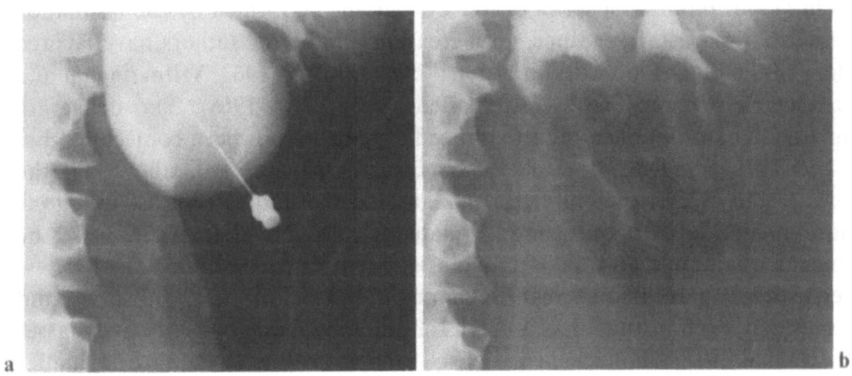

Fig. 2. a Cystogram: huge cyst in hilar region of the left kidney with mild ectasia of renal pelvis. **b** Cyst after voiding of 160 cc fluid: Reduction of pelvic ectasia.

Kakiailalu (1978) discovered 24 renal cysts on the intravenous pyelograms (IVPs) of 300 men with bladder outlet obstruction (mean age 71.5 years). Being most common in adults in their 5th and 6th decades, cysts are thought to be aquired rather than congenital.

The simple solitary unilateral cyst is most common and probably outnumbers all other renal masses combined (Lang 1971; Pollack et al. 1974). A significant difference in location in the right or left kidney does not appear to exist, but the lower pole seems to be the preferential site. In 150 patients, we saw 54% of the cysts on the right side, 40% on the left and 6% in both kidneys. Fifty-six percent of all cysts were found in the lower pole, 34% in the upper pole, and 10% in the midportion.

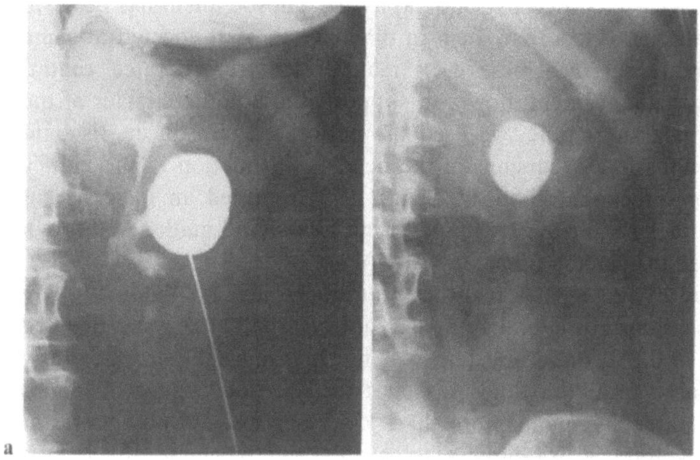

Fig. 3. Cystograms: same cyst in 1977 (a) and 1980 (b).

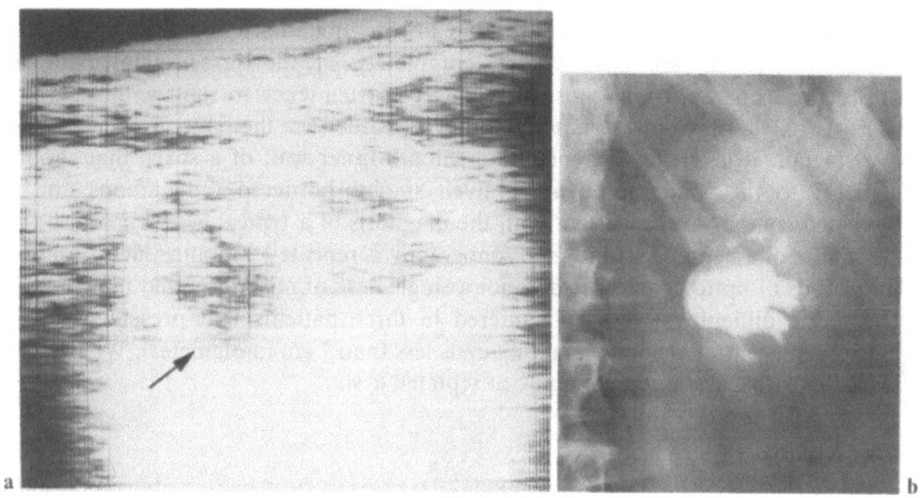

Fig. 4. a Sonography of right kidney (longitudinal section): lobulated sonolucent mass (*arrow*) with scattered central echoes and dorsal echo enhancement. b Cystogram: finger-like extensions of cyst consistent with sonographic mass.

A galaxy of studies, diagnostic demands, and hints have been advocated for differentiation of renal space-occupying lesions, e.g., nephrotomography, compressibility of mass on retrograde pyelography, arteriography, phlebography, CT scan, and routine surgical exploration of all masses. With the wider use of sonography, the following stategy has been generally accepted: a transonic liquid mass is aspirated; a dry tap and echogenic solid masses require arteriography.

The aspirating needle may be guided both by fluoroscopy and ultrasound; since 2 years ago, we have preferred sonographic guidance. Its special virtues include ease of performance, rapidity, freedom from X-ray exposure, economy, and possibility of exact location of cysts down to 1–1.5 cm in diameter. Cysts of more than 2 cm width can easily be needled under sonographic guidance. Liquid masses and solid tumors are well separated by sonography. Diagnostic dilemmas occur in obese patients and masses of less than 2 cm in diameter that are located at some distance from the body surface; these cysts may present reverberated central echoes. A dorsal echo enhancement, however, supports the liquid character of the mass (Fig. 1a, b). For a short time, we used the perforated transducer. Its rigid system, however, inhibits free excursions of the needle with motion of the kidney due to respiration or directional changes. Lang (1977) reported an incidence of major complications of 1.1% for the technique using ultrasound guidance through transducer (as opposed to 0.4% for a flexible system).

The cyst is located by means of a real-time transducer, and the landmarks are identified. We prefer a dorsal or lateral approach, but eventually the cyst is needled ventrally. A cannula of 0.7–0.9 mm in external diameter is injected percutaneously without local anesthesia until the fluid is aspirated. The thin caliber precludes lesions of bowel or parenchyma; in more than 150 cases we saw no significant complications. The aspirate is examined cytologically and biochemically (LDH, cholesterine, triglycerides). The absence of tumor cells and lack of fat support the diagnosis of renal cysts. If any of these parameters is not entirely typical for cyst or if bloody fluid is aspirated, it is our policy to recommend arteriography or surgical exploration. Cysts are only voided completely in the presence of pain or obstruction (Fig. 2a, b), as most of them have a tendency to refill within several weeks (Fig. 3a, b). Contrast material (30%) is instilled via the puncture needle, and a cystogram is taken to demonstrate a smooth inner wall of a space that should conform to the sonographic mass. Even smooth-bordered indentations and a lobulated contour are consistent with the diagnosis of a typical cyst (Fig. 4a, b). If all criteria of a benign cyst are met, sonography is repeated 3 months later. Follow-up periods of up to 5 years yielded not a single case of misinterpreted malignoma. Diagnostic difficulties were encountered in three patients that presented liquid masses with central echoes (excluding cysts less than 2 cm in diameter). We present two cases with a cystic conglomerate or septated cyst.

Case Reports

Case I (B.R.): A 45-year-old male was admitted for an osteoclastic lesion in the fifth lumbar vertebra. Urinalysis and blood chemistry were normal, ESR was 7/22 mm, and blood pressure was measured at 140/80 mm Hg. Urography (Fig. 5a) showed flattening of a left lower calyx. At sonography (Fig. 5b), a liquid mass of 5×5 cm at the lateral spect of the left kidney was found with septa and a solid portion in its center. The cystogram (Fig. 5c) revealed a space with concave borders not consistent with the liquid mass. A Papanicolaou smear of the aspirated fluid was negative and no cholesterine or triglycerides could be demonstrated. At computer tomography (Fig. 5d), a liquid septated mass with solid walls was encountered. Selective arteriography (Fig. 5e) identified a reticular neovascularity at the margin of a hypovascular mass. At surgical exploration, there was a conglobate of cherry- to plum-sized cysts, partially containing hemorrhagic fluid. A smear of one of the cysts yielded Papanicolaou IV. Frozen section histology described an unidentifiable tumor. Final histologic diagnosis was renal carcinoma with massive central necroses and pseudocystic cavities.

Case II (H.K.H.): A 51-year-old male presented with atypical left flank pain. Urinalysis was normal, creatinine was 120 μmol/liter. ESR was 8/16 mm, and blood pressure was measured at 130/80 mm Hg. Urography (Fig. 6a) revealed a nonfunctioning kidney on the right and a questionable mass at the left upper pole. Sonography (Fig. 6b) showed a primarily sonolucent mass with a somewhat complex pattern. A cyst puncture yielded a hemorrhagic aspirant, and

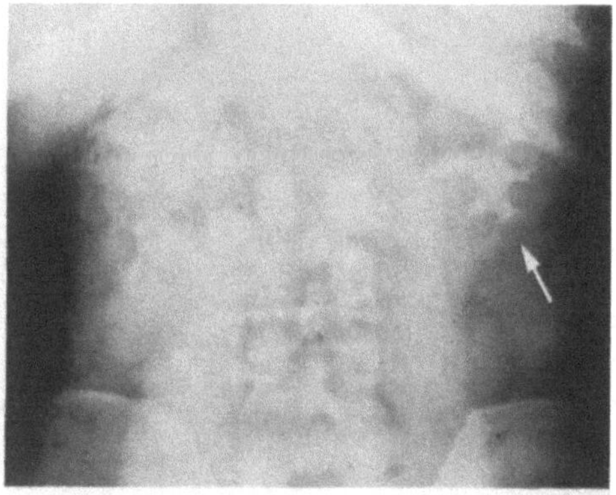

a

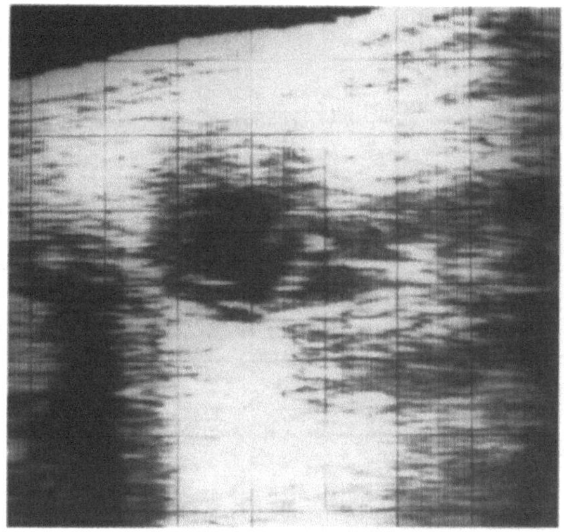

b

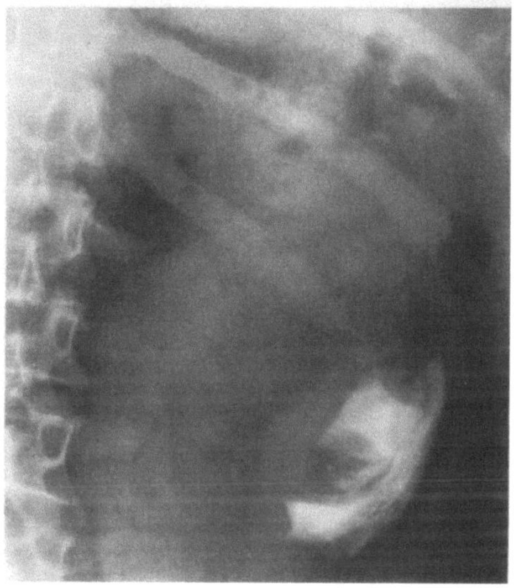

c

Fig. 5. **a** Urogram: discrete flattening of a left lower calyx (*arrow*). **b** Sonography (longitudinal section of lower half of left kidney): sonolucent mass protruding beyond the normal renal outline with linear echoes and solid portions. **c** Cystogram: concave-bordered space with some extravasation, not consistent with sonographic mass. **d** Computer tomography: liquid mass with septa and solid walls. **e** Selective left-sided arteriography: fine neovascularity caudal to a hypovascular mass.

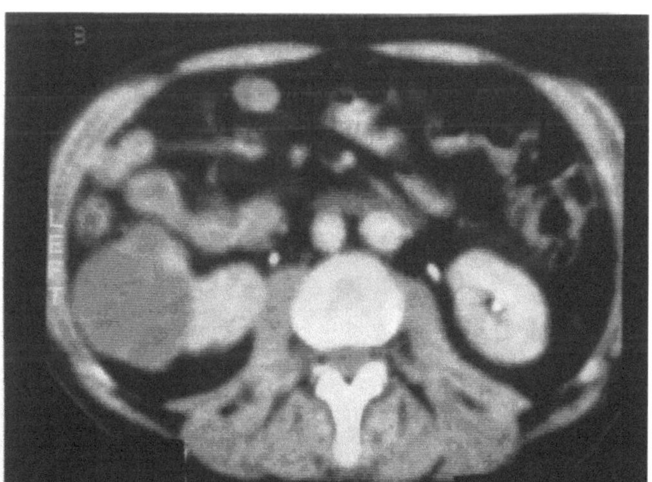

d

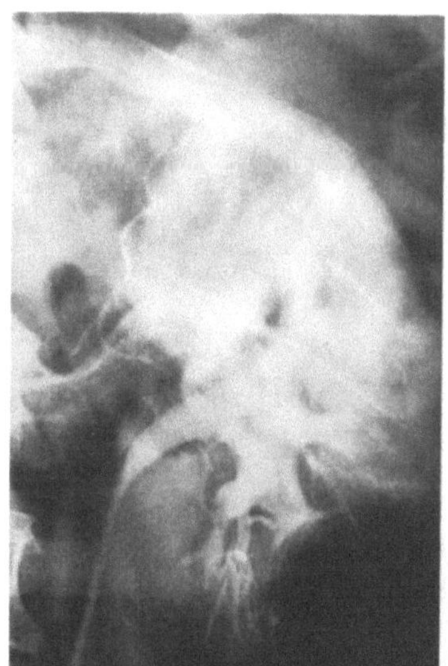

e

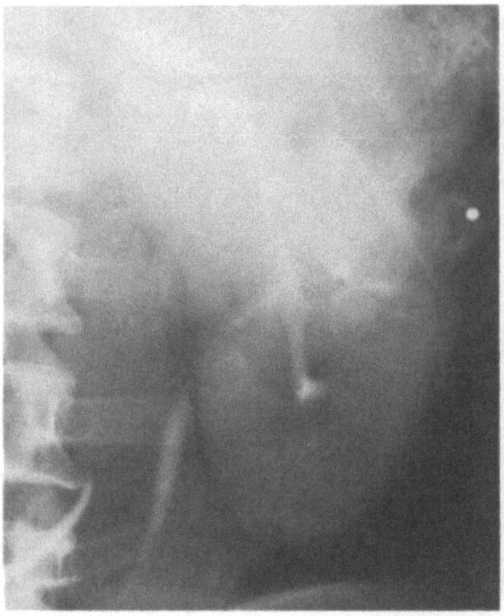
a

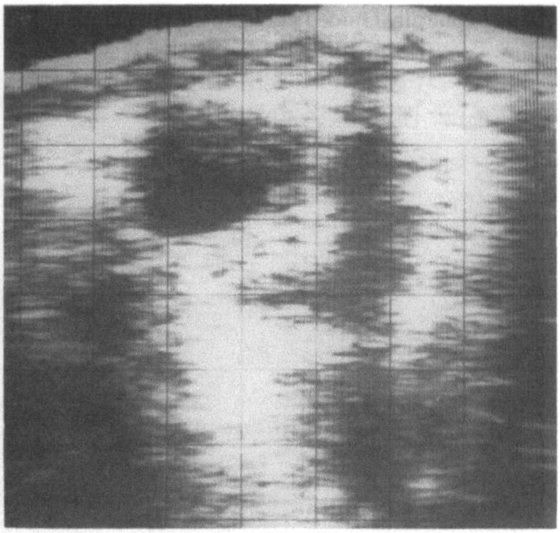
b

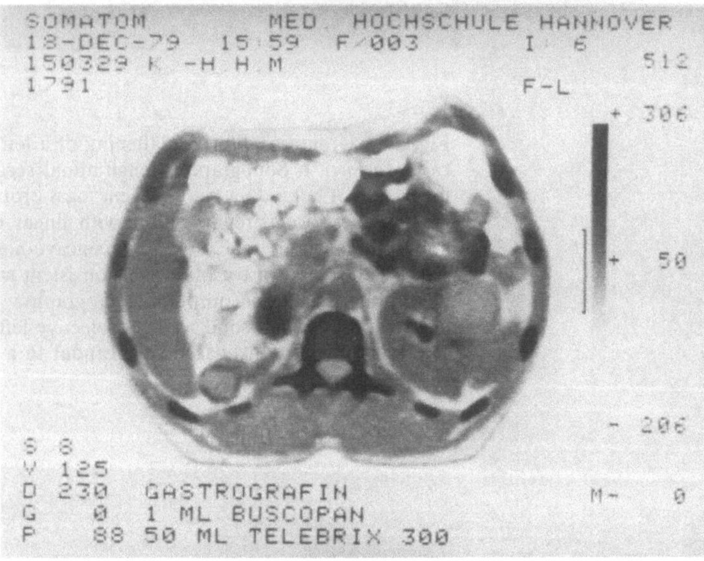

c

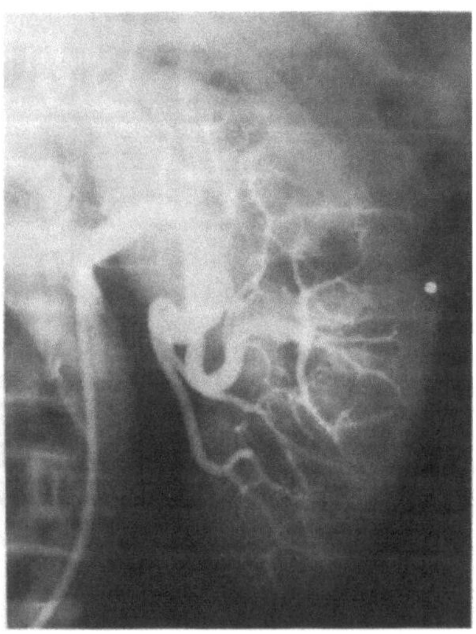
d

Fig. 6. a Urogram: nonfunctioning right kidney, ill-defined mass at left upper pole. **b** Sonography (oblique section of left upper pole): sound absorption by a rib, 4×3 cm mass with 2×2 cm liquid portion. **c** Computer tomography: cystic mass with internal septa. **d** Selective left-sided renal arteriography: hypovascular mass in lateral upper portion of kidney.

the cytologic preparation was negative. Computer tomography (Fig. 6c) gave the impression of a septated cyst. Arteriography (Fig. 6d) exhibited a hypovascular mass without tumor vessels. At the time of operation, a chambered cyst with grossly bloody, murky, and clear fluid was encountered. Histologic diagnosis of the removed cyst walls was cystic disease with chronic inflammatory changes.

Septated cysts are rather rare; Emmett et al. (1963) encountered 24 "cystic" renal carcinomas in 579 tumors. Computer tomography (CT) and sonography, in our two cases, gave some hints as to the chambered character of the liquid mass, but the contrast cyst study allowed a more definite judgment of the lesion. Cytology is not reliable in these cases as the tumor cell content of the individual cysts may vary. A histochemical assay of the aspirant may also fail to indicate a malignancy, as intact cyst lining may preclude the entry of cells or tumor breakdown products. Arteriography is known to be ineffective in the diagnosis of hypovascular tumors, though some fine neovascularity was seen in the patient with the cystic carcinoma. Macroscopic inspection at surgical exploration cannot separate a conglomerate of cysts from a cystic carcinoma. Even the frozen-section microscopic investigation was not too reliable. Only a through histologic workup supplied the definite diagnosis.

McLennan et al. (1979) recently suggested that renal cyst aspiration need not be performed when lesions meet all CT criteria for a benign cyst. X-Ray exposure, cost effectiveness, and availability of CT scanning has led us not to support this concept for the time being. Besides, modern gray scale ultrasound evaluation of patients with renal cysts is almost as accurate as CT scanning. The question must be raised, however, whether with continuing technical improvement of sonographic instruments aspiration is necessary in cases of *unequivocal* renal cysts.

Summary

Ultrasound is generally recommended as the first diagnostic procedure once a space-occupying lesion has been detected on IVP. In conjunction with aspiration and contrast studies, renal cysts can be diagnosed with a confidence rate of almost 100% without surgical exploration. Sonographically unequivocal cysts may even turn out not to require puncture. Diagnostic difficulties are raised by septated cysts, where histologic investigation is the only safe diagnostic procedure.

References

Branch CF (1929) Some observations on solitary cysts of the kidney. J Urol 21:451–453

Buttarazzi PJ, Poutasse EF, Devine CJ jr, Fiveash JG jr, Devine PC (1968) Aspiration of renal cysts. J Urol 100:591–593

Dean AL (1939) Treatment of solitary cyst of the kidney by aspiration. Am Ass Genito Urin Surg 32:91–95

Devine CJ jr, Buttarazzi PJ, Devine PC, Fiveash JG, Poutasse EF (1968) Aspiration or exploration to confirm diagnosis of renal masses. JAMA 204:758–762

Donker PJ, Kakiailatu F (1978) Preoperative evaluation of patients with bladder outlet obstruction with particular regard to excretory urography. J Urol 120:685–686

Emmett JL, Levine SR, Woolner LB (1963) Coexistence of renal cyst and tumour: incidence in 1007 cases. Br J Urol 35:403–410

Fish GW (1939) Large solitary serous cysts of the kidney. Report of thirty-two cases, including two cases cured by aspiration and instillation of 50 per cent dextrose solution. JAMA 112:514–517
Goldberg BB, Pollack HM (1971) Differentiation of renal masses using A-mode ultrasound. J Urol 105:765–771
Klosterhalfen H (1963) Zur Differentialdiagnose Nierentumoren-Nierencyste mit Hilfe der Renocystographie. Z Urol Nephrol 56:419–422
Lang EK (1966) The differential diagnosis of renal cysts and tumor. Cyst puncture, aspiration and analysis of cyst content for fat as diagnostic criteria for renal cysts. Radiology 87:883–888
Lang EK (1971) Renal cystic disease. In: The roentgenographic diagnosis of renal mass lesions. Green, St. Louis, pp 68–124
Lang EK (1977) Renal cyst puncture and aspiration: a survey of complications. Am J Roentgenol 128:723–727
Lindblom K (1946) Percutaneous puncture of renal cysts and tumors. Acta Radiol (Paris) 27:66–72
McClennan BL (1979) CT of the renal cyst: Is cyst aspiration necessary? Am J Roentgenol 133:671–675
Pearman RO (1966) Percutaneous needle puncture and aspiration of renal cysts: a diagnostic and therapeutic procedure. J Urol 96:139–145
Phillips DEH (1963) The percutaneous aspiration of renal cysts. Proc R Soc Med 56:928–930
Pollack HM, Goldberg BB, Bogash M (1974) Changing concepts in the diagnosis and management of renal cysts. J Urol 111:326–329
Sanders RC (1975) Renal ultrasound. Radiol Clin North Am 13:417–434
Wheeler BC (1942) Use of aspirating needle in diagnosis of solitary renal cysts. N Engl J Med 226:55–57
Witherington R, Rinker JR (1966) Percutaneous needle puncture in the diagnosis of renal cysts. J Urol 95:733–737

Sonographic Findings in Blunt Renal Trauma

G. Kunit, H. Schmoller, and J. Frick

The kidneys are ideally suited for sonography because of their location and characteristic shap with sharp acoustic boundary. No preparation of the patient is necessary. The examination itself takes only a short time and is not invasive. It was therefore of interest to prove the diagnostic value of nephrosonography in renal trauma.

Material and Method

The ultrasonic examination was done by Vidoson 735 and RA 1 with a frequency of 2.25 MHz or 3.5 MHz. An intravenous urogram or, better, an infusion urogram must be carried out fore since a coordinated evaluation is more effective.

From 1 January 1976 to 31 December 1979, 27 patients with blunt renal trauma were subjected to sonographic examination. Pathologic findings were ascertained in 17 of these cases. In ten cases there was no pathologic evidence.

Results and Discussion

The pathologic findings were subcapsular and pararenal hematomas, rupture of the kidneys, lesions of the renal pedicle, and pretraumatically affected kidneys such as cysts, hydronephrosis, and tumors. The latter kidneys are especially predisposed to trauma.

1) Sonographic findings in subcapsular and pararenal hematomes: Whereas old blood has the consistency of fluid, an old hematoma is without reflection and echohomogeneous. A fresh one on the other hand consists of coagula which have boundary surfaces and are therefore echogenic (Figs. 1, 2).

2) Sonographic findings in ruptured kidneys: Ruptured kidneys are mostly combined with hematomas. The extent of the rupture and the displacement of the parts can be seen exactly by sonography. Between the fragments more or less echogenic, mostly mushroom-shaped areas can be found, corresponding to the hematoma (Fig. 3).

3) If one finds a nonvisualized kidney after a blunt renal trauma in the urogram and if there is a sonographically normal or enlarged kidney, one has to think about an injury of the renal pedicle. In these cases only an angiogram gives the exact diagnosis.

4) Pretraumatic affected kidneys are preadominantly cysts, cystic kidneys, hydronephrosis, and also tumors. The sometimes minimal lesions in such pretrau-

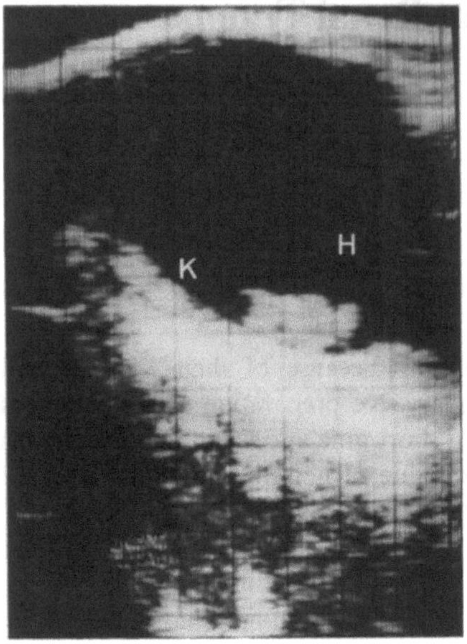

Fig. 1. Sonogram of the left kidney (longitudinal section, posterior-anterior). Subcapsular hematoma around the lower pole of the left kidney. *H,* Hematoma. *K,* Kidney.

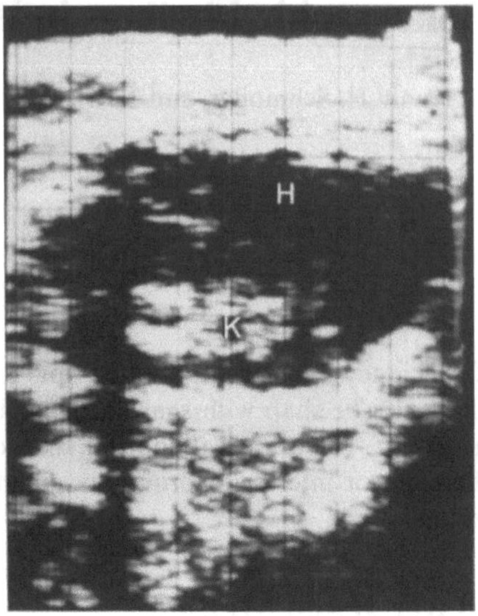

Fig. 2. Sonogram of the left kidney (longitudinal section, posterior-anterior). Huge, old, nonechogenic, subcapsular hematoma of the left kidney. *H*, Hematoma. *K,* Compressed kidney.

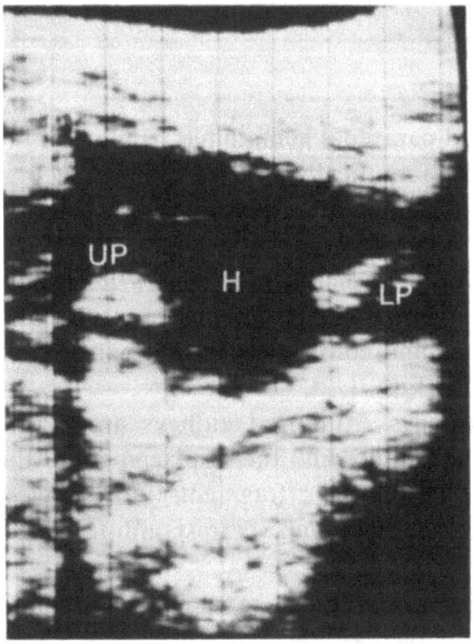

Fig. 3. Sonogram of the left kidney (longitudinal section, posterior-anterior). Ruptures left kidney with a broad, mustroom-shaped hematoma between the upper and lower poles of the kidney. *UP*, Upper pole. *LP*, Lower pole. *H*, Hematoma.

matic affected kidneys often cannot be detected sonographically but one will find of course the pretraumatic changes. Only in cases with a parapelvic cyst can it be difficult to differentiate it from an enlarged collecting system. This differential diagnosis must be done by intravenous urogram. Also a badly damaged kidney with organ fragments and blood clots may be difficult to differentiate from tumor tissue.

Summary

In cases of blunt renal trauma sonography is an excellent method for examing the degree of lesion of the kidneys. The examination should be based on an intravenous excretory urogram. The sonographic accuracy is about 100%. The diagnostic sequence as applied in our institute is as follows: After exact clinical evaluation an intravenous urogram with nephrotomography is done. Even when these examinations are negative nephrosonography is performed. A negative sonogram concludes the examination procedure. If the urogram and sonography are positive, an angiogram is performed, but only in cases with multitrauma and in those patients with a nonvisualized kidney in the urogram. The adoption of this diagnostic sequence is not only the most economic way, but also the one which provides the clearest findings and is the least irksome for the patients.

References

Beduhn D (1970) Angiographischer Nachweis einer traumatisch bedingten Intimaeinrollung an der Nierenartierie. Fortschr Röntgenstr 112:829

Kratochwill A (1977) Ultraschalldiagnostik in der Inneren Medizin, Chirurgie und Urologie. Thieme, Stuttgart

Kyle KF, Deane PR, Morley P, Barnett E (1971) Ultrasonography of the urinary tract. Br J Urol 43:709

Lenz P, Meridies R (1971) Unfallbedingte, einseitige Nierenarterienthrombose mit akuter Hypertonie. Unfallheilkunde 74:338

Lutz H (1978) Ultraschalldiagnostik (B-Scan) in der Inneren Medizin. Springer, Berlin Heidelberg New York

Lutz H, Rettenmaier G (1973) Sonographische Nierendiagnostik. Dtsch Med Wochenschr 58:361

Micksy LV, Radkousky MA, Heker I, Firnby W (1974) Optimal diagnosis of renal masses in children by combining and correlating diagnostic features of sonography and radiography. AJR 120:438

Mück G, Schmoller H (1973) Traumatische Intimaeinrollung einer Nierenarterie. Unfallheilkunde 76:335

Remond A, Dieval M, Grumbach Y, Petit J, Delamarre J, Trinez G (1979) Wert der Sonographie bei der dringlichen Diagnostik von Nierenverletzungen. Ein Bericht über 12 Fälle. Ann Radiol (Paris) 22:579

Rosenberg J, Weiss B, Hernberg J (1971) Nephrosonography – a new diagnostic tool. J Urol 106:127

Sanders RC (1975) Renal ultrasound. Radiol Clin North Am 8:417

Sanders RC, Bearman S (1973) B-Scan ultrasound in the diagnosis of hydronephrosis. Radiology 108:375

Schmoller H (1978) Ultraschalldiagnostik als Zusatzuntersuchung zu radiologisch-diagnostischen Maßnahmen. Wien Med Wochenschr [Suppl] 49, Jg. 128

Weitzel J, Bahlmann J, Otto P (1974) Die Wertigkeit der Sonographie für die Diagnostik von Zystennieren. Dtsch Med Wochenschr 99:1587

Evaluation of Lower Urinary Tract Pathology by Ultrasonography

L. Denis

Introduction

Recent improvements of ultrasonographic techniques of the lower urinary tract have provided clues to early diagnosis and exact staging of prostatic tumours and have brought additional benefit to a host of other diseases (Resnick and Sanders 1979; Watanabe et al. 1980). In a slow evolution of 5 years, ultrasonography has become a clinical technique straight from the clinical laboratory in the evaluation of lower urinary tract pathology (Declercq and Denis 1978; Denis et al. 1980; Denis 1979) on patients from the Department of Urology. This review relates the different techniques employed to evaluate the clinical benefit or the practical limitations on these patients to the few but lasting advances made in this field.

Methods and Materials

Ultrasonography sends short bursts of ultrasound waves into the body and displays the echoes received from the reflections in tissue or tissue interfaces. Although sound waves have special characteristics, they can be roughly compared to light waves to make it clear that these waves are absorbed, attenuated, scattered and reflected and that only the reflections are displayed. Ultrasound equipment consists basically of two parts, the tranducer system, which emits and recieves ultrasound waves, and the display system, which processes the echo information into visual systems. Our first equipment consisted of a manual compound scanner (Aloka MSU-12) attached to a cathode ray display system (Aloka SSD. 60C) and a memoryscope, which allowed manual transabdominal A and B scans. In 1975 a transrectal B scan became possible by attaching a transducer to a transrectal probe (Aloka ASU-8L). This probe allowed rotational and longitudinal movements (Fig. 1). A tomographic reconstruction of the obtained radial B scans or transverse sections was possible. Minor variations in the display of this system where most reflecting dots were represented with equal intensity allowed for gross resolution of the bladder and the prostate. Substantial improvement was made by the introduction of the grey scale display where reflecting dots are represented with variable intensity. The addition of an improved amplifier provided finer resolution of the examined tissues, especially the prostate. We also used a transrectal probe fixed in a chair-type device (ASU-8R-C). The use of this radial scanner was discontinued because of patient discomfort with this technique and the fact that the short probe did not always reach the prostate in our overweight patients.

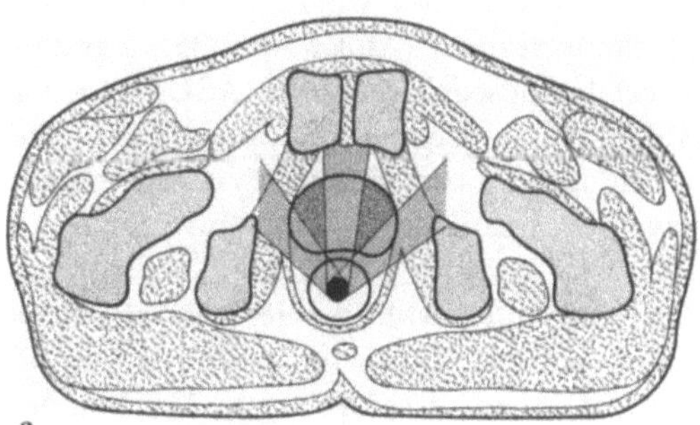

a

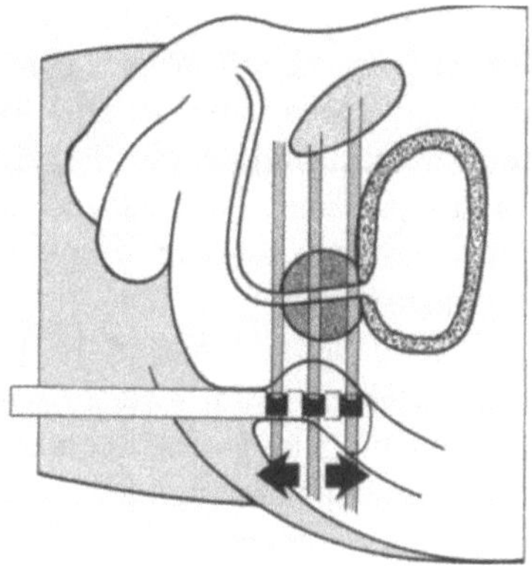

b

Fig. 1 a, b. Transrectal compound scan. **a** Transverse sections. **b** Longitudinal movement (*arrows*) provides step sections.

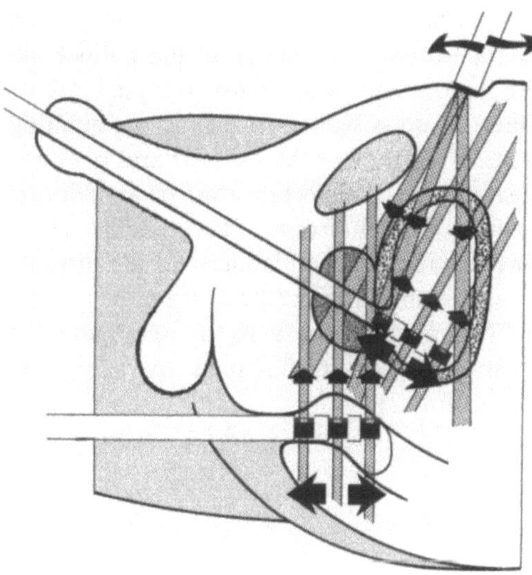

Fig. 2. Real-time scans via transabdominal, transrectal and transurethral ways provide complementary information on the bladder and prostate.

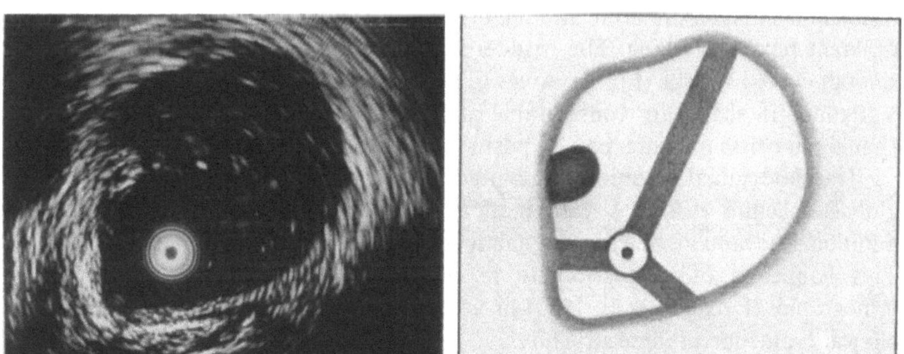

Fig. 3. Real-time transurethral sonogram is the preferred method for the staging of bladder tumours by perpendicular sonic analysis.

Multipurpose B mode equipment (Aloka USI. 51) where real-time sector scanning is possible with a mechanical handy scanner (Aloka ASU-25), a pistol-type high-speed radial scanner for transrectal endoscopic real time (ASU-51) or for transurethral endoscopic real time (ASU-52) has been utilized since 1980. The latter equipment is introduced into the bladder as a conventional cystoscopic unit. The real-time observation unit is displayed on a cathode ray tube and stored in a TV video system.

The patient is placed in left lateral decubitus with the legs flexed for a transrectal sonogram with the compound radial scan. This is our preferred method for obtaining transverse sections of high resolution of the prostate. The bladder neck forms the baseline. Step sections up are numbered positively every 0.5 cm and down are numbered negatively, e.g. –2 (×0.5 cm). Patient preparation consists of an enema to clean the rectum and a full bladder. The presence of a balloon catheter can serve as a useful landmark for starting the prostatic scan. Ultrasound propagation is enhanced by placing the probe in a condom filled with water inside the rectum. More than 1500 sonograms were performed in this way with only minor problems for the patients. For a transabdominal sonogram the patient lies supine with a full bladder. A parallel longitudinal and transverse scan allows visualization of the bladder and prostate. A cross-sectional scan is a minimum requirement for provideing the two largest diameters of the bladder and prostate. With the patient in the lithotomy position the transrectal scanner and/or the transurethral scanner are properly placed for ultrasonic examination. These techniques allow extensive ultrasound investigation of the bladder and the prostate from different directions (Fig. 2). In males the transurethral scanner is only introduced under general anaesthesia. The main purpose is to investigate the invasion of bladder tumours. The best resolution is obtained by a straight perpendicular ultrasonic beam on the tumor (Fig. 3).

Results

Bladder

The full bladder is an ideal and easy object for sonographic visualisation. The distinction between the urine and the bladder wall is clear and easy to follow in the different phases of filling. The bladder wall reflects as a uniform structure with a smooth curved surface (Fig. 4). Areas of fixation can be followed during the filling. Variations in shape are considerable and are due to the total amount of urine, changes in pelvic pressure, patient position and probe location.

Transabdominal scanning in longitudinal and transverse directions reveals this global structure easily. A combination of experience and patience offers the additional advantage of exposing enlarged pelvic lymph nodes or other structures. This happened only occasionally in our series since we rely on computed tomography (Declercq et al. 1980) or accepted surgical staging procedures for the clinical evaluation of these structures.

Variations in the smoothness of the bladder wall by hypertrophy and trabeculation, or atrophy by ureteroceles or diverticulae are easily recognised. These problems, however, are normally solved by standard urological procedures such as intravenous urography, cystography and/or cystoscopy. Visualisation of the bladder contours by ultrasound can be utilised in the percutaneous aspiration of urine and/or the placement of a suprapubic catheter by ultrasonically guided puncture, a technique which we apply in very obese patients, patients with small bladders or children. Transrectal ultrasonography provides transverse scans. Step sections make tomographic reconstruction possible. A detailed visualisation of the bladder wall is possible and tumours are readily identified as mass lesions located within the lumen adjacent to the bladder wall. The total tumour mass and/or the number of tumours can be determined by the layout of the total number of step sections. The differential diagnosis with bladder stones or blood clots depends on echogenic variations and altered locations with patient position.

Superficial and non-invasive tumours have a well-defined base without distortion or fixation of the bladder wall (Fig. 5). Infiltration is characterised by disruption of the bladder wall and extension in the surrounding tissues or neighbouring organs such as the prostate or the seminal vesicles. A problem with the transrectal examination is the tumours located in the dome or the trigone since they reflect the echogenic pulses sideways. Also the distinction between T2 and T3a tumours (Harner 1978) with minimal extravesical involvement is nearly impossible. Even with these technical limitations in mind we find the transrectal technique a useful diagnostic adjunctive technique to our clinical staging technique, which includes intravenous urography, bimanual examination, transurethral resection and multiple biopsies. It provides a guideline for avoiding extensive transurethral resections where cystectomy is the preferred treatment and offers a baseline for following tumour regression or progression under radiation therapy or chemotheraphy with subsequent appropiate treatment (Fig. 6).

The technical problem of a bladder pushed out of the 10 cm reach of the transrectal probe can be solved by transurethral ultrasonography. Measurement of tumour infiltration by an intraluminal approach seems promising for the resolution of detail of tumour invasion (Fig. 3). The procedure, however, involves the introduction of the transurethral probe. Additional advantages are obtained by longitudinal scanning methods, which provide a better approach for tumours located on the trigone.

Seminal Vesicles

The normal sonogram of the seminal vesicles is represented by a bilateral, symmetrical structure at the base of the bladder wall. The transrectal approach exposes minor variations in size and relationship to the prostate by a succession of transverse sonograms. The walls of the seminal vesicles are usually well defined with no distortions from internal echoes (Fig. 4).

Primary pathology of the seminal vesicles is extremely rare but cysts as fluid collections under ultrasonic observation can be easily demonstrated (Walls and Lin 1975). Secondary infiltration of tumours from the bladder and especially the prostate is frequently observed (Fig. 7). The echo-free zone of the seminal vesicle is replaced by a dense mass of reflections that are frequently continuous with a proven tumour in the prostate. In selected instances of endocrinological pathology a rare absence of a seminal vesicle or a bilateral atrophy in cases of Klinefelter's syndrome was observed.

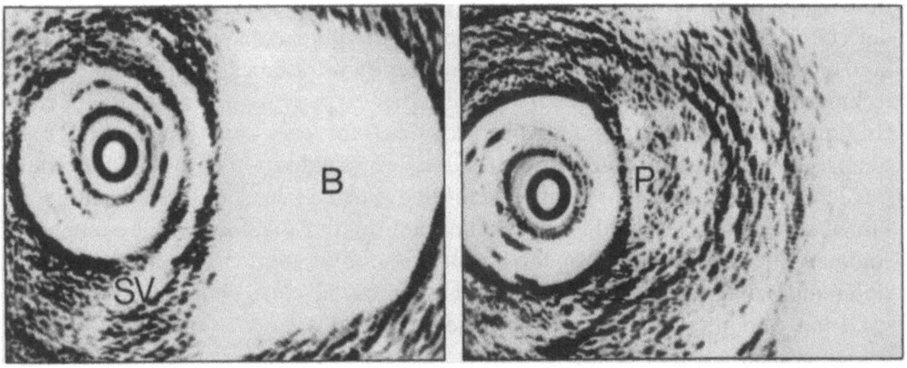

Fig. 4. Transrectal compound scan of normal seminal vesicles (*SV*), normal bladder (*B*) on transverse section +1 (*left*) and of a normal prostate (*P*) on transverse section −2 (*right*).

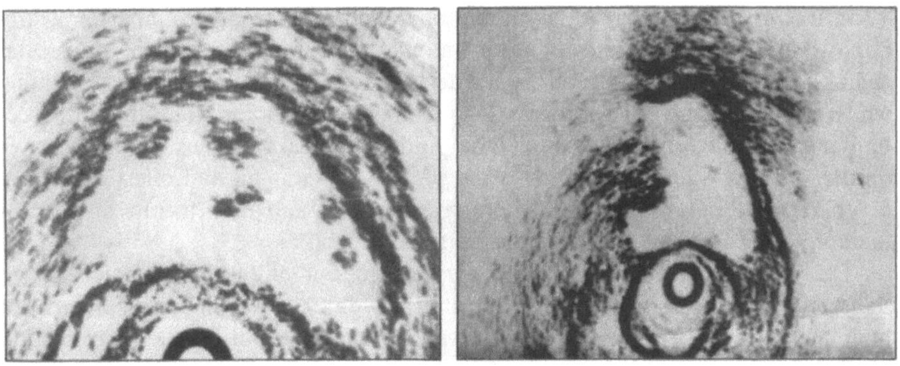

Fig. 5. Demonstration of T1(m) (*left*) and T3 (*right*) bladder tumours by transrectal ultrasound.

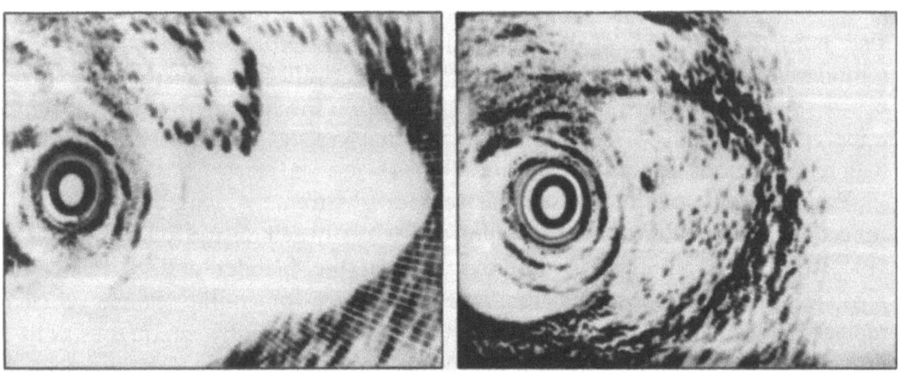

Fig. 6. A clinical routine sonogram on a 60-year-old male patient reveals a T1 bladder tumour on section +2 (*left*) and a peri-urethral adenoma on section −1.5 (*right*).

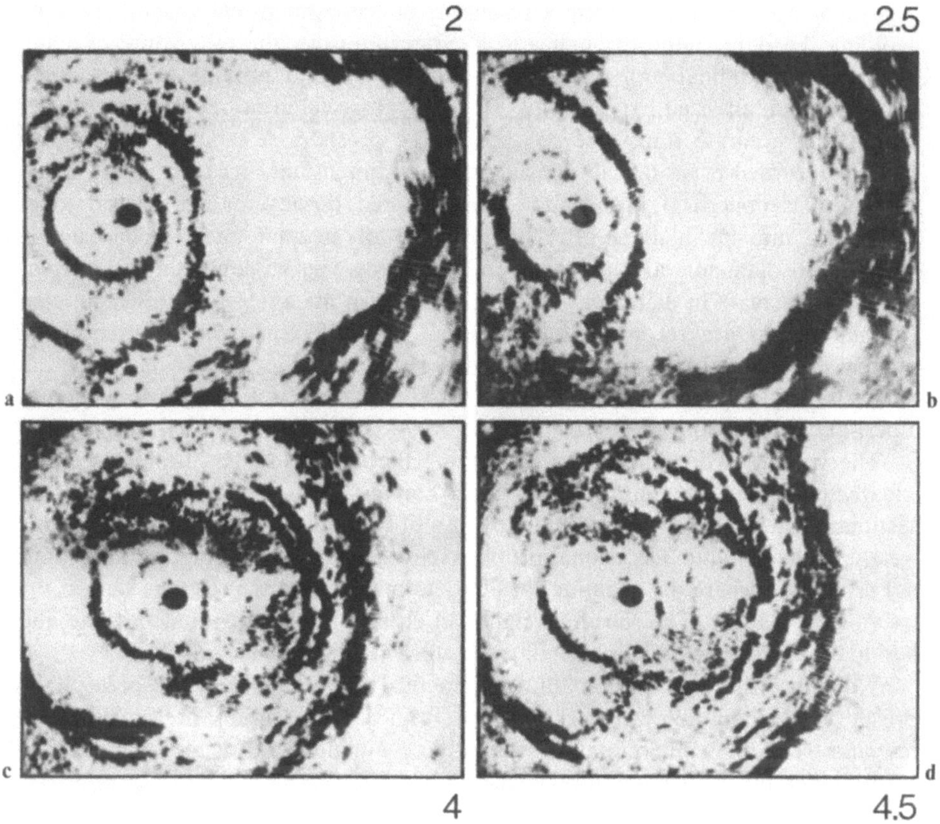

Fig. 7a–d. Transverse scans show infiltration of left seminal vesicle by prostatic carcinoma T3 tumour at different levels (2, 2.5, 4, 4.5).

Prostate

The normal sonogram of the prostate shows a regular capsule and is of a triangular or semi-lunar form. Scattered and aspecific echopatterns are present and representative for the glandular pattern.

Ultrasonography has been shown to provide important information in the clinical diagnosis of peri-urethral adenoma, the diagnosis and staging of prostatic cancer and the evaluation of prostatic infections and lithiasis (Watanabe et al. 1975; Harada et al. 1979; Denis et al. 1980).

Peri-urethral Adenoma. Benign enlargement of the peri-urethral glands is one of the most common problems in urology. Two important questions in this disease are: Is there a problem of obstruction and how big is the prostate?

Obstruction is a problem to be solved by a clinical and urodynamical approach. Volume is a problem that can be solved by ultrasonography. Indeed numerous techniques, most of which are radiological, have not been able to give a satisfactory approximation of prostatic mass. Most urologists rely on the rectal examination with its well-known errors and an endoscopic examination. Transabdominal ultrasonography is able to bring a resonably fair assessment of prostatic mass by avoiding the pubic bone through angulated scanning by the easy route of a full bladder. Longitudinal and transverse scans are able to provide the two main diameters in a fair-sized hypertrophy (Fig. 8). Transrectal ultrasonography provides remarkably accurate transverse sections of the prostate. A series of consecutive sections recorded every 0.5 cm allows a good tridimensional reconstruction. Small prostates, asymmetrical forms and overdeveloped cervical or subcervical lobes protruding into the bladder offer no problem for an anatomical reconstruction (Fig. 9). All diameters are increased and the transverse sections adapt a circular form. The increase in diameter is most noticeable in the anteroposterior diameter. Internal echoes are recorded that represent the different areas of adenomata, microcysts, fibrous and myomatous tissue reactions. The grey scale sonogram allows for a subdivision into solid, cystic and mixed areas in a transverse section of a peri-urethral adenoma.

The volume is determined by calculating the surface of the different sections usually by planimetry, multiplying by 0.5 cm and adding the total number of sections. The weight is determined by multiplying the volume by the specific weight of the prostate. Occasional problems are encountered in the cephalad–caudal estimation where the examiner has to determine where the sections start at the base of the bladder. The specific weight can change in an individual prostate and add to the error of the final weight figure as obtained by surgery.

We utilise this information for two practical purposes. The mere size of the prostatic adenoma allows a choice for surgical enucleation or transurethral resection. The mass determination makes the evaluation of a therapeutic effect of medical therapy on a peri-urethral adenoma possible.

Prostatic Cancer. The exact determination of primary tumour mass as obtained by transrectal ultrasonography is a prime parameter for the assessment of response to therapy or for the detection of relapse after a period of tumor regression. The measurement of the usually irregular tumour mass is more difficult to assess with transabdominal ultrasonography.

The diagnosis of prostatic cancer is based on the nature of the intraprostatic echoes and the regularity of the prostatic capsule. The intraprostatic echoes in a normal prostate or in a peri-urethral adenoma fade away with increase of the field strength. In irregular and dense sonic areas the presence of cancer should be suspected (Fig. 10). The grey scale application in the compound scan has been extremely helpful in this respect. The capsule is often asymmetrical, distorted and interrupted by tumour extension into the periprostatic tissue or the seminal vesicles (Fig. 7). These results could not be reproduced by real-time transabdominal or transrectal ultrasonography where suspicion is primarily based on asymmetrical findings and sonically dense irregular areas. Where the overall correlation hovers around 90% we found false negative (four) and false positive (two) results in 1979 on 84 newly diagnosed patients with prostatic cancer. No attempt was ever made to diagnose microscopic cancer and all these patients consulted for urological problems. A small focus of well-differentiated cancer less than 0.5 cm in diameter can be easily missed by our actual methodology. Transrectal ultrasonography indicates the need for a prostatic biopsy.

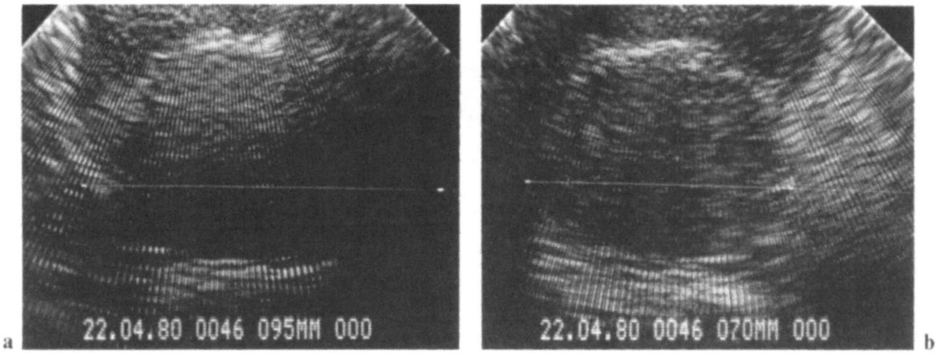

Fig. 8a, b. Transabdominal ultrasound brings a quick volume estimation by cross-sectional scanning (length 95 mm, width 70 mm). Longitudinal scan (**a**) and transverse scan (**b**).

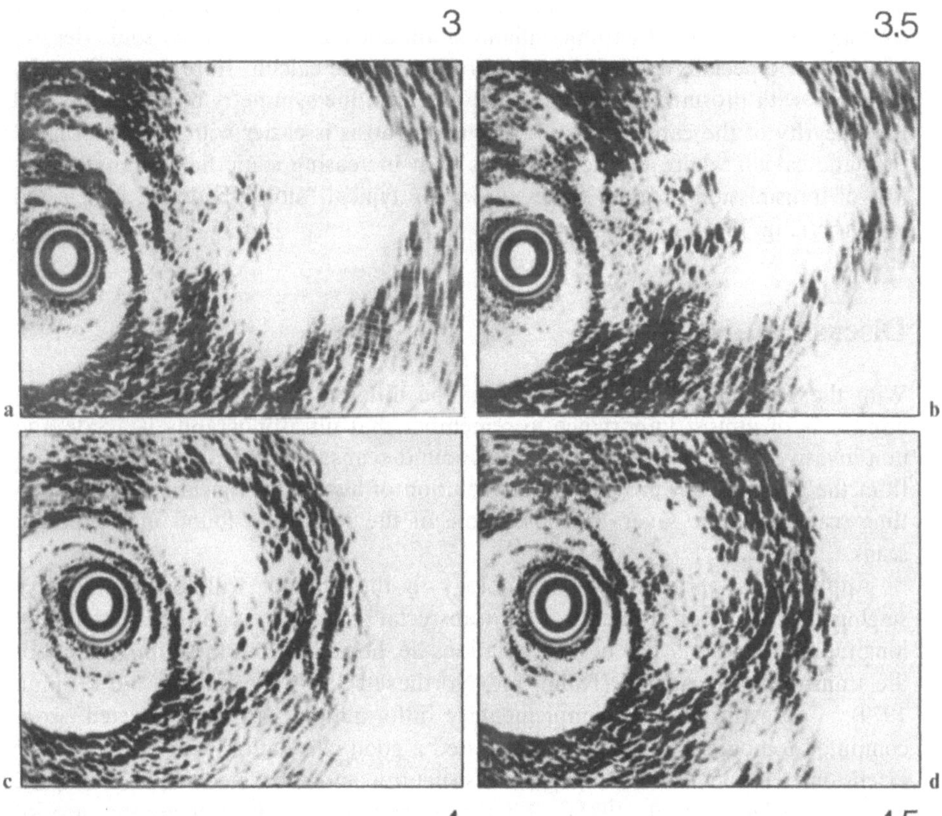

Fig. 9a–d. Transrectal step sonograms produce reliable reconstructions of adenomatous variations, e.g. median lobe.

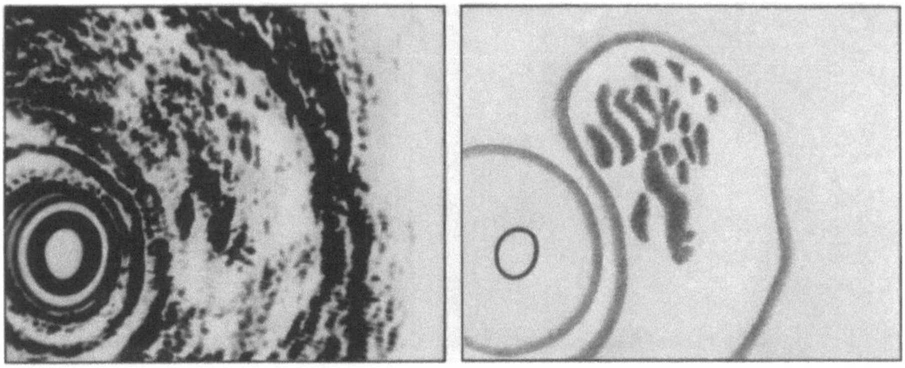

Fig. 10. Prostatic carcinoma T2 tumour. Irregular and dense sonic areas and capsule distortions point to the possible presence of tumour tissue.

Prostatic Infections and Prostatic Lithiasis. Inflammation of prostatic tissue presents on ultrasonography as diffusely enlarged glands with a decrease in sonic density. At times the formation of a prostatic abscess is clearly delineated (Fig. 11). On the contrary, the scarring of chronic inflammation adds to the increased sonic density of the area especially in the presence of microscopic calculi. Here the differential diagnosis with prostatic cancer has to be based on the symmetry of the lesions and the integrity of the capsule (Fig. 12). This diagnosis is easier with aggregations of prostatic calculi where the density stays with increasing sonic field strength. The loss of transmission of sonic waves shows the typical "stone shadows" in selected instances (Fig. 13).

Discussion

With the possibilities and limitations of the different sonographic techniques in mind it is of utmost importance to remember that ultrasonography is a safe and non-invasive diagnostic technique. Compound scans demand a lot of experience from the operator but provide good resolution of histopathological changes. Real-time scans are time savers but lose some of the resolution found in compound scans.

Applications of ultrasound technology in the bladder will focus on cancer staging. The inherent problems of the transrectal technique might be overcome by longitudinal scanning. The best expectations lie, however, with the improvement of the transurethral scanners (Holm and Northeved 1974; Nakamura and Niijima 1979). Competition and complementary information can be expected from computed tomography, which demonstrated a good correlation with extravesicular extension, relation to other intrapelvic structures and the detection of metastatic lesions (Declercq et al. 1981). Other applications of ultrasonography are of secondary interest to the urological clinic. Bladder sonography, however, forms an ideal training ground for the apprentice to appreciate the capricious nature of sound waves and the patience needed to avoid ghost reflections.

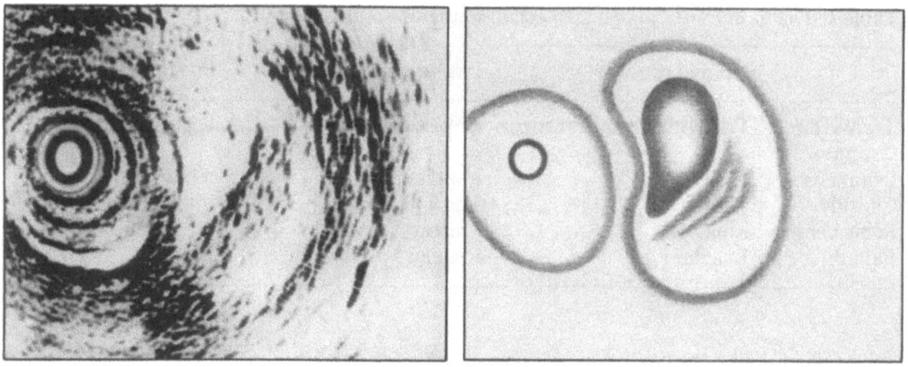

Fig. 11. Abscess formation in left lateral lobe of the prostate (*left*). Abscess drained (*right*).

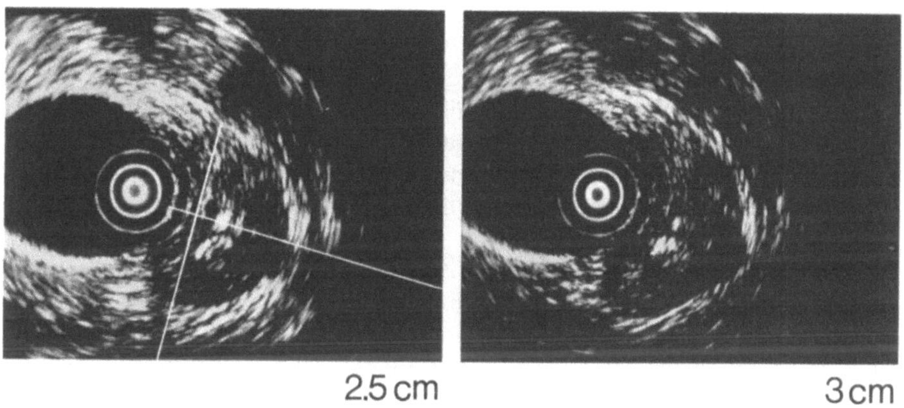

Fig. 12. Real-time transrectal sonogram representing a chronic prostatitis.

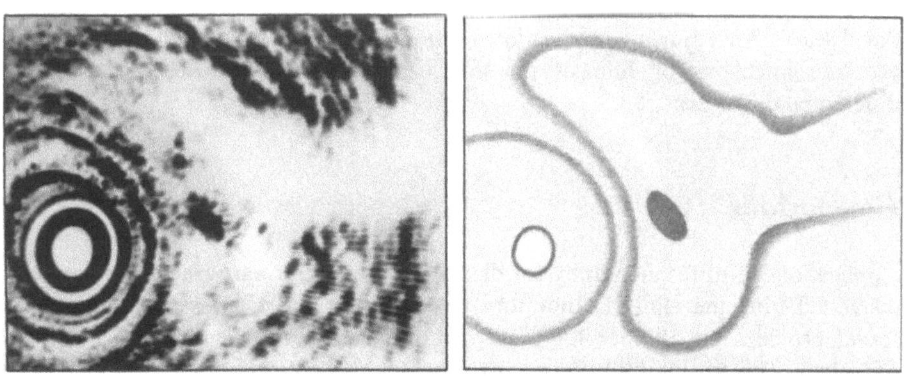

Fig. 13. Prostatic stone fragments do not fade with increasing field strength and cast a sonic shadow.

Table 1. Diagnostic criteria of a transrectal sonogram of the prostate.

	Normal prostate	Peri-urethral adenoma	Prostatic cancer
Transverse section	Triangular/semi-lunar	Half/full circle	Deformations
Symmetry	Present	Usually present	Absent
Capsule	Thin	Thick/regular	Interrupted/distorted
Sonic density	Minimal	Present	Increased
Pattern	Regular	Regular	Irregular

The cinical observation of the seminal vesicles is easiest by transrectal ultrasonography. The diagnosis of prostatic cancer invasion is by far the most promising application. Local disease control is certainly jeopardised by this observation and it may avoid the need for surgical staging procedures such as pelvic lymph node dissection. Additional interest lies in the rare primary disorders of the seminal vesicles and the variations in certain endocrinological problems. The main application of ultrasonography remains the evaluation of prostatic mass and the diagnosis and staging of prostatic cancer. It is especially in this application that we are ready to convert from a laboratory diagnosis procedure to a clinical procedure. No clinical procedure, computed tomography included, has been found to produce such reliable data on prostatic mass as transrectal ultrasonography. These data will make possible reliable investigations on the therapeutic effects of drugs on the size of peri-urethral adenomas.

The diagnosis of prostatic cancer by this non-invasive technique is also a step forward in the clinical approach to this disease. It should be remembered, however, that except for a straightforward interrupted capsule by tumour formation all the signs, especially in the early stages of the disease, merely represent the different echogenicity of prostatic cancer tissue. A sonogram suggesting prostatic cancer indicates the site to be biopsied and a repeat biopsy is required if the first one is negative. The criteria for a sonographic diagnosis of prostatic cancer are listed in Table 1. Once the diagnosis is established we find the sonogram an extremely useful parameter in the follow-up of these patients after therapy. The total mass or the density of the echoes reflects the regression or the subsequent reactivation of the disease. An adjuvant application of transrectal ultrasonography is found in prostatic infections or lithiasis for the localisation of focal disease or for a differential diagnosis.

Conclusions

Applications of ultrasonography for diagnosis of lower urinary tract pathology are converted from the clinical laboratory to clinical practice. Transabdominal ultrasound provides possibilities for mass determinations and the diagnosis of gross pathology. Transrectal ultrasonography provides excellent mass determinations and detailed diagnosis on a histopathological basis. Transurethral ultrasound provides the possibility for non-invasive staging procedures of bladder tumours.

References

Declercq G, Denis L (1978) Ultrasonic assessment of prostatic mass. Acta Urol Belg 46:74–79

Declercq G, Denis L, Broos J, Appel L (1981) Evaluation of lower urinary tract by computed tomography and transrectal ultrasonography. J Comput Assist Tomogr (accepted for publication)

Denis L (1979) Transrectal ultrasonography: Staging of bladder tumours. In: Pavone M, Smith Ph, Edsmyr F (eds) Bladder tumours and other topics in urological oncology. Plenum, New York, pp 97–100

Denis L, Appel L, Broos L, Declercq G (1980) Evaluation of prostatic cancer: Transrectal ultrasonography and CT scan. Acta Urol Belg 48:71–77

Harada K, Igari D, Tanahashi Y (1979) Gray scale transrectal ultrasonography of the prostate. J Clin Ultrasound 7:45–49

Harner MH (1978) TNM classification of malignant tumours. UICC, Geneva

Holm HH, Northeved A (1974) A transurethral ultrasonic scanner. J Urol 3:238–241

Nakamura S, Niijima T (1979) Ultrasonic cystoscopy – Clinical application for staging bladder cancer. In: 4th World Congress on Ultrasonics in Medicine. Scimed, Tokyo, p 339

Resnick ML, Sanders RC (1979) Ultrasound in urology. Williams & Wilkins, Baltimore

Walls WJ, Lin F (1975) Ultrasonic diagnosis of seminal vesicle cyst. Radiology 114:693–695

Watanabe H, Igari D, Tanahashi Y, Harada K, Saitho M (1975) Transrectal ultrasonography of the prostate. J Urol 114:734–739

Watanabe H, Holmes SH, Holm HH, Goldberg BB (1980) Diagnostic ultrasound in urology and nephrology. Igaku Shion, Tokyo

Transrectal Ultrasonography in the Evaluation of Cancer of the Prostate

P. J. Brooman, G. J. Griffiths, E. E. Roberts, W. B. Peeling and K. T. Evans

Introduction

Cancer of the prostate is now the second most common cause of death from malignant disease in Western males. Accurate assessment of the disease is essential for planning patients' treatment and also for clinical trials. Yet most clinicians still rely upon the time-honoured method of digital palpation for assessment of primary prostatic cancer. It is well known that this method is inaccurate both in diagnosing and staging this disease. Therefore, an objective method is required and imaging of the prostate by transrectal ultrasonotomography has recently been introduced. This paper reports our experience in South Wales using the Aloka chair-mounted probe.

Equipment and Methods

The Aloka probe contains a 3.5 MHz rotating transducer, which is coupled to a Searle Phosonic 'B' Mode Scanner, incorporating a microprocessor and digital scan converter. Photographs of the scans are obtained using a Birchover Multiformat camera back. The probe is gently introduced into the rectum (Fig. 1) until the bladder base is visualised on the scanner, usually at a distance of 7 or 8 cm. Sequential scans are then made as the probe is withdrawn in 0.5 cm steps. The whole process occupys around 25 min.

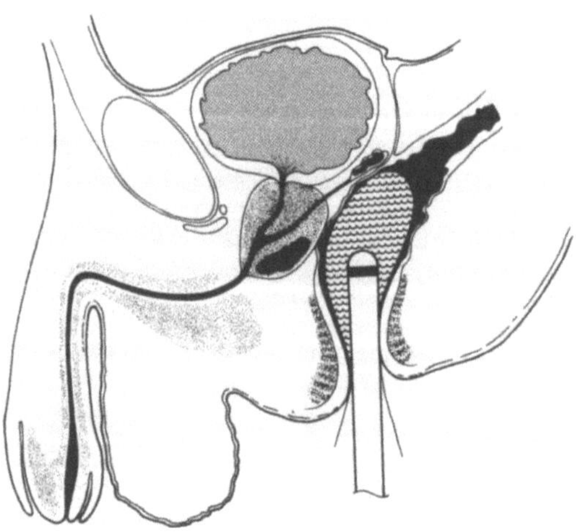

Fig. 1. Diagramatic representation of a sagital section through the pelvis showing the transducer in the rectum. This is surrounded by a water-filled balloon, which acts as a transonic coupling medium between the transducer and the prostate, bladder base and seminal vesicles.

Ultrasonic Features of the Prostate

Normal Prostate

The normal prostate has a crescent shape in cross-section (Fig. 2). The capsule appears to be intact at all levels and the internal echoes are homogenous.

Benign Hyperplasia

In benign hyperplasia (Fig. 3), the capsule adopts a more circular shape whilst the internal echo pattern is typically homogenous. Sometimes, large nodules are demarcated by thin transonic lines (Fig. 4).

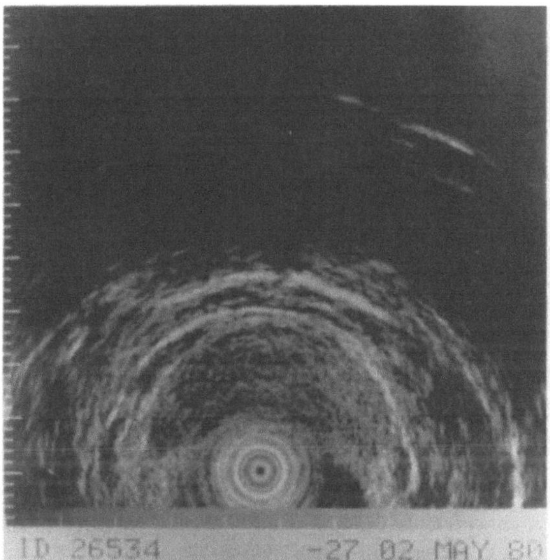

Fig. 2. Normal prostate. This ultrasonotomogram shows the characteristic crescent shape of the capsule, which is intact. The internal echoes are homogeneous.

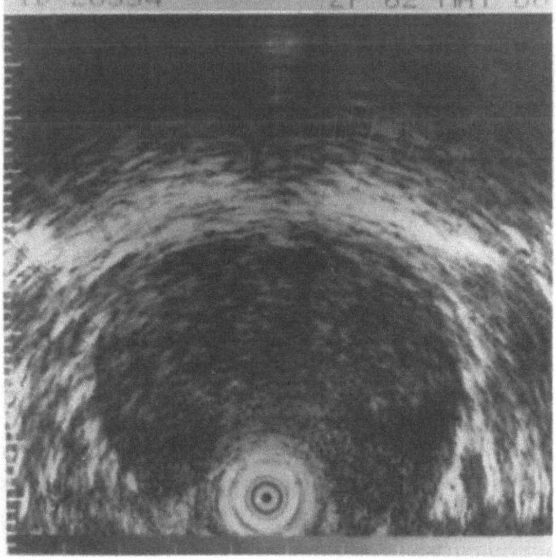

Fig. 3. Benign hyperplasia. The prostate is circular in shape. The capsule is intact. The internal echo pattern is homogeneous.

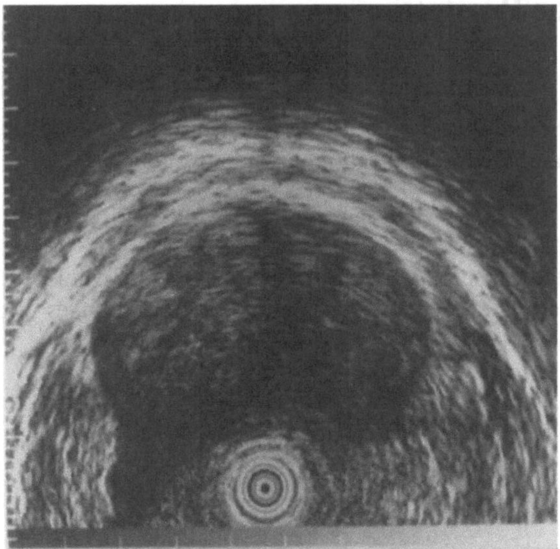

Fig. 4. Benign hyperplasia. The large nodule seen in the right lobe is clearly demarcated by a transonic margin.

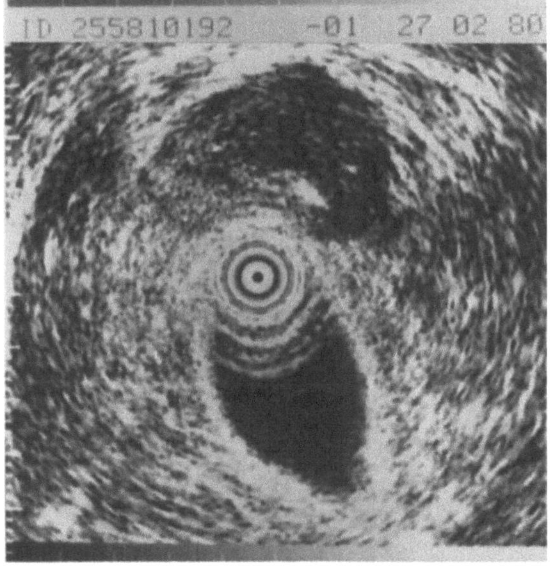

Fig. 5. Confined prostatic cancer. The internal echo pattern is heterogeneous, with increase in the strength of echoes in the right lobe. Highly reflective echoes indicating calcification are seen in the midline, in the posterior part of the gland. The capsule is intact.

Prostatic Cancer

In prostatic cancer, the internal echo pattern is usually heterogeneous, containing irregular echoes of relatively increased density. The most reliable signs of prostatic cancer are distortion or penetration of the capsule by the growth. If the capsule is seen to be intact at all levels, the cancer is described as 'confined' (Fig. 5) whereas evidence of a breach in the capsule means that the cancer is 'unconfined' (Fig. 6) and has started to invade the surrounding tissues.

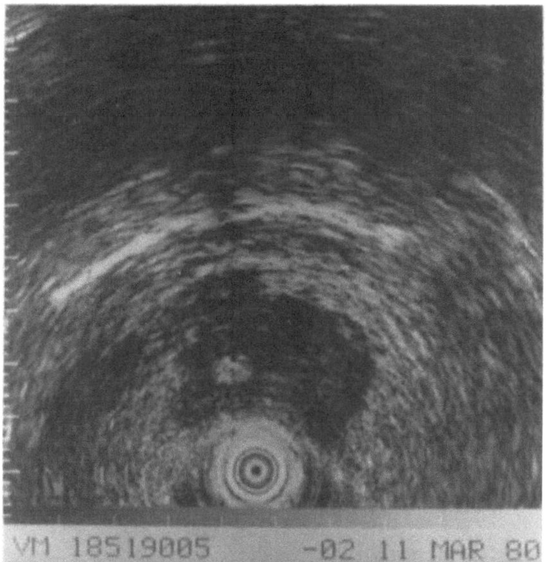

Fig. 6. Unconfined prostatic cancer. There is a breach in the right anterolateral part of the capsule. The internal echoes are heterogeneous, with a small area of increased echo density in the right lobe.

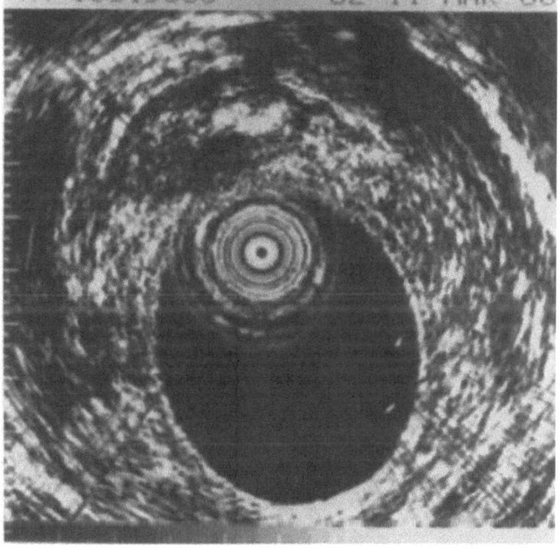

Fig. 7. Chronic prostatitis. The capsule is intact. The internal echoes are heterogeneous. The highly reflective echoes are produced by calcification.

Prostatitis

Areas of chronic prostatitis (Fig. 7) produce irregular areas of increased echo density similar to that of carcinoma; however, capsular distortion or penetration is absent. Differentiation between prostatitis and the confined carcinoma may only be possible by surgical biopsy.

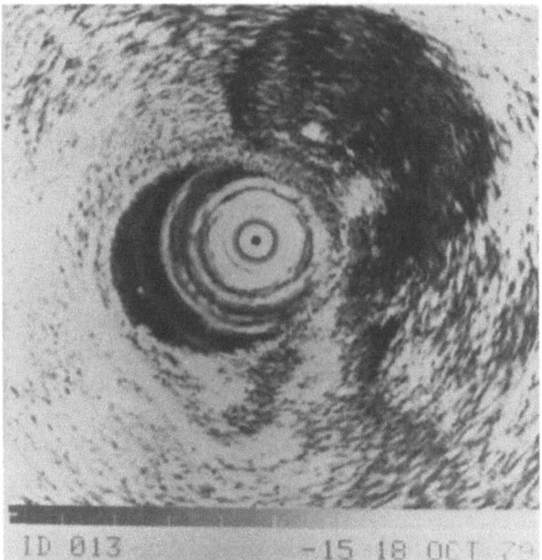

Fig. 8. Calculi. Two areas of highly reflective echoes produced by calculi are seen lying posteriorly. The prostate has the typical appearance of benign hyperplasia.

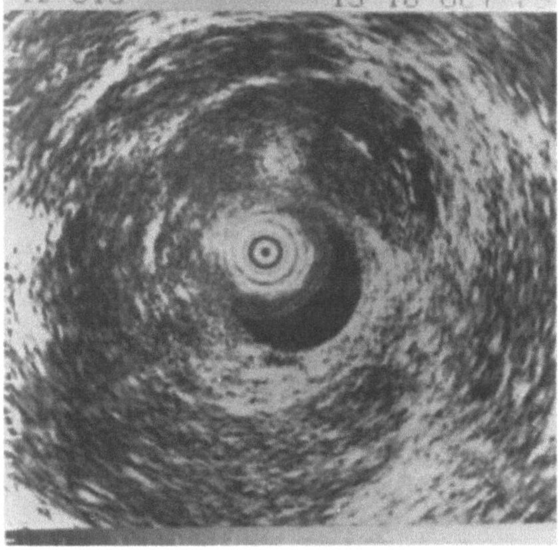

Fig. 9. Confined prostatic cancer. There is an abnormal area with increased strength and number of echoes in the midline posteriorly.

Calculi

Calculi (Fig. 8) produce areas of bright echo density, which may be easily differentiated from the slightly less intense echoes of carcinoma or prostatitis. In difficult cases, differentiation can be helped using the technique of post-image processing with expansion of the strong echoes (Figs. 9, 10).

Seminal Vesicles

These are usually visualised as curved transonic areas lying behind the base of the bladder (Fig. 11).

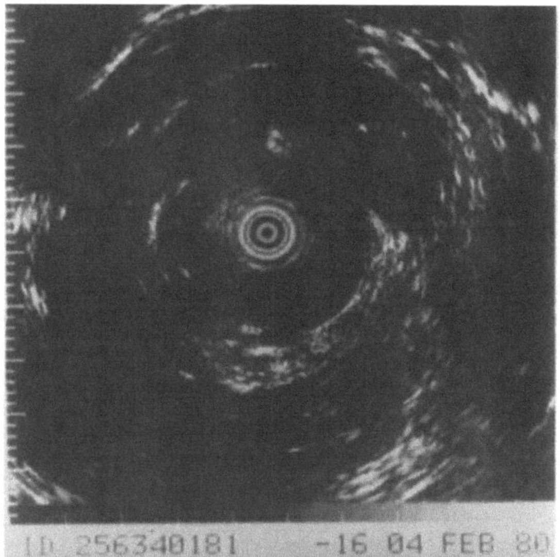

Fig. 10. Post-image processing. Expansion of the strong echoes in Fig. 8 shows the abnormal area to consist of highly reflective echoes due to calcification with slightly weaker echoes due to carcinoma.

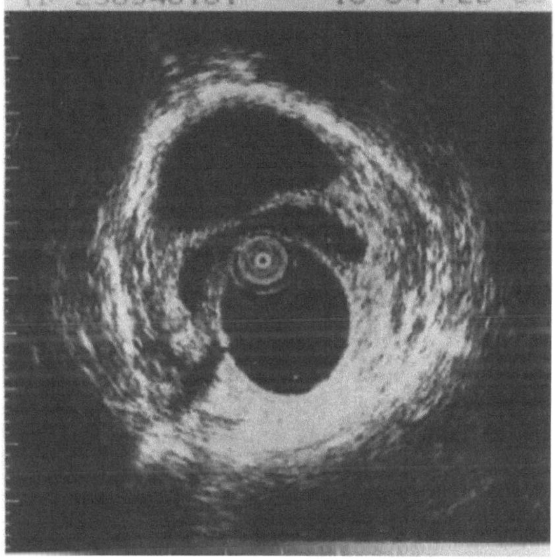

Fig. 11. Seminal vesicles and bladder base. The seminal vesicles are demonstrated as curvilinear transonic areas posterior to the bladder.

Cadaver Studies

To prove that the ultrasonic features of the prostate in living subjects are a true representation of the clinical situation, the prostate, bladder and rectum were removed as a single unit from a number of cadavers at autopsy. They were mounted in a special tank in their normal anatomical relations, and then scanned with the Aloka probe (Fig. 12). The prostates were then sectioned at all levels of scanning, and examined histologically for comparison with the ultrasound scan.

In the first ten specimens that we have studied, the ultrasound diagnosis agreed with the histological findings, four with benign hyperplasia and six with carcinoma

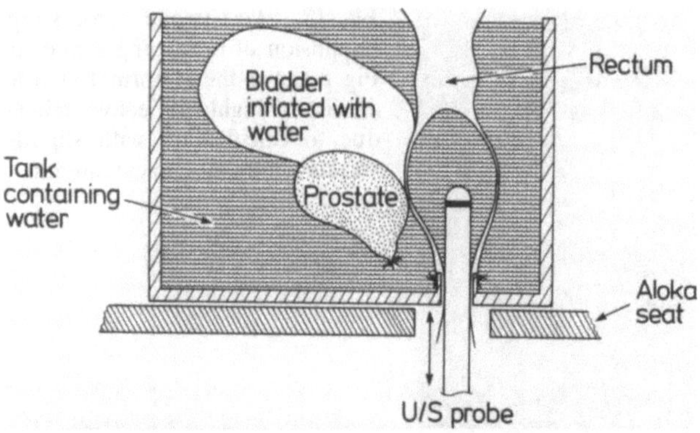

Fig. 12. Diagram of apparatus used to study cadaver prostates. *U/S probe,* Ultrasonic probe.

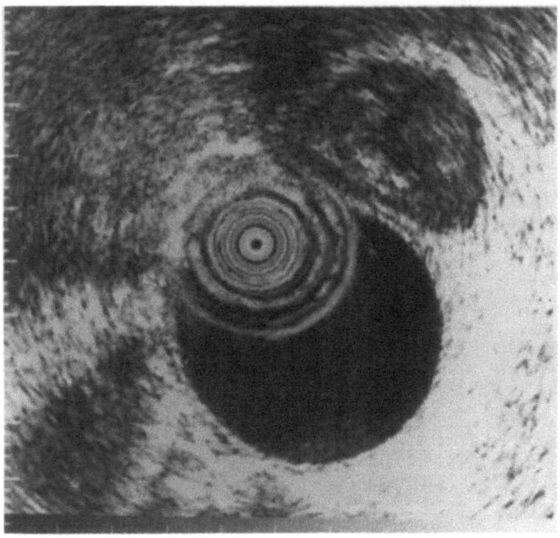

Fig. 13. Ultrasonotomogram of a cadaver prostate. Confined cancer. The echo pattern is heterogeneous. The capsule appears intact. Highly reflective echoes due to calcification are seen in the midline posteriorly.

Table 1. Comparison between ultrasound and histological findings of cadaver prostates. *U/S,* ultrasound.

Case no.	Diagnosis		Staging (UICC)	
	U/S	Histology	U/S	Histology
1	BPH	BPH		
2	BPH	BPH		
3	BPH	BPH		
4	BPH	BPH		
5	CaP	CaP	T2	P2
6	CaP	CaP	T2	P2
7	CaP	CaP	T2	P2/3
8	CaP	CaP	T2/3	P3
9	CaP	CaP	T2/3	P3
10	CaP	CaP	T3	P3

(Table 1). Of the six specimens with cancer, three were thought ultrasonically to be confined within the capsule (Fig. 13), which was confirmed histologically, whilst three were thought ultrasonically to be unconfined tumours which had breached the capsule, and this was also shown to be the case on histological examination.

Transrectal Ultrasonography in Prostatic Cancer

In our clinical series we studied 200 patients. All the ultrasound scans were evaluated by one of us (Griffiths) without any knowledge of the clinical diagnosis or symptomatology. The initial digital examination of the prostate suggested that 68 men had benign hyperplasia, 68 men had cancer confined to the prostate and 33 men had prostatic cancer that was locally invasive (Table 2). Ultrasound examination detected incidental confined carcinomas, which were proved histologically in three of the men with clinical benign hyperplasia. Of the 68 patients with suspected localised prostatic cancer, only 30 were proved histologically to have the disease; in 28 this was detected accurately by ultrasound. However, 14 of these cases had ultrasonic evidence of locally invasive cancer, mostly through the anterior part of the capsule, and had therefore been clinically understaged.

Of the 33 men with clinically invasive cancer, 31 had histological proof of the tumour; this was detected ultrasonically in 30. In this group, the ultrasound scan showed that six of these patients had been clinically overstaged by rectal palpation and that when capsular perforation had occurred, it was usually in a posterolateral situation, where it could be felt by the examining finger.

Table 2. Detection and staging of carcinoma of the prostate (CaP) by the Aloka transrectal ultrasonic probe. ( ) indicates histological confirmation of CaP.

Clinical diagnosis made by digital palpation	No.	Ultrasound findings of CaP		
		Diagnosis	Confined	Unconfined
Benign hyperplasia	68	3 (3)	3	
Confined CaP	68	28 (30)	14	14
Unconfined CaP	33	30 (31)	6	24

Conclusion

We consider that transrectal ultrasonography of the prostate with the Aloka probe is a most promising, safe and easy technique that can be used to increase accuracy of diagnosis and staging of prostatic cancer.

Computer Evaluation of Ultrasound Imaging of the Prostate for the Early Detection of Cancer *

P. H. Walz, G. Hutschenreiter, G. Wessels, U. Scheiding, and W. von Seelen

Tissue characterization by means of a noninvasive technique must still be considered wishful thinking. The now widespread use of computed tomography with determination of tissue density has not changed the situation much.

Yet the use of ultrasonics for tissue characterization seems to be possible in combination with computer-aided methods of pattern recognition. In a first step, pathologic alterations of tissue areas have to be recognized. This seems to be possible only by using a B picture. When a physician has recognized such an area, special methods of signal analysis can be applied to differentiate between benign and malignant lesions, for example, between benign prostatic hyperplasia (BPH) and prostatic carcinoma.

Purely visual evaluation of the prostate by the B scan using the suprapubic-transvesical approach (Fig. 1) clarifies quite a number of different problems. The examination is not harassing compared with transrectal or transurethral scanning. The patient is in a prone position, the bladder filled with not less than 80–100 cc.

The size of the prostate is determined with great accuracy, thus facilitating the preoperative indication for transurethral resection or prostatectomy in cases with BPH (Fig. 2). Adenomas show a well-defined capsule and a characteristic echo pattern with few internal echos of identical intensity. In contrast, carcinoma of the prostate shows typical areas of irregular structure and high echo return (Fig. 3). Local extension of the carcinoma can be estimated and infiltration of the capsule (Fig. 4) or of the seminal vesicles (Fig. 5) are easily seen.

Nevertheless, for a primary diagnosis of a prostatic tumor, sonography without computerized analysis is not accurate enough. The scan contains a lot of information that, due to the characteristics of the human visual system, cannot be evaluated by the eye. To improve upon simple visual evaluation of the ultrasonic picture of a prostate, a technique was developed which utilizes computer evaluation. The method consists of the following procedures:

1) Transvesical examination of the prostate;
2) digitization and storage of B pictures in a computer;
3) preprocessing of the picture;
4) feature extraction;
5) classification.

By preprocessing the pictures, the physician's eye can be aided in recognized tissue alterations; thus the "readability" of the scan is improved by bringing out or

* Supported by the BMFT, Bonn, West Germany

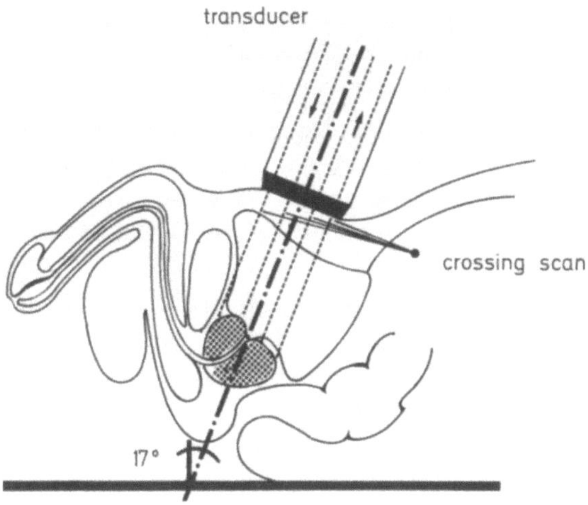

Fig. 1. Schematic illustration of the suprapubic-transvesical method for ultrasonic examination of the prostate with a commercialy available nonmodified compound scan.

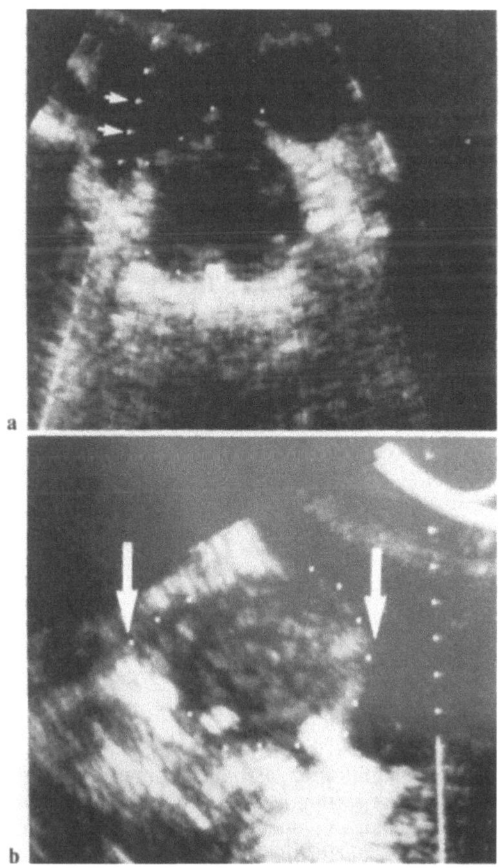

Fig. 2 a, b. Prostatic adenoma. **a** Transverse section; **b** longitudinal section. The *small arrows* in **a** indicate a distance of 1 cm; the *large arrows* in **b** indicate the length of the prostatic urethra. [From Walz et al. Ultraschall (1), 1980, 158–164, Georg Thieme Verlag, Stuttgart, New York]

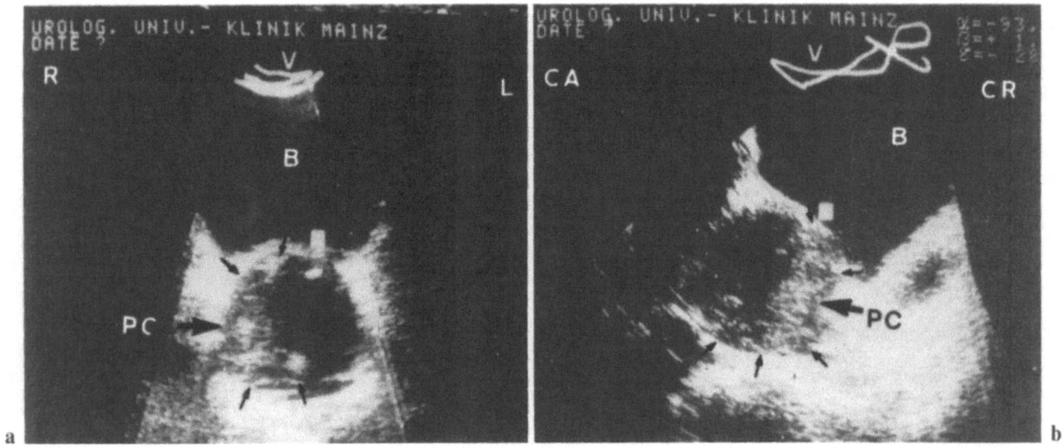

Fig. 3a, b. Noninvasive adenocarcinoma of the prostate (*PC*). **a** Longitudinal section; **b** transverse section. The carcinoma presents as an area of irregular structure and increased echo ratio on the right side and dorsocranially in the prostate. *B*, Bladder; *CR*, cranial; *CA*, caudal; *V*, ventral. [From Walz et al. Ultraschall (1), 1980, 158–164, Georg Thieme Verlag, Stuttgart, New York]

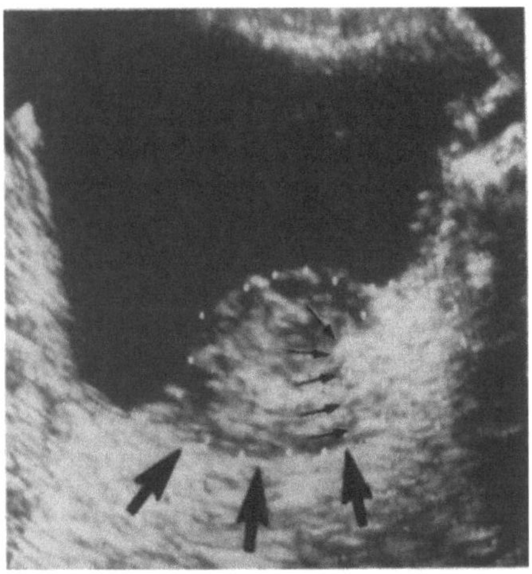

Fig. 4. Infiltrating prostatic adenocarcinoma on the left side in a transverse section. Dorsally the prostate is sharply outlined (*large arrows*); on the left side there is no clear separation from the surrounding tissue. Inside the prostate there is an area of high echo return (*small arrows*) indicating the region of the carcinoma. [From Walz et al. Ultraschall (1), 1980, 158–164, Georg Thieme Verlag, Stuttgart, New York].

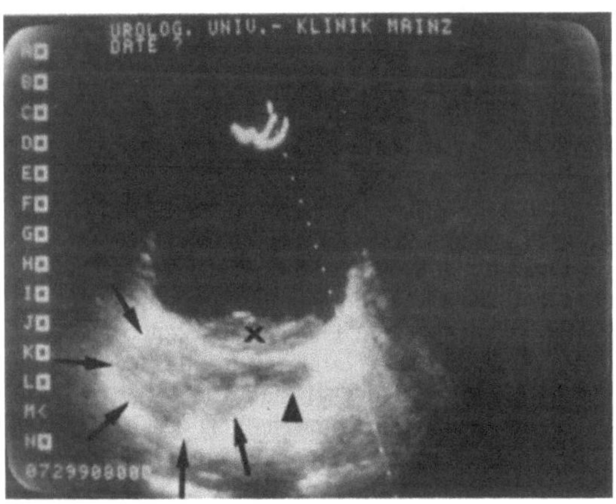

Fig. 5. Infiltration of right seminal vesicle in transverse section. Dorsal to the cranial part of the prostate (*X*), the normal left seminal vesicle (*triangle*) and the right seminal vesicle with wide tumor extension (*arrows*).

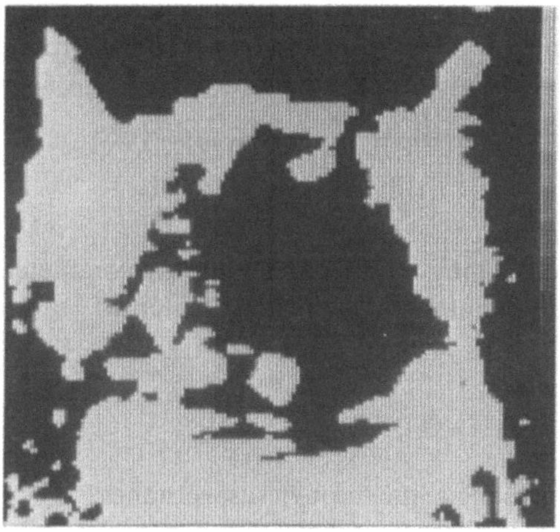

Fig. 6. Threshold operation. Only echoes above a given level are depicted; thus the contour of the prostate is more easily outlined. On the right side there might be a gap in the capsule (filtered version of Fig. 3a).

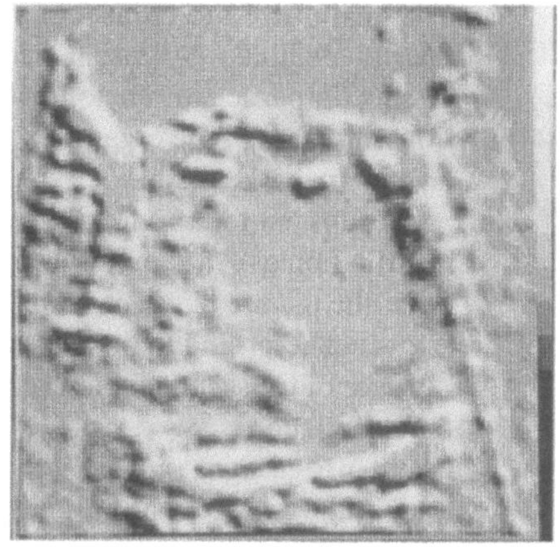

Fig. 7. Phase-dependent filtering (pseudo-three-dimensional). By this transformation, small intensity modulations can better accentuated. The apparent angle of "incidence of light" can be varied, thus sharpening the contrast (filtered version of Fig. 3a).

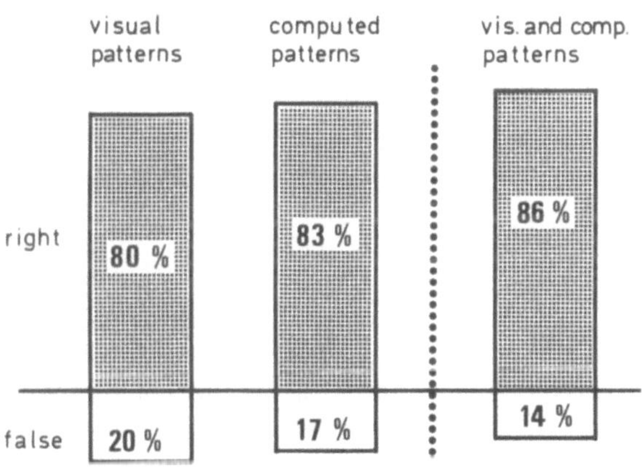

Fig. 8. Results of computer-aided B scan classification in differentiating carcinoma versus noncarcinoma.

emphasizing information not normally seen. Furthermore, preprocessing of the picture serves to prepare the pictures for a computer-aided feature extraction by analyzing measurable parameters so that objective data are obtained from the picture. Finally, the computer-aided feature extraction and calssification assists the physician with the diagnosis.

The equipment consists of a compound scanner (Combison 200, Kretz Technik), a specially developed interface, a transient recorder, and a computer PDP 11/34 (Digital Equipment).

Symmetric, matched, or phase-dependent filtering helps to eliminate disturbances and distortions in the pictures, improves the signal-to-noise ratio, and exposes relevant tissue patterns (Figs. 6, 7).

The analysis of the ultrasonic picture refers to global and local features, which are partly obtained by visual scrutiny of the screen and partly by computer processing. In particular, the following visual features are quantified:

1) Measurement of the organ;
2) symmetry of the organ;
3) local gaps in the capsule;
4) distribution of echo sounds in organ area.

After the picture has been transferred to the computer, the following parameters are extracted according to the physician's definition of the region of interest:

5) Surface of the sectional picture;
6) autocorelation;
7) standardized signal power in the region of interest;
8) amplitude density distribution;
9) curve of the autocorrelation function along a line through suspect zones;
10) coherence width and relative extremes of the autocorrelation function along a line through suspect zones;
11) power and energy above a threshold or within an amplitude window, respectively.

By two steps – (a) visual analysis of both the original and preprocessed picture and (b) extraction of specific technical features – the computer aids the eye of the physician in recognizing pathologic patterns and objectivying subjective impressions while the physician "shows" the computer the regions of interest, thus directing the analysis.

The validity of all parameters mentioned is being tested with an adapted classifier.

Results

Computerized classification of visual data in distinguishing carcinoma versus noncarcinoma had a false negative rate of 15.3% and a false positive rate of 21.4%, corresponding to a total error of 20% (Fig. 8). The classification of computer-processed data had a false negative rate of 8.5% and a false positive rate of 20.7%, corresponding to a total error of 17.4%. A combination of both procedures increased the accuracy rate to 86% (false negative 10.2%, false positive 15.1%).

Conclusion

Our results show that ultrasonic tissue characterization of the prostate is possible. Computer-aided B scan analysis improves the visual image of the B scan. This preliminary study, however, cannot determine all the possibilities offered by this method.

Computed Tomography of the Kidney

C. C. Schulman, G. Kuhn, and J. Struyven

Computed tomography (CT) is the reconstruction by computer of a tomographic section of the body using multiple X-ray absorption measurements. The first attempts at medical application of image reconstruction were carried out by Aldendorf in 1961, Cormack in 1963, and Kuhl and Edwards in 1968. The development of the first clinical unit (head unit) was accomplished by Hounsfield (1973). The first total body scanner was developed by Ledley et al. (1974).

Principle of CT

Computed tomography scan equipment includes a patient-handling table, an operator, a viewing console, a computer, the X-ray generator, and a scanning gantry. Presently, most of the X-ray scanners are so-called third-generation scanners. The scanner consists basically of a X-ray tube rigidly mounted opposite a detector array (fan beam). In the order of 300 to 500 detectors are located within the fan angle. The X-ray beam, finely collimated, passes through the body and is recorded by the X-ray detectors (attenuated X-rays). The system rotates in a 360° motion.

The computer is used to process the data in an appropriate algorithm (computer program) to generate an image representing the pattern of attenuation coefficients in the cross section of the patient. The thickness of a slice (collimated beam) is 2–13 mm.

The computer displays the matrix on a video monitor using varying shades of greys or colors to represent the computed attenuation coefficients [CT numbers or Hounsfield Units (HU)]. This image reflects anatomic structures. A special display is used to measure the CT numbers (density) of any region of interest in numeric data. The TV monitor is photographically recorded to provide a permanent record.

Investigations were performed using a third-generation scanner which obtains two simultaneous 8-mm-thick slides in 4–5 s. The scanner has an image matrix of 256×256. A cursor circle, variable in size and location, can measure attenuation numbers of any region of interest. Special programs provide histograms, surfaces, volumes, etc.

Patients are scanned in dorsal decubitus position. A first series of plus or minus eight sections is performed without contrast medium. The scanning is repeated after intravenous injection of 50–100 ml contrast medium in a bolus. Most patients are referred to CT scan because of IVP abnormalities or a nonfunctioning kidney. Other patients are investigated for hematuria, clinically suspected neoplasm, or unproven renal pathology.

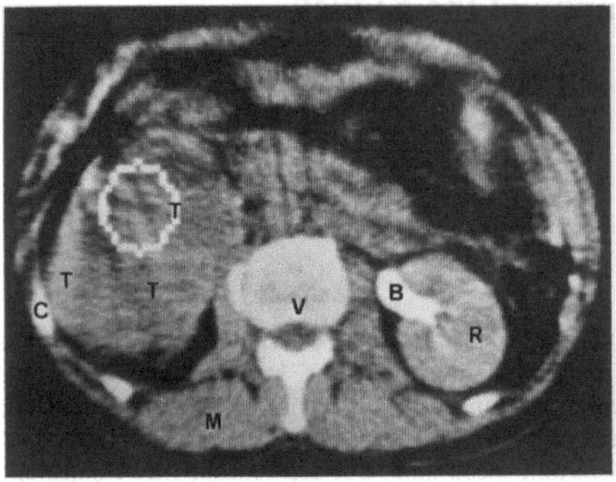

Fig. 1. Left renal tumor (*T*) with extension to the costal margin (*C*) outside the renal capsula. The right kidney (*R*) is normal after injection of contrast medium which appears in a normal renal pelvis (*B*). *V*, Vertebra; *M* posterior muscles.

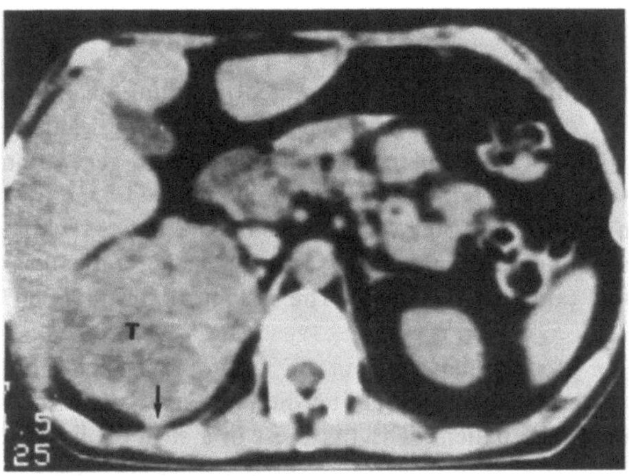

Fig. 2. Left renal tumor (*T*) extending outside the capsula (*arrow*).

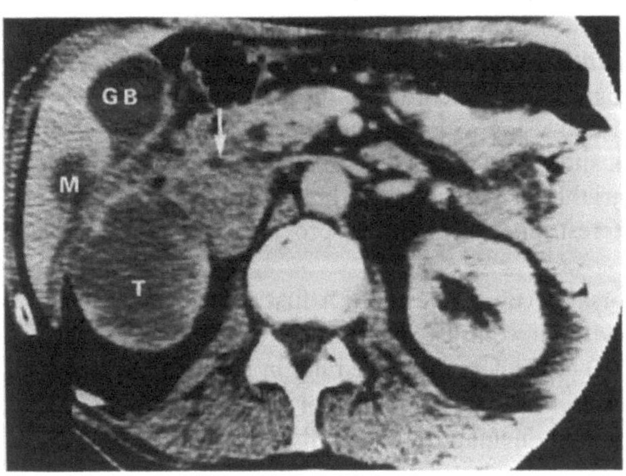

Fig. 3. Left renal tumor (*T*) with extension toward the renal hilus (*arrow*) with metastasis in the liver (*M*). *GB*, Normal gallbladder.

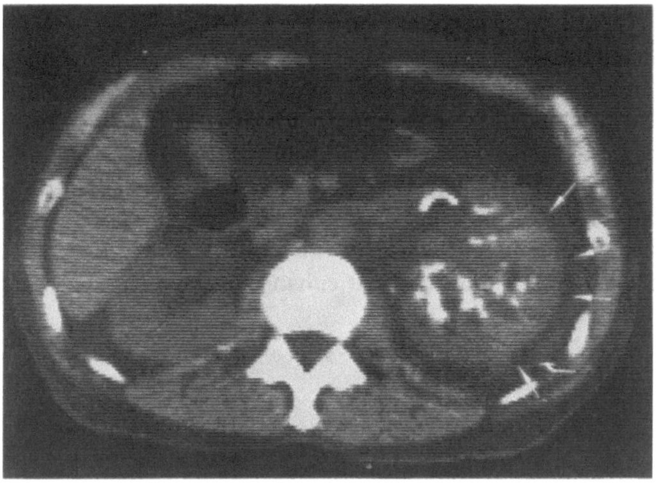

Fig. 4. Right renal tumor after embolization with Gelfoam mixed with contrast medium. A plane of cleavage is clearly delineated around the tumoral kidney (*arrows*).

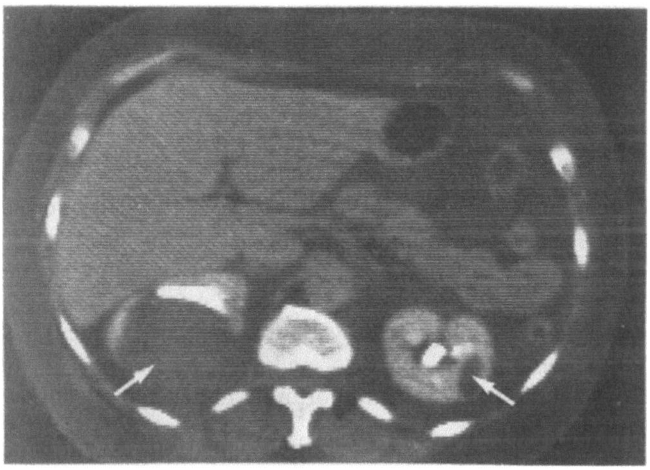

Fig. 5. Bilateral renal cysts. Huge cyst on the left side and small intraparenchymal cyst on the right side (*arrows*).

Diagnostic Criteria

The diagnostic criteria employed in the CT evaluation of the kidney are:

1) Alteration of the normal contour,
2) visualization of a renal mass,
3) disappearance of perinephric outline, and
4) measurements of the attenuation coefficient in a region of interest.

Normal Kidney

The kidneys are well defined by CT scan because of the presence of perinephric and sinus fat which provides a clear outline of renal parenchyma. The renal contour is smooth and well delimited from peritoneal structures. A break occurs at the hilus when the vascular pedicle is directed anteromedially toward the aorta and the inferior vena cava. The renal parenchyma is homogeneous. After administration of contrast media the shape of the calices and renal pelvis is sharply defined. Without contrast media, normal parenchyma has an attenuation coefficient of 50–70 HU and rises to 100–120 HU after contrast enhancement. Renal veins and arteries are usually seen.

Renal Neoplasms

A renal neoplasm may alter the outline and usually enlarges the kidney. The neoplastic parenchyma is not homogeneous and has an attenuation value approximately equal to the normal tissue, but after contrast the tumor enhances far less than the surrounding normal parenchyma. If the normal attenuation equivalent rises from 60 to 100 HU, neoplastic tissue reaches 70–80 HU. Another useful sign is the loss of the fat surrounding the kidney which most likely represents infiltration by the neoplasm. This sign is reliable in normal patients but less significant in very thin patients. An involvement of the hilus will be easily recognized. Accuracy of the technique is about 95% (Figs. 1–4).

Cysts

Renal cysts have sharp margins and are rounded structures on CT scan. Their attenuation value is −10 to +10 HU and does not increase after injection of contrast medium. Renal cysts are a very common finding in patients evaluated by axial tomography. Cysts of 1 cm are easily seen, especially when projecting beyond the cortex (Fig. 5).

Polycystic renal disease is correctly diagnosed by bilateral enlarged kidneys with lobulated contours, multiple cysts of variable size, and distortion of calices and parenchyma. The same examination allows the opportunity to detect cystic disease of the liver (Fig. 6).

Benign Lesions

An adenoma usually presents as a lobulated parenchymal lesion with strong contrast enhancement which does not occur in neoplasm. Hamartomas are easily recognized by their fatty component identified as a very low density structure (−100 HU).

Hydronephrosis

Urography cannot detect a hydronephrotic, nonfunctioning kidney, even on delayed films after injection of high doses of contrast medium. Obstructive uropathy is easily recognized by axial tomography. The kidney is enlarged and attenuation value measurement shows low densities. If there is still any excretion,

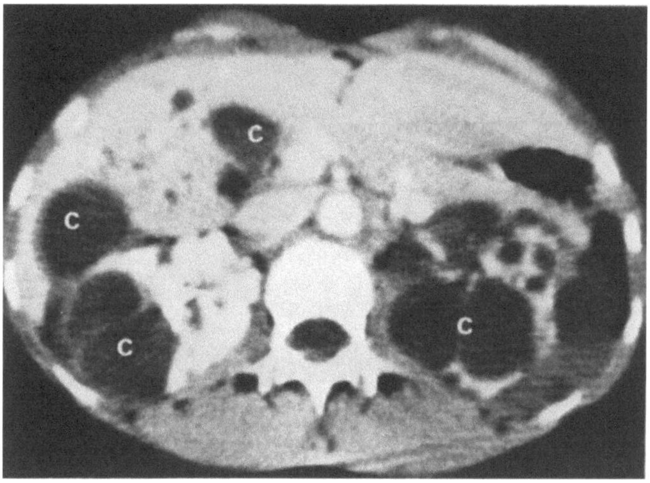

Fig. 6. Polycystic disease with cysts (*C*) involving both kidneys and the liver.

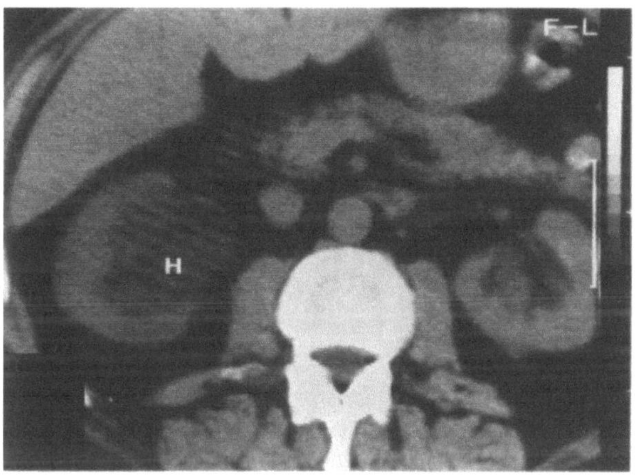

Fig. 7. Left hydronephrosis: the renal pelvis is slightly dilated (*H*).

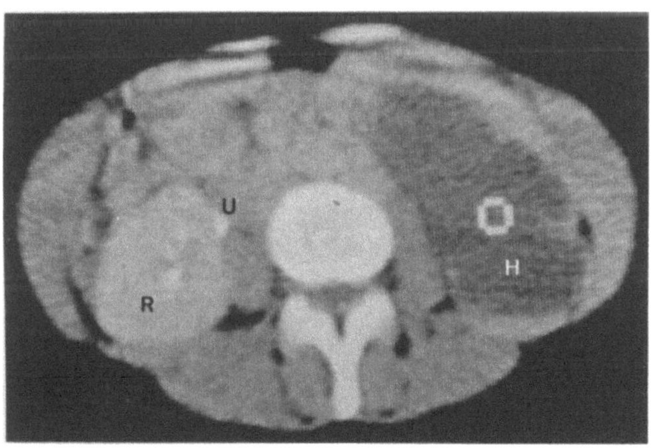

Fig. 8. Nonfunctioning right kidney with huge hydronephrosis (*H*) and complete destruction of the kidney with disappearance of the renal cortex (*H*). The left kidney (*R*) is normal and the ureter (*U*) is clearly visualized after injection of contrast medium.

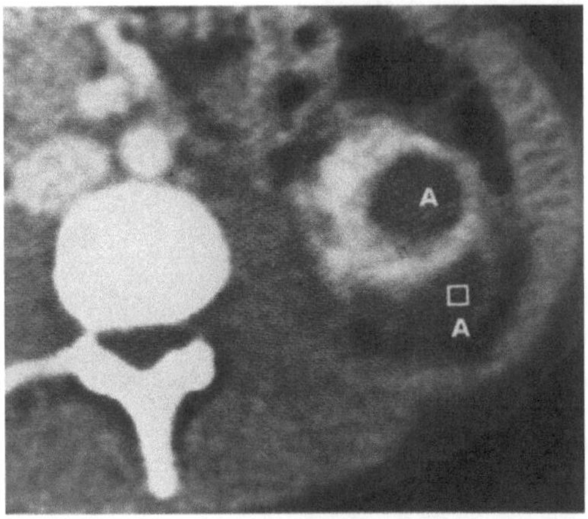

Fig. 9. Renal abscess (*A*) deforming the shape of the right kidney.

Fig. 10. Right hydronephrosis (*H*) after injection of contrast medium with abscess outside the renal margin (*arrow*).

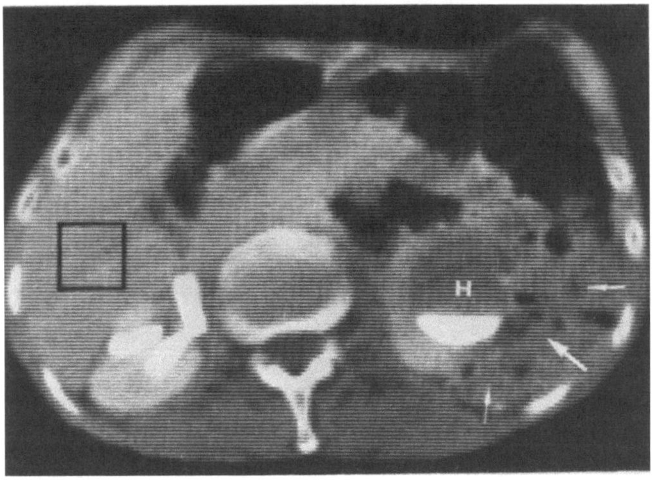

levels of contrast media can be seen in dilated calices. CT is often able to recognize the origin of obstruction, for example, by neoplastic involvement or calculus (Figs. 7, 8).

Inflammatory Lesions

Intrarenal abscesses are demonstrated by CT as lower density lesions (20–35 HU) with less sharp delimitation than renal cysts. There is no contrast enhancement of the pathologic area. Evolutive abscesses are not distinguishable from xanthogranulomatous pyelonephritis (Figs. 9, 10).

Other Pathologic Processes

Computed tomography aids in the diagnosis of renal atrophy or aplasia. Focal infarction is characterized by a marginal area which does not show contrast enhancement, and the kidney seems normal prior to contrast injection (Fig. 11).

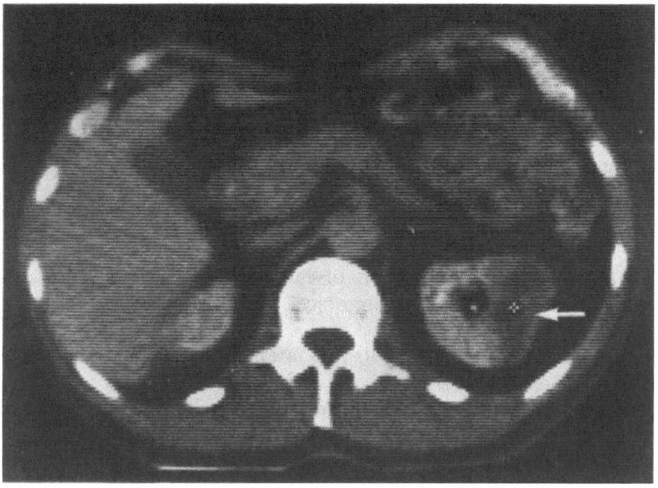

Fig. 11. Right renal infarct with absence of enhanced density in the infarcted portion of the kidney (*arrow*).

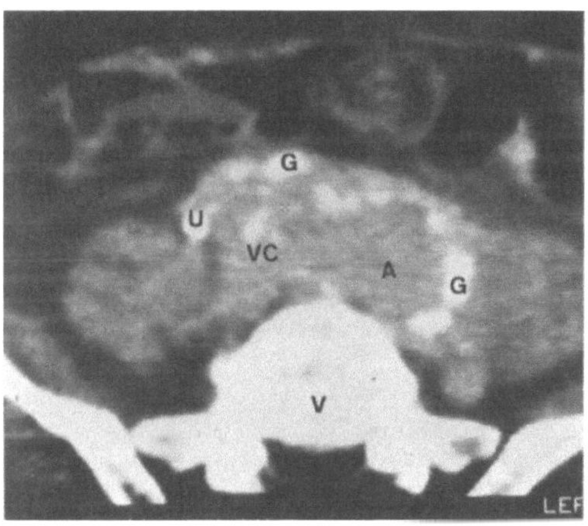

Fig. 12. Retroperitoneal infiltration by a lymphomatous process. The ganglia are contrasted after lymphangiography (*G*) and surround the aorta (*A*), the vena cava (*VC*) and the ureter (*U*).

Changes from the normal anatomy of the retroperitoneum can easily be recognized. Tumor masses are well profiled by surrounding fat. Muscles, aorta, and inferior vena cava are well-defined structures, and any malignant process will obliterate the tissue plane and obscure normal clear delineation of the retroperitoneal structures (Fig. 12).

Conclusions

Experience shows that CT can diagnose most morphological diseases of the kidney. It is a noninvasive technique and obviates the need for arteriography in a significant number of cases. The diagnostic accuracy of computed tomography is excellent when compared with ultrasound and selective renal arteriography. CT scan provides a diagnosis and defines the extent of neoplastic processes; it is considered an excellent screening procedure, since it has a high level of accuracy. The cost of the procedure remains quite high, but where it is available it should become part of the urologic armamentarium for the diagnosis in selected cases.

References

Aldendorf WH (1961) Isolated flaying spot detection of radiodensity discontinuities displaying the internal structural pattern of a complex object. IRE Trans Biomed Electron 8:68–72

Cormack AM (1963) Representation of a function by its line integrals with some radiological applications. Appl Phys 35:2722–2727

Hounsfield GN (1973) Computerized transverse axial scanning (tomography). Br J Radiol 46:1016–1033

Kuhl DE, Edwards PQ (1968) Reorganizing data from transverse section scan of the brain using digital processing. Radiology 91:975–983

Ledley RS, Di Chiro G, Luessenhof AJ, Twigg HL (1974) Computerized transaxial X-ray tomography of the human body. Science 186:207

Love L, Churchill R, Reynes C, Schuster GA, Moncada R, Berkow A (1979) Computed tomography in staging of renal carcinoma. Urol Radiol 1:3–10

Malinger AD, Ostrum BJ (1978) Computed tomography in the diagnosis of renal masses. Radiology 126:715–718

Sagel S, Stanley RJ, Evens RG (1977) Early clinical experience with motionless whole-body computed tomography. Radiology 124:359–370

Struyven J, Brion JP, Frederic N, Schulman CC (1977) Computed tomography of the kidney. Br J Urol 49:583–588

The Value of Angioscan with Density Curves in CAT Scan for Renal Tumors

H. Botto, J. C. Bornes, B. Lecudonnec, N. Vasile, and J. Auvert

This is a technique that provides additional dynamic information to conventional CAT scan.

Procedure

After location of the suspicious area on unprepared conventional CAT scan sections injection occurs emblous within 6 s of 60 ml iodized water-soluble opacifier for urinary excretion (with the help of a pump). CAT scan sections are then performed every 15 s. All sections are made in the same plane and marked when the examination started. Thus eight sections are made within about 2 min. This technique can only be used with third-generation CAT scan. The present one is a Siemens 2C Somaton that makes 4–8-mm thick sections within 2 to 4 s.

Results

They are of two types: static results allowing construction of denseness histograms and dynamic results with a survey of denseness development in terms of time.

Static Results with Density Histogram

For each section, the observed denseness values are carried to a curve plotted by writing the densities on the x-axis and the number of points measured for each denseness on the y-axis.

The kidney cortex: on the unprepared section, a renal cortical area provides a narrow, pointed curve (between 30 and 40 units in this instance) (Fig. 1). On the negative taken 15 s after injection of the contrast material (according to the above procedure), the curve is still narrow but shifted to the right with no distortion between 127 and 150 units (in this instance) (Fig. 2).

This lump shifting without distortion after injection of the contrasting material is typical of a healthy homogenoeus tissue (Fig. 3). This aspect was constantly found on more than 50 cases investigated.

If the denseness variations of a renal area that is both cortical and medullary is now considered under the same conditions as above (unprepared exposure and exposure at the 15th s), a narrow denseness curve is first obtained (Fig. 4) but on the 15th s exposure the curve shows two regular but separate peaks (Fig. 5).

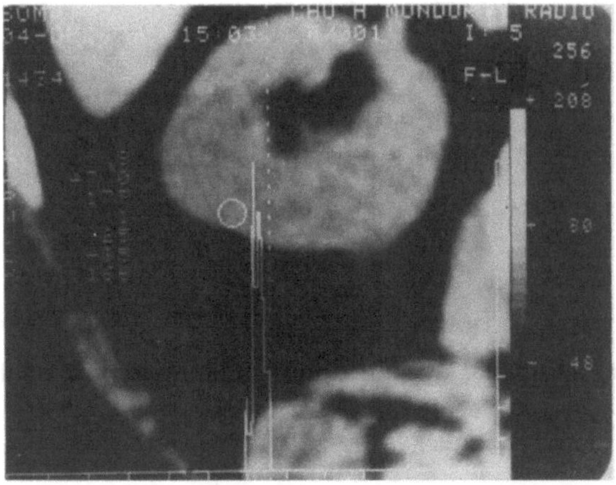

Fig. 1. Kidney cortex: density histogram on the unprepared section.

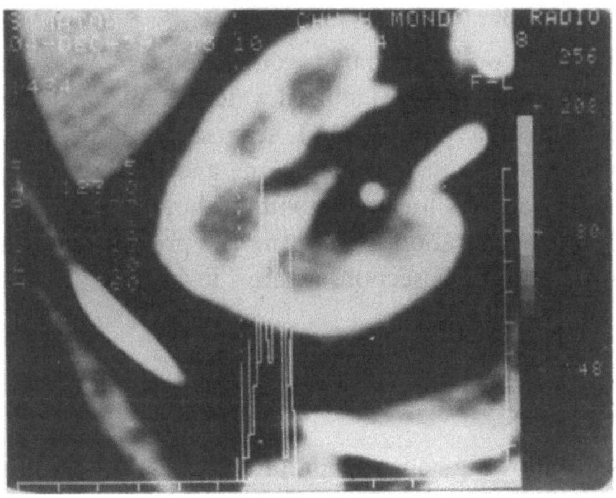

Fig. 2. Density histogram on the negative taken 15 s after injection of the contrast material (according to the procedure).

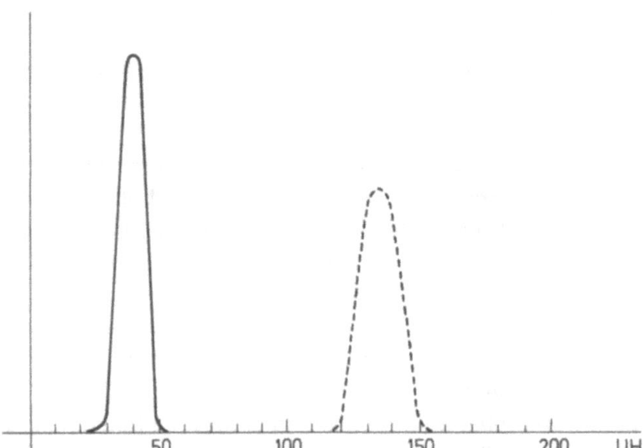

Fig. 3. Kidney cortex. ——, Density histogram on the unprepared exposure. ······, Density histogram on the 15th s exposure.

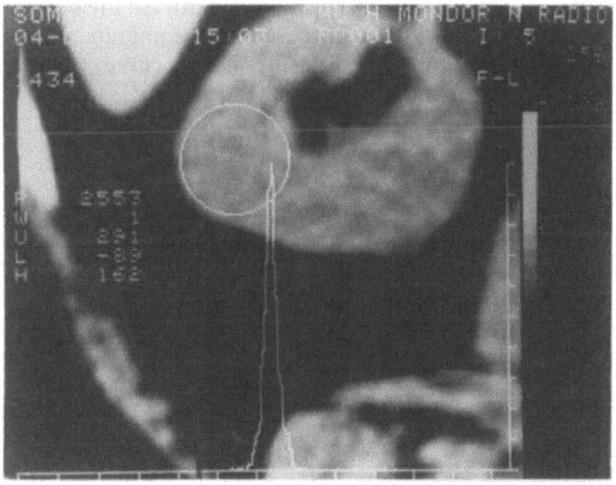

Fig. 4. Renal area that is both cortical and medullary. Density histogram on the unprepared section showing a narrow denseness curve.

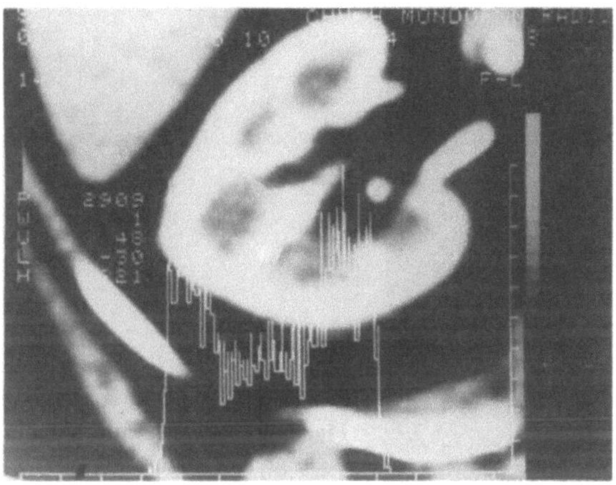

Fig. 5. Renal area that is both cortical and medullary. The density histogram on the exposure at the 15th s shows two regular but separate peaks.

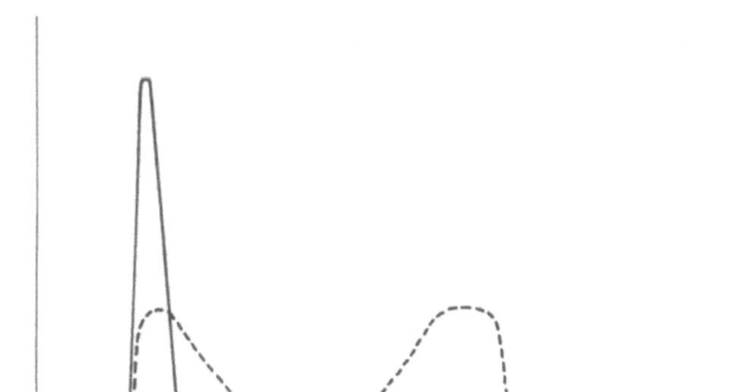

Fig. 6. Renal area that is both cortical and medullary. ——, Density histogram on the unprepared exposure. ······, Density histogram on the 15th s exposure.

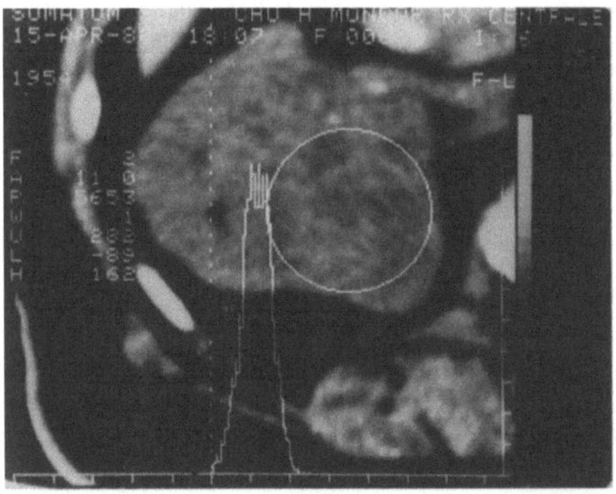

Fig. 7. Renal cancer: the density histogram on the unprepared exposure shows a curve much more spread.

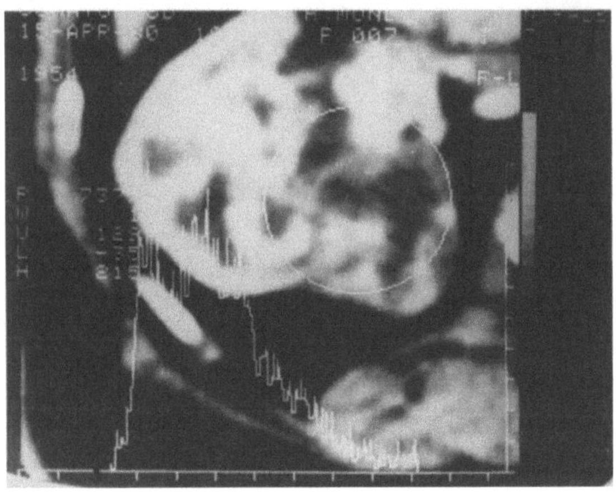

Fig. 8. Renal cancer: the spreading is greater on the 15th s exposure.

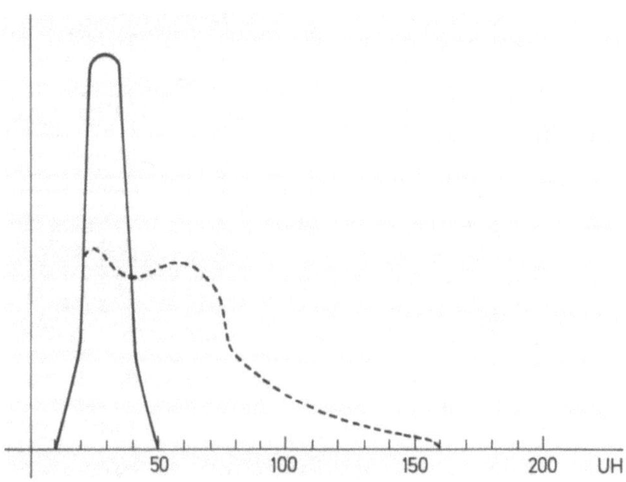

Fig. 9. Renal cancer. ——, Density histogram on the unprepared exposure. ······, Density histogram on the 15th s exposure.

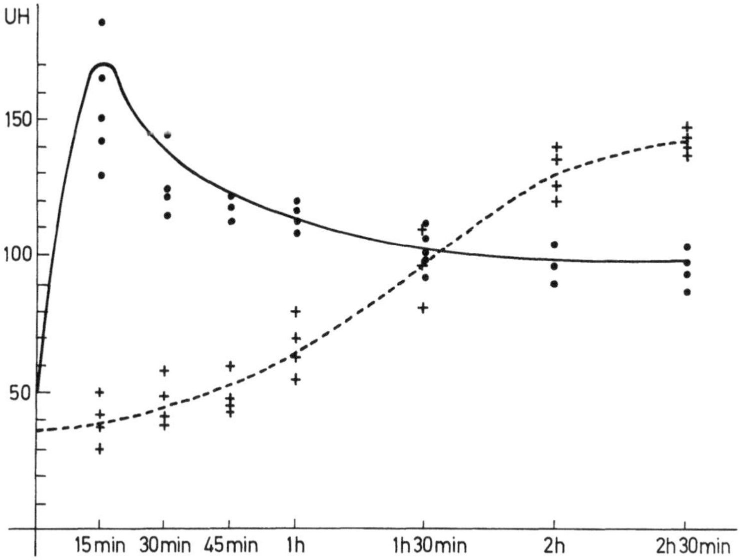

Fig. 10. Survey of denseness: development with time. —, Vascular area; ·····, renal medullary area.

The first peak corresponds to the cortical and the second, to the medullary. The two peaks, however, are very regular, showing the homogeneousness of the two parenchyma with different dynamics (Fig. 6). Indeed, the denseness depends on vascularization, and, in the present case, the two parenchyma have different dynamics. At the 15th s the cortex is very opacified, while the medullary opacification is less contrasted. On an exposure made after 1 min, the denseness opacity is equalized.

The curves obtained in the case of a renal cancer are entirely different. On the unprepared exposure, the curve is already much more spread (between 10 and 25 units in this example) (Fig. 7). The spreading is even greater on the 15th s exposure: between 10 and 170 units (Fig. 8). This widening before and after injection of the contrasting material is typical of a very heterogeneous tissue (Fig. 9). It was always found on ten renal cancers investigated by this process

Dynamic Results with a Survey of Denseness Development with Time

This survey makes it possible to investigate the contrasting material dynamics in each tissue by plotting a curve the time on the x-axis and the denseness of the tissue on the y-axis.

Those curves show an initial, upward portion that corresponds to the absorption of the contrasting material by the tissue. The denseness goes to a maximum before decreasing and reaching a value that it will keep to the end of the investigation.

The vascular area (arterial area or cortical renal arteries and Bertin's column) is characterized by a denseness increasing phase with very deep slope, the apex being reached early about the 15th s. Inside the parenchyma, is such as hepatic parenchyma, for example, the increase in denseness is slower, the apex being reached about the 45th s to 1 min.

As for the renal medulla, it has a very special dynamic, corresponding to the gradual concentration of the contrast material and appearing as a regular increase in concentration (Fig. 10).

In the case of renal cancers, which is a very heterogeneous tissue, each point shall evolve in a very peculiar way; some will have a vascular-type dynamic and some (necrosis) will show no change in denseness with any possible intermediate aspects. A kidney cyst that is not vascularized will have a constant denseness to the nearest test dubiousness.

The Use of Computed Tomography in the Diagnosis of Renal Abscess

C. C. Abbou, C. Cordonnier, J. Carlet, D. Larde, D. Chopin, T. Nebout, and H. Botto

Renal abscess (RA) is a rare and frequently severe affection. During renal sepsis, with or without obstruction, or during a sepsis of unknown origin, the discovery of RA may dramatically modify therapeutic strategy. However, the diagnosis of RA is often difficult by conventional investigations. So, the potential contribution of a noninvasive, precise, and rapid procedure such as computed tomography (CT) must be studied. The diagnosis of RA was made in patients with severe renal sepsis, usually after a failure of conventional investigations. The aim of this study is to comment on those cases, to discuss the radiologic aspects and the indications for CT in the diagnosis of RA, and to compare this procedure with conventional methods of diagnosis.

Method

We used a third generation CT (Somatom 2C Siemens) with a scanning time of 4 s. The interspace between two "slices," jointed or not, is 7–9 mm. Opacification of the gastroduodenal tract was accomplished with Gastrografin (Dilution 3%–4%).

Two or three slices were made initially, and then, an opacification of the vessels was made with a bolus of intravenous water soluble contrast media (60%, 1 mg/kg). The total duration of the procedure was 15 to 30 min.

Clinical Study

Case 1

A 75-year-old woman was admitted with a febrile left flank pain. The urine and blood cultures were positive for *Escherichia coli.* The first urography showed an obstructive lithiasis of the ureteropelvic junction. Fever remained despite antibiotic therapy and spontaneous elimination of the calculus. The kidney was enlarged, but the cavities were not distended on the second urography. CT has demonstrated a very heterogeneous parenchyma, with numerous 5- to 10-mm defects, irregularities of the cortex, and a voluminous cystic formation (Fig. 1). Complete recovery resulted after 2 weeks of antibiotic treatment.

Case 2

A 73-year-old man was admitted with a septic shock and a septicemia due to *Escherichia coli.* Nothing indicated that sepsis might be due to renal infection,

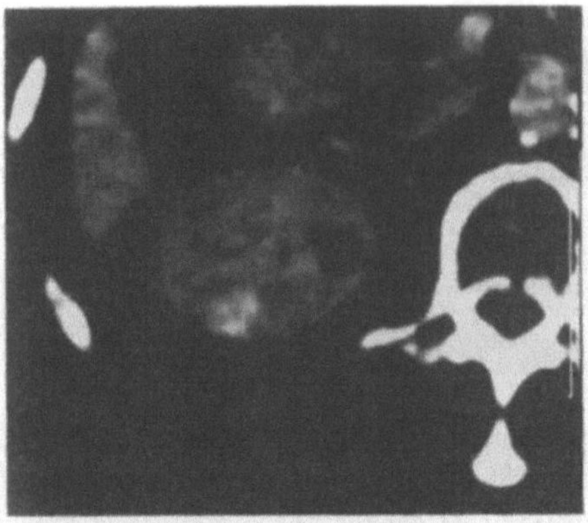
1

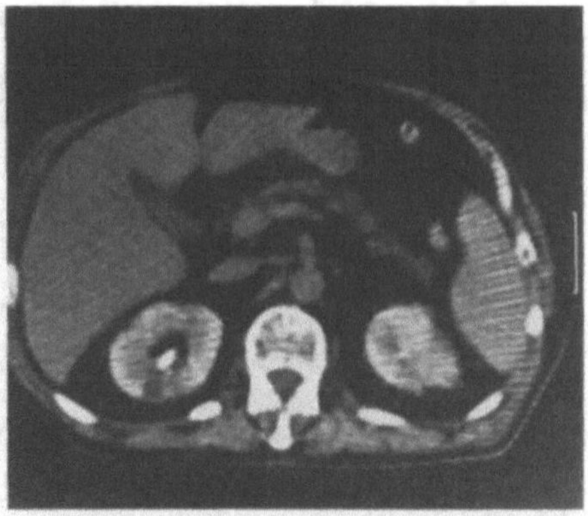
2

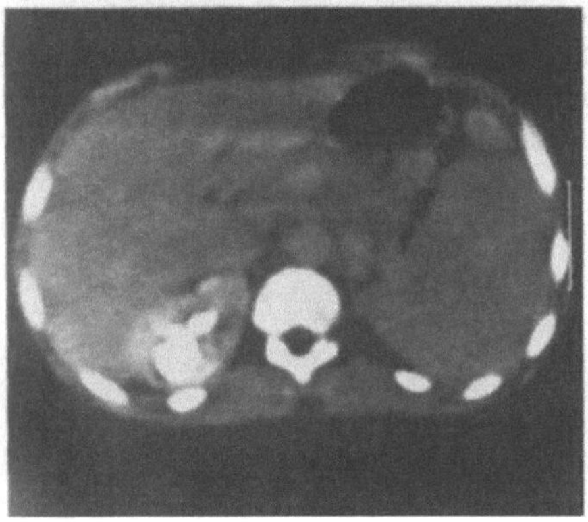
3

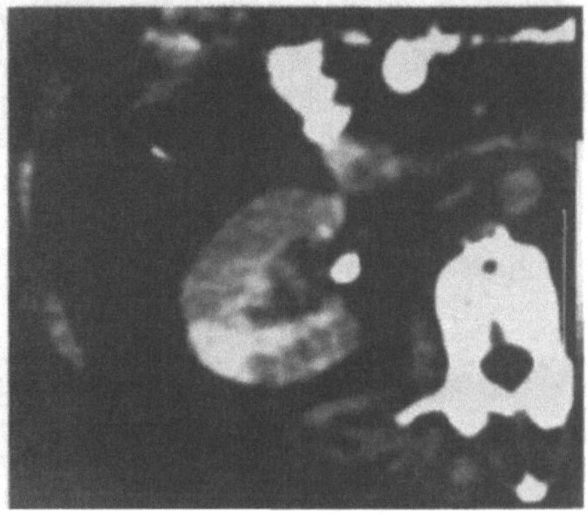
4

Fig. 1. A left pyelonephritis pursuing after ureteral lithiasis obstruction elimination.
Fig. 2. Bilateral renal abscesses with a septicemia as a complication of a subphrenic abscess.
Fig. 3. A right primitive renal abscess with spontaneous drainage in the urinary tract.
Fig. 4. A right pyelonephritis with obstructive lithiasis.

except that the same bacillus grew in the urine and in the blood. The urography showed a bilateral delay in the secretion, especially on the left. Retrograde ureteropyelography (RUP) was normal. CT was scheduled because of the persistence of a severe septic state. The renal parenchyma was heterogeneous in both kidneys, but in the left one numerous small defects were present, associated with a larger cavity (diameter 20 mm) just under the cortex (Fig. 2). A left side nephrectomy confirmed the presence of multiple RA. The septic state remained and the patient died 2 weeks later. The necropsy demonstrated a subphrenic abscess of unknown origin and a pyelonephritis of the remaining kidney.

Case 3

A 37-year-old man was admitted with hematuria, fever, right flank pain, and septicemia due to *Escherichia coli.* The urography showed a tumoral aspect of the upper part of the right kidney. Arteriography demonstrated that this formation was a nonvascular one. CT, performed immediatly after, showed an isolated cavity, with

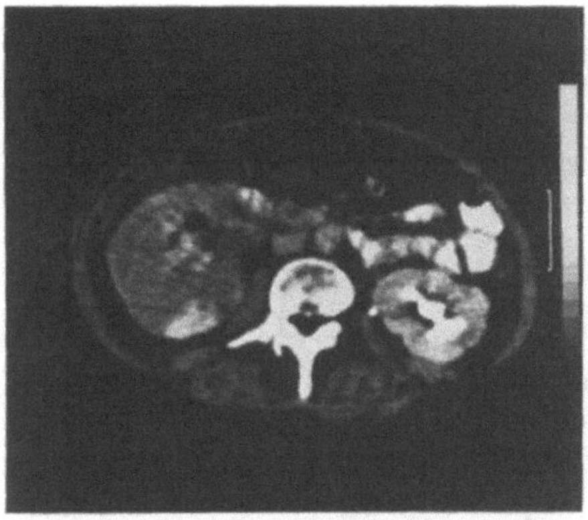
5

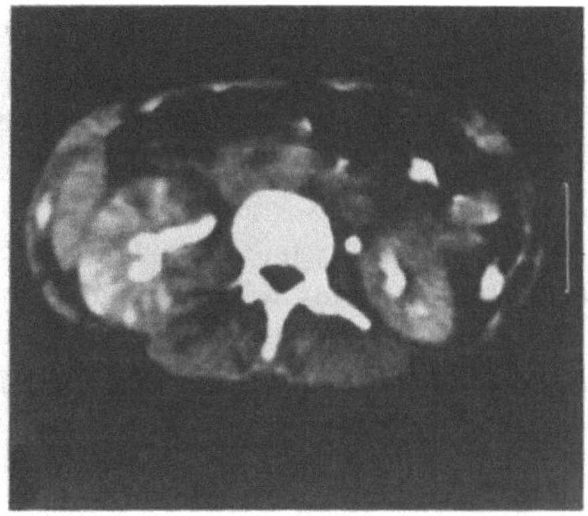
6

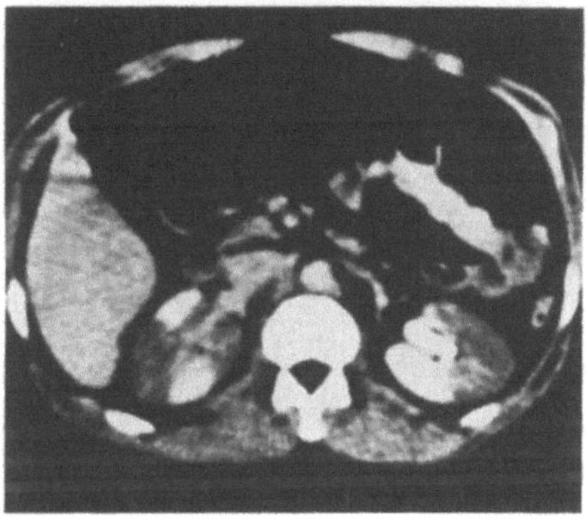
7

Fig. 5. A right pyelonephritis with Cacchi-Ricci disease.
Fig. 6. A right pyelonephritis with ureteral obstructive lithiasis.
Fig. 7. A bilateral pyelonephritis as a complication of a renal biopsy with a septicemia.

a diameter of 25 mm, which was very dense and connected with the renal cavities (Fig. 3). Antibiotic therapy allowed a complete recovery.

Case 4

Case 4 involved a 57-year-old woman with hyperparathyroidism. A pyelotomy had been performed for a "coraliform" calculus 5 years ago. She was hospitalized for right flank pain, septicemia, and urine infection due to *Escherichia coli.* Urography showed distension of the right cavities due to a ureteral calculus. An ureteral catheterization failed to pass beyond the calculus and a right lumbar ureterotomy had to be performed. Despite drainage of the cavities, the septic status remained unchanged. The CT demonstrated a heterogeneous aspect of the right kidney parenchyma, with alternating zones of very low and very high density (Fig. 4). Two defects (10 mm) were discovered. Antibiotic therapy allowed a complete recovery and a CT performed 2 months later showed a normalization of the kidney.

Case 5

A 53-year-old woman with Cacci and Ricchi disease was hospitalized for right flank pain and fever. The urine and the blood cultures were positive for *Enterobacter cloacae.* On the urography, the right kidney did not show any secretion, and there was a suspicion of a septic formation in the lower pole of the left kidney. The septic state remained, and a CT was scheduled. The right kidney was enlarged, the cortex was irregular, and the parenchyma was very heterogeneous with a lot of small defects (Fig. 5). The contrast media remained abnormal in the defects. The formation in the left kidney seemed to be a cyst. Antibiotic therapy allowed recovery.

Case 6

A 31-year-old woman was hospitalized for right flank pain and fever. The urine was infected with *Escherichia coli.* Urography showed a late secretion on the right, and an enlarged kidney with a lower pole which was difficult to see. The cavities were not distended. CT was performed to explain the persistence of the fever. The septic state was severe, with circulatory disorders. The cortex of the right kidney was irregular (Fig. 6). Numerous defects with a low density and smaller than 15 mm were disseminated in the lower half of the parenchyma. Triangular zones in the parenchyma had an abnormally high density, with persistence of the contrast media. A total recovery was obtained with antibiotic therapy. A control CT performed 1 month later was normal.

Case 7

Case 7 involved a 52-year-old man. Two weeks previously a closed renal biopsy had been performed for glomerulopathy. The patient was hospitalized for right lumbar pain, fever, and chills. The right kidney was not visualized on the urography. The retrograde ureteropyelography was normal. CT showed an irregular vascularization bilateraly, with zones of very low and very high density, and in the right kidney a rounded, small, hypodense defect, with a diameter smaller than 10 mm (Fig. 7). A total recovery was obtained with antibiotic therapy. A second urography, performed a few days later, showed a normal secretion of the right kidney.

Discussion

Radiologic Pattern of RA in CT

The elementary lesion is a round defect with a variable size and is always smaller than 25 mm in our study. Its density (10–28 in Hounsfied Units) is spontaneously smaller than the normal renal parenchyma. The density is, however, higher than the liquid one and increases slighty after the bolus of intravenous water-soluble contrast. We have never seen the peripheral shell as described in intraperitoneal abscesses (Callen 1979) nor hydroaeric aspects (however, we do not have any anaerobic infection in this study). The abscesses were single in one patient, multiple in six patients, unilateral in five patients, and bilateral in two patients. This small and rounded defect seems to be very characteristic of RA but not really pathognomonic, and it is imperative to correlate the radiologic, clinical, and bacterologic patterns. In a patient not included in this study the diagnosis of RA was suspected, due to the discovery of multiple small defects with low density. On the other hand, central temperature was normal and the bacteriologic data were negative. The patient died a few months later and the necropsy showed a bronchial cancer with multiple and bilateral renal metastases, without any infection. A defect, discovered in CT, may be either RA, a primary cancer of the kidney, metastases with necrosis, hematoma, or an infected cystic formation. The multiplicity of the defects and a central position in the parenchyma are, however, strong arguments for RA. In our experience, the coexistence of some other radiologic aspects seems to be very discriminative:

1) Irregularities of the cortex, due to peripheral microabscesses, an aspect that we have noted three times.
2) Thickening and heterogeneity of the parenchyma, noted four times. This aspect may be due to pyelonephritis or to microabscesses impossible to individualize by CT.
3) We have noted five times alternating zones of low and high density, usually triangular, with a medullary top in which the contrast media persisted for an abnormally long time.

This last aspect is difficult to interpret at present but may suggest abnormalities of the renal vascular tone due to parenchymal sepsis. In one patient, a central CT performed a few weeks later was entirely normal. However, to discuss this finding it would probably be important to define the tomodensitometric aspect of acute tubulonephritis with acute renal failure.

In case 7, the absence of any bacteriologic data, the paucity of defects in the parenchyma, and the bilateral disorders in the vascularization suggest care in the diagnosis of RA. A recent prospective study emphasizes the frequency of perirenal hematoma after renal biopsy (85%), usually without any clinical symptoms (Rosenbaum et al. 1978). However, none of the 20 patients of this study had intraparenchymal hematoma in CT. We consider that in this septic patient the diagnosis is probably RA of the right kidney, secondary to renal biopsy. The aspect of the left kidney is likely to be due to vascularization disorders secondary to septicemia, with or without renal abscesses.

Value of CT Comparison to Other Available Procedures in the Diagnosis of RA

Comparison with Urography. The superiority of CT over standard radiography is due to its greater ability to discriminate the densities (0.5% for CT and 5%–10% for usual radiography) (Abrams and McNeil 1978). If the contrast is strong enough, CT is able to discriminate defects 3 mm in diameter. CT is nonaggressive and does not require more contrast media than urography.

In our study, the urography shows:

1) A nonvisualization of the kidney in two patients,
2) a tumoral aspect in one patient,
3) an enlarged kidney, with a late secretion in three patients,
4) a normal kidney in one patient.

Urography allowed the diagnosis of RA only in two cases (3 and 6). In the five other cases it was impossible to make the diagnosis. In one patient CT demonstrated bilateral abscesses while the clinical signs indicated unilateral ines (case 7). In another patient (case 3) the clinical examination was normal and the CT showed bilateral RA.

Even if RA is suspected upon urography, the superiority of CT is evident, particularly in case of a nonvisualization of the kidney, demonstrating the exact size of the kidney, its functional state, and any radiotransparent calculi. CT visualizes precisely abscesses with a 5-mm diameter, their uni- or bilateral localization, and any possible communication with the renal cavities. CT easily demonstrates hydronephrosis (Sagel et al. 1977) and, avoids ureteropyelography, which may be a dangerous investigation. Finally, CT because of its noninvasive character may be repeated. In our study a second CT was performed in two patients, attesting a total recovery. Thus, CT seems to be more helpful than urography in the diagnosis of pyelonephritis with or without obstruction of the cavities. Arteriography is more dangerous and may be avoided altogether in most cases.

Comparison with Echography. A recent study of 13 patients underlines the advantages of this method in the diagnosis of RA (Plainfossé et al. 1980). We did not use this investigation in our study. However, in comparison with the study of Plainfossé the following points seem to appear: echography is less expensive, easily repeated, and without any irradiation. CT is able to show very small abscesses with a diameter less than 15 mm (which is frequently the case in our study) and appreciate the functional state of the kidneys. CT is not complicated by obesity. CT may demonstrate the nature and the exact localization of an obstruction. CT is less dependent on the operator than echography. Finally, both methods permit a transcutaneous drainage of a hydronephrosis (Haaga et al. 1977; Plainfossé et al. 1980) and perhaps of abscesses, but we do not have any personal experience with those techniques.

Indications and Therapeutic Implications of CT in RA

The detection of RA is a very important step in the investigation of septicemia, a renal septic state, or a septic state of unknow origin.

In our study CT was performed for the following clinical patterns:

1) Severe septic state with septicemia of unknown origin requiring an immediate diagnosis (case 2),
2) renal septic state persisting in spite of correct antibiotic therapy and often in spite of drainage of the distended cavities (case 1, 4 and 6),
3) sepsis and absence of secretion in the urography (case 5 and 7),
4) tumoral Mass (case 3).

The absence of any parallel between the anatomic and clinical pattern is well known during renal sepsis (Cukier et al. 1971; Simonin 1980). Some patients exhibit a severe septic state with shock due to microabscesses, and other patients present a mild fever coexisting with irreversible damage of the kidney, such as pyelonephrosis. The drainage of the cavities, if they are distended, is always an emergency, but the management of the infected parenchyma is not clearly specified. In some patients the antibiotic treatment allows a total recovery and on the contrary, the presence of microabscesses may explain the persistence of a severe septic shock in other patients. In the latter an immediate nephrectomy should be considered. CT may be extremely useful in such an emergency situation. However, the therapeutic management must be based not on the radiologic pattern of RA but on the clinical pattern (Simonin 1980). In fact, the presence of RA is probably very common during any acute obstruction of the cavities and the constatation of RA using CT must not increase therapeutic aggressivity.

Practical Implications of CT

The study of these seven cases underlines the importance of CT in the three following conditions:

1) Severe septic state with unilateral renal symptomatology. The correlation between clinical pattern and CT constatations may be very useful in deciding whether immediate nephrectomy is necessary (Cukier et al. 1971; Aubert and Cukier 1974; Kurth et al. 1976; Simonin 1980).
2) Septic state of renal origin, without any obstruction, or persisting despite drainage of the cavities. CT may prove essential in the decision between antibiotic therapy, drainage of the abscess, and nephrectomy.
3) Severe septic state of unknown origin. CT permits the localization of the sepsis (kidney, liver, intraperitoneal, extra-abdominal, etc.)

Conclusion

Computed tomography seems to be the most logical approach in the diagnosis of RA. This is due to the vascularization of the kidney, to its position among fatty formations which increases the contrast of the images, and to the innocuity of the procedure. Presently, the main obstacle is economic. However, it is logical to assume that CT will dramatically modify the classical hierarchy of radiological procedures and, thus, the future cost of this examination.

References

Abrams HL, McNeil BJ (1978) Medical implications of computed tomography. N Engl J Med 298:255–318

Aubert J, Cukier J (1974) La rétention purulente dans le haut appareil urinaire. J Urol (Paris) 3:237–256

Callen PW (1979) Computed tomographic evaluation of abdominal and pelvic abcesses. Radiology 31:171–175

Cukier J, Aubert J, Broc A (1971) Les pyonéphroses. Etude de 50 cas. J Urol Nephrol (Paris) 9:737–754

Haaga JR, Zelch MG, Alfidi RJ, Stewart BH, Daugherty JD (1977) CT-guided antegrade pyelography and percutaneous nephrostomy. AJR 128:621–624

Kurth K, Skoluda D, Hohenfellner R (1976) Septicémie rénale. Expériences sur le traitement chirurgical et l'antibiothérapie. J Urol Nephrol (Paris) [Suppl 2] 82:220–225
Magilner AD, Ostrum BJ (1978) Computed tomography in the diagnosis of renal masses. Radiology 126:715–718
Plainfossé M Ch, Mercier-Pageyral B, Bacques O, Vital JL (1980) Apport de l'échographie dans le diagnostic des abcès du rein. Ann Radiol (Paris) 23:7–13
Rosenbaum R, Hoffsten PE, Stanley RJ, Klahr S (1978) Use of computerized tomography to diagnose complications of percutaneous renal biopsy. Kidney Int 11:87–92
Sagel SS, Stanley RJ, Levitt RG, Geisse G (1977) Computed tomography of the kidney. Radiology 124:359–370
Segal AJ, Spataro RF, Linke CA, Frank IN, Rabinowitz R (1978) Diagnosis of non opaque calculi by computed tomography. Radiology 129:447–450
Simonin D (1980) Les états infectieux graves à point de départ urinaire. Thèse, Paris

Computer Tomographic Scanning of Adrenal Tumors

E. J. Zingg and M. Haertel

Between 1978 and 1980, 96 patients with adrenal tumors confirmed at operation or autopsy were investigated by computer tomographic (CT) scanning (Table 1). Hormonally active adrenal tumors suspected on clinical grounds can be confirmed by biochemical investigation. Exact anatomic localization is of course mandatory if surgical treatment is to be undertaken. In our opinion whole body CT scanning is the most useful diagnostic method available. It has the obvious advantage of being noninvasive and in over 90% of cases is the key investigation providing the diagnosis at an early stage. Only in ectopic pheochromocytoma and in carcinoma of the adrenal with extension of invasive growth into surrounding tissues of a questionable degree are selective angiography and hormone measurements on venous effluent indicated.

The 14 pheochromocytomas were all demonstrable as unilateral tumors up to 10 cm in diameter, and occasionally necrotic areas were identified. The CT

Table 1. Breakdown of adrenal tumors.

Pheochromocytoma	14
Hormonally active adrenal adenoma (including Cushing's syndrome)	21
Conn's syndrome	2
Adrenal cysts	3
Adrenal neuroblastoma	8
Carcinoma of the adrenal	3
Adrenal metastases	45
Total	96

Table 2. Sources of diagnostic difficulty in CT scanning of the adrenal gland.

- Paucity of retroperitoneal adipose tissue: margins of the adrenal gland obscured.
- Overlying dorsomedial hepatic lobe: right-sided adrenal tumor obscured.
- Prominent blood vessels near the adrenal glands: misleading evidence of an adrenal tumor.
- Inadequate examination technique: false negative findings.

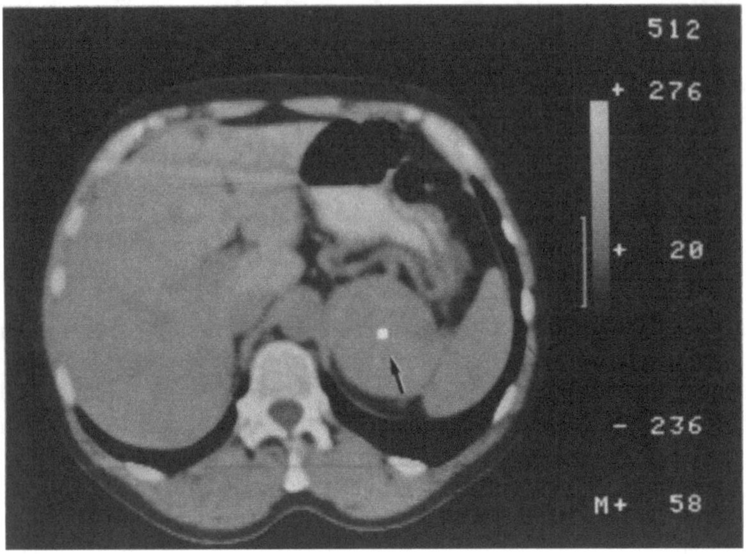

Fig. 1. Left pheochromocytoma.

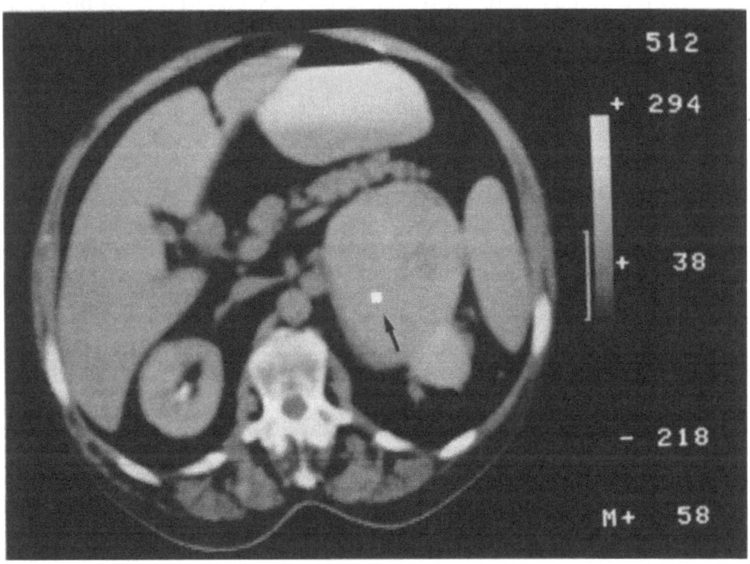

Fig. 2. Metastasis in the adrenal gland from a bronchus carcinoma.

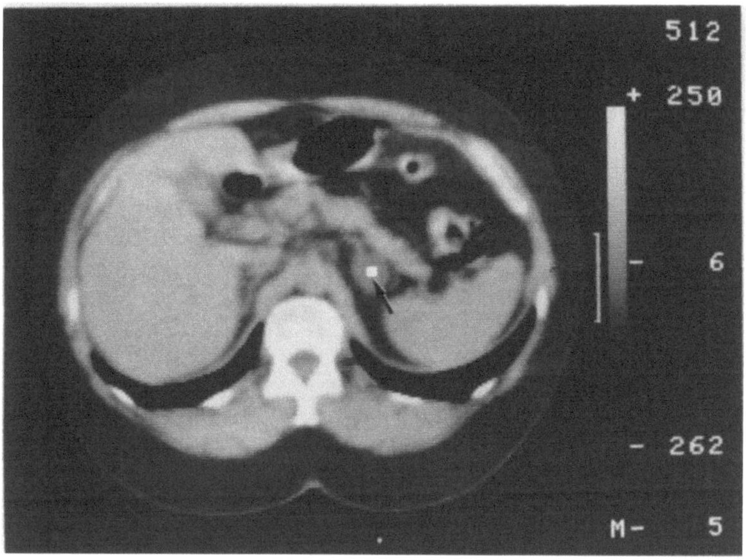

Fig. 3. Metastasis from a renal adenocarcinoma in the left adrenal gland.

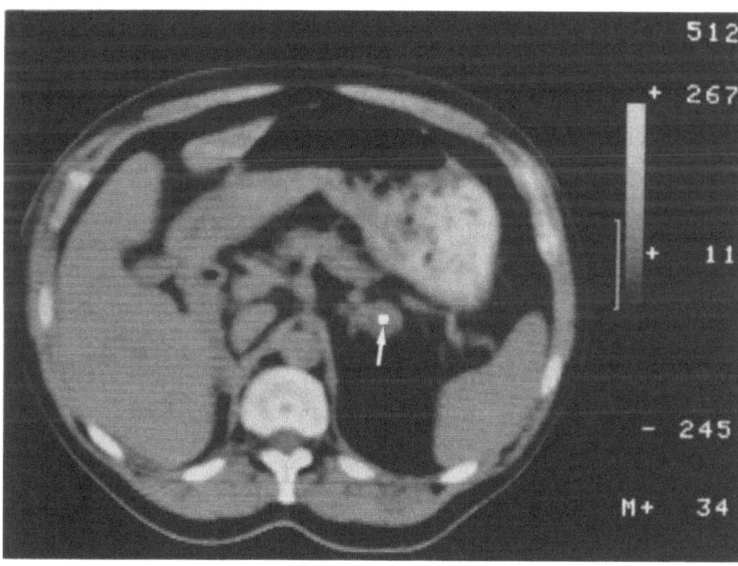

Fig. 4. Adenoma of the left adrenal gland with Conn's syndrome.

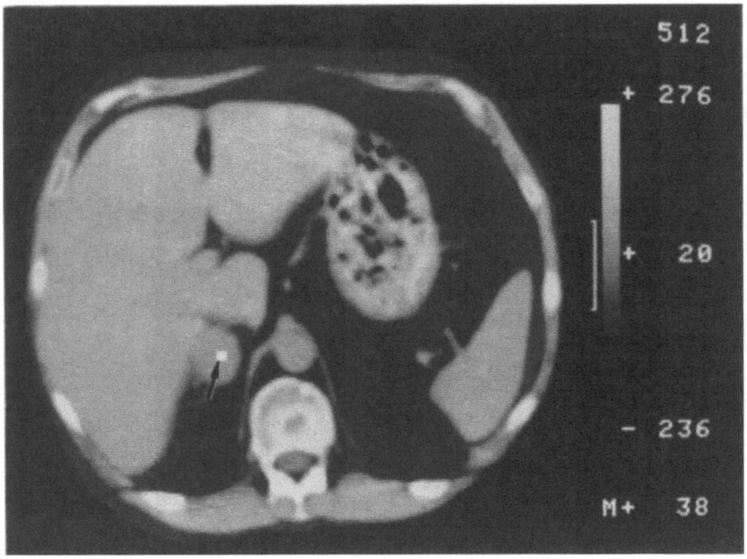

Fig. 5. Right suprarenal adenoma with Cushing's syndrome.

appearances of adrenal adenomas were striking in always showing well-circumscribed changes in the contour with increase in the volume of the adrenal. In each case the diameter exceeded 1 cm. These caused few diagnostic difficulties.

Adrenal metastases formed by far the commonest group of adrenal tumors. Neuroblastomas as a rule showed intratumoral calcification. A diffuse increase in the size of the adrenals on the CT scan was difficult to interpret. Normal variation in adrenal morphology could only be distinguished from hyperplasia by reference to clinical features (Table 2, Figs. 1–5).

Computed Tomography for Staging Bladder Tumors

L. Giuliani, G. Carmignani, E. Belgrano, P. Puppo, and A. Cichero

The preoperative staging of bladder tumors has a fundamental importance for prognostic evaluation, surgical indication, and evaluation of results. The current standard procedures for assessing this are cystoscopy, biopsy, and bimanual examination under anesthesia, together with radiographic studies as fractionated cystography, arteriography, and so on.

Kenny et al. (1972) at Roswell Park Memorial Institute stated that there is a 56% degree of inaccuracy in clinical staging of bladder cancer when compared to the pathologic staging. Computed tomography (CT) seems to offer additional useful information in the staging of bladder tumors.

On the basis of our experience of 72 bladder patients studied with CT, we try to make a balance between what the urologist would know from CT scan, i.e., an exact preoperative staging according to UICC, and what CT can actually offer to the urologist.

Material and Methods

Seventy-two consecutive unselected patients with bladder cancer underwent CT scanning for preoperative staging. The clinical staging was performed according to the suggestions of UICC, without considering the results of CT. The therapy was radical cystectomy in 42 cases, transurethral resection in 14 cases, transurethral resection plus radiotherapy in 12 cases, and radiotherapy only in four cases.

The pathologic staging was available in 68 cases. It was pT1 in nine cases, pT2 in 15 cases, pT3 in 19 cases, and pT4 in 25 cases.

For bladder scanning we use a *EMI Total Body Scanner CT 5005/12* with scanning interval of 27″. No particular preparation of the patients was performed. In female patients, whenever possible, a tampon was inserted to identify the vagina (Cohen et al. 1977).

In seven patients the bladder was filled by forced diuresis by intravenous glucose in water. However, the difference in density between the urine and the bladder was not sufficient to define the small tumors.

In 24 patients the double contrast method suggested by Seidelmann et al. (1977b, 1978) was used. This technique has the only defect of causing artifacts in a considerable percentage of cases.

In 15 patients the bladder was contrasted by intravenous pyelography. This method has the advantage of making evident the upper urinary tract, and therefore it can be associated with the other techniques for a more complete evaluation.

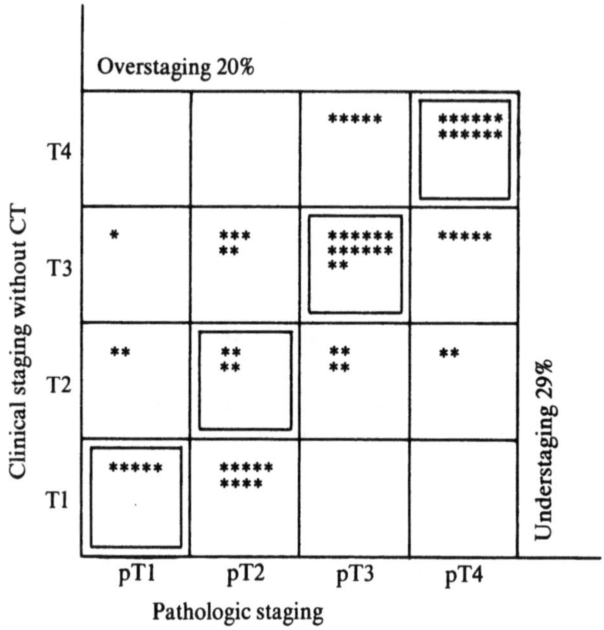

Fig. 1. Comparison of the clinical staging (without CT) versus the pathologic staging in 68 cases of bladder tumors.

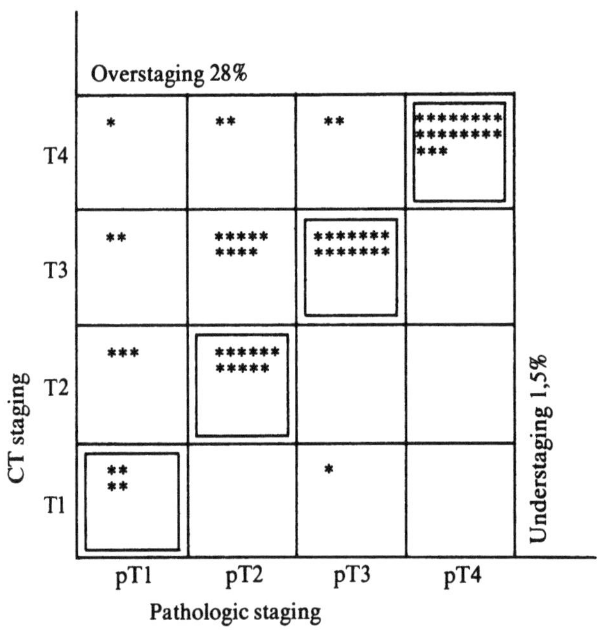

Fig. 2. Comparison of the CT staging versus the pathologic staging in 68 cases of bladder tumors.

In 26 patients the bladder was filled with extremely diluted contrast medium (0.6%) according to Hamlin and Cockett (1979). This technique is very useful in deliminitating small intravesical tumors.

Results

Figures 1 and 2 compare the clinical and CT staging with the pathologic staging. The clinical staging had an accuracy rate of 51% with a 20% degree of overstaging and a 29% degree of understaging. In low stage tumors (intravesical tumors) (Fig. 3a, b) the percentage of errors of clinical and CT staging is nearly the same. In fact, in the stages pT1, pT2, and pT3 the percentage of inaccuracy of CT, due to overstaging, was very high (28%).

a 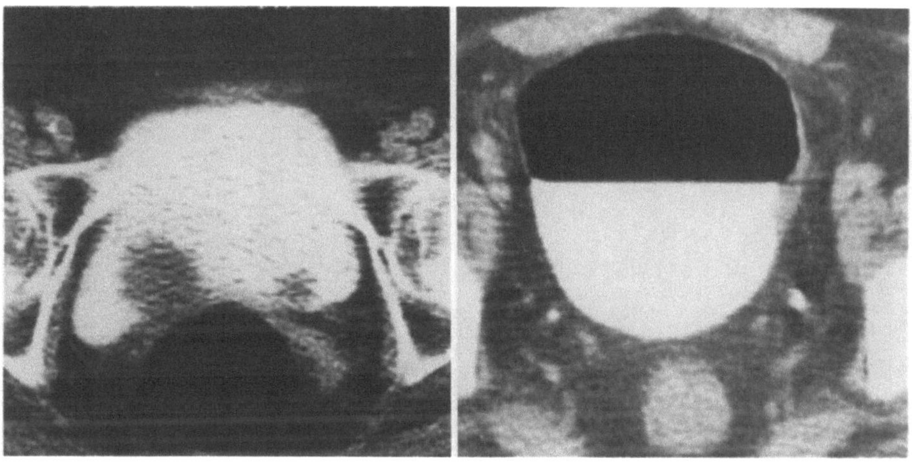 b

Fig. 3. **a** Intravesical low-stage tumors. The lack of parietal infiltration (pT1) is evident. **b** Localized thickening of the bladder wall with preservation of the perivesical fat (infiltrating intravesical carcinoma; pT3 or less).

On the contrary in advanced stage tumors CT showed the highest degree accuracy (100%) in making evident the extravesical spreading of the tumors. From this point of view the CT scanning is much more accurate, because it showed extravesical spreading of the tumor in all the cases in which it was confirmed by the pathologic examination. The clinical staging in the same cases showed a 26.6% degree of understaging.

Discussion

The analysis of our data shows that presently CT scanning cannot solve all the problems of preoperative staging of bladder tumors. The bladder wall is too thin and the power of discrimination of CT scanning between normal and tumoral tissue too little to make possible any preoperative assessment of low stage tumors (T1 versus T2 and T2 versus T3). In these tumors CT tends to increase the stage compared with

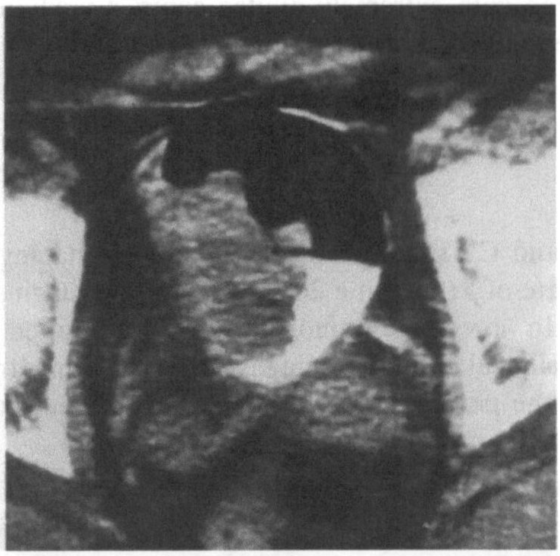

a

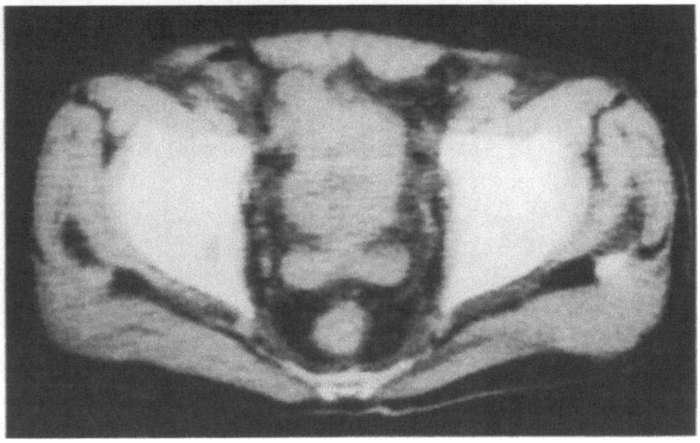

b

Fig. 4. a Spready of the tumor out of the bladder with infiltration of the right seminal vesicle, as demonstrated by the obliteration of the right seminovesical angle (pT4a). **b** Advanced extravesical tumors with infiltration of the anterior muscular wall of the abdomen (pT4b).

clinical examination. This overstaging is usually due to localized thickening of the bladder wall being interpretated as tumor invading deep muscle (Seidelman et al. 1977a, 1978).

This could be the case if an open intervention or a transurethral resection has been performed previously or if the patient has been irradiated.

Computed tomography overstaging, if not recognized, would exclude some patients from undergoing radical cystectomy, a potentially curative procedure. Therefore, when clinical staging suggests a low stage, it is probably useless to perform CT scanning. On the contrary, when there is also a minimal suspicion of extravesical infiltration, CT scanning can solve the diagnostic problem with great accuracy. As far as concerns the diagnosis of infiltration of the pelvic organs, it is practically impossible to reveal with CT a neoplastic infiltration of the prostate and of the rectum, because there does not exist a well-defined fat plain between the bladder and these organs. On the other hand, it is easy to show neoplastic invasion of the seminal vesicles (Fig. 4a) because of the presence of a small definite space occupied by fat in the corner between bladder and seminal vesicles. Also the neoplastic spreading towards the anterior muscular wall of the abdomen is easily seen (Fig. 4b).

Finally, we can state that CT scanning is a valuable diagnostic aid in the preoperative study of bladder cancer patients, provided that one wants to know if a tumor is still intravesical or is already infiltrating the perivesical fat or the adjacent organs. Further investigations are required to state whether CT scanning will give any long-term benefit as a result of improved preoperative selection of treatment and whether the cost–benefit ratio in this particular case will suggest its introduction in routine management of bladder cancer patients.

References

Cohen WN, Seidelmann FE, Bryan PJ (1977) Use of a tampon to enhance vaginal localization in computed tomography. AJR 128:1064–1065

Hamlin DJ, Cockett ATK (1979) CT of bladder: staging of bladder cancer using low density opacification technique. Urology 13:331–337

Kenny GM, Hartoner GJ, Moore RM, Murphy GP (1972) Current results from treatment of stage C and D bladder tumours at Roswell Park Memorial Institute. J Urol 107:56–59

Seidelmann FE, Cohen WN, Bryan PJ (1977a) Computed tomographic staging of bladder neoplasm. Radiol Clin North Am 15:419–440

Seidelmann FE, Temes SP, Cohen WN, Bryan PJ, Patil U, Sherry RG (1977b) CT of gas filled bladder: method of staging bladder neoplasm. Urology 9:337–344

Seidelmann FE, Cohen WN, Bryan PJ, Temes SP, Kraus D, Schoenrock G (1978) Accuracy of CT staging of bladder neoplasm using gas-filled method: report of 21 patients with surgical confirmation. AJR 130:735–739

The Value of Pelvic Computed Tomography in Prostatic Carcinoma

F. Pagano, A. Lembo, F. Zattoni, L. Laurini, D. De Faveri, and M. Vigo

For many years bimanual examination was the primary diagnostic technique in the evaluation of pelvic and prostatic pathologic. Computerized tomography provides a useful noninvasive method of demonstrating the prostate and surrounding tissues. The accuracy was believed comparable to that achieved in the skull. The facility with which the prostate, bladder, seminal vesicles, pelvic musculature, and bony structures can be imaged by CT should help in tumor staging (Redman 1977; Seidelmann et al. 1977; Sukov et al. 1977).

Patients and Methods

We considered a group of 16 patients with prostatic cancer which had been proved histologically. All the patients were classified following the UICC system. In every case, traditional staging investigations were performed and the CT finding was compared to the other parameters. The patients were positioned within the scanning gantry so that the first CT scan was done at the level of the fifth lumbar or the first sacral vertebra. Sections were performed moving in caudal direction, just below the symphysis pubis. In the prostatic area both the 13-mm and 8-mm rings were used, even in overlap, without any noticeable difference in the final scan quality. Because it was sometimes difficult to delineate the prostate from the bladder, air (100 cc) and moderately diluted iodinated solutions (100 cc) were instilled into the bladder

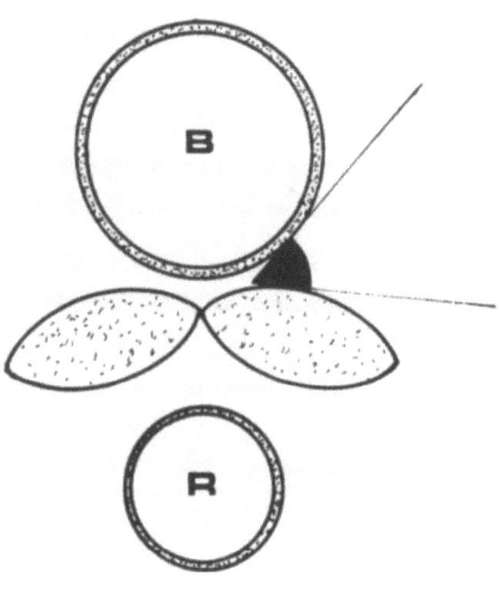

Fig. 1. Examination of patient in lateral decubitus position for a more accurate investigation of the vesicoseminal angle. *B*, Bladder; *R*, rectum.

through a Foley catheter with a little air-filled balloon. The patients were always investigated in a supine and afterwards in a prone position: this provided excellent visualization of the bladder contour and configuration and allowed for identification of the prostate as a separate organ.

Sometimes the examination was done with the patient in a right or left lateral decubitus for a more accurate investigation of the vesicoseminal angle (Fig. 1). To stop the bowel movement, immediately before the exame all the patients received 1 cc glucagon intravenously. In order to avoid false vesicoseminal angle obliteration, in every case an evacuating enema was performed.

Results

The aforementioned 16 patients were considered to have tumors strictly localized to the prostate gland. We were confirmed in our opinion by traditional investigations and by CT results. Six of these patients underwent a radical excision: histologic studies confirmed intraglandular, perfectly localized tumors. Lymph nodes, in every case, were tumor free. The other patients, in whom surgical excision was not possible because of age or other causes, were submitted to vesiculography which attested to uninjured seminal vesicles.

Discussion

Although CT accurately displays gland morphology, it does not appear that the densities of the prostate, prostatic adenoma, prostatitis, and small prostatic carcinoma are sufficiently different to be consistently separated on the basis of the attenuation values (Redman 1977; Seidelmann et al. 1977; Sukov et al. 1977; Haaga and Reich 1978).

Meanwhile it offers no advantage in evaluation of intraglandular extension. It must be emphasized that CT reveals extreme accuracy in evaluation of the vesicoseminal angle, whose obliteration represents a very important indication of extraglandular tumor extension. Moreover, CT investigation allows one to explore lymph nodes in those areas which, primarily involved in prostatic cancer pathology, are not commonly visualized during traditional lymphography (hypogastric–obturator–presacral areas) (Bonney et al. 1978). These lymph nodes are not seen by CT scans, but if enlarged an/or metastatic, they may become evident in pelvic fat: if they are not recognized, it may mean a limited or absent tumor diffusion. CT investigation also reveals initial metastatic involvement of pelvic bones.

Conclusion

In our experience, we believe in advanced stages of prostatic tumor CT is useless. Our findings, on the other hand, suggest that preoperative pelvic and prostatic CT is a very useful staging parameter in early prostatic cancer. Therefore, it should be added to the accepted staging modalities prior to a planned radical prostatectomy (Table 1).

Table 1. Capabilities computed tomography in prostatic cancer.

- ■ CT cannot differentiate tumoral from normal prostatic tissue.
- ■ CT does not reveal the infiltration of prostatic capsula; it can show seminal vesicle involvement.
- ■ CT identifies tumors infiltrating pelvic floor and evaluates their extension more accurately than rectal examination.
- ■ CT could show hypogastric–presacral lymph node involvement not visualized by pedidial lymphography.

Summary

Preoperative pelvic and prostatic computerized tomography (CT) is a very useful staging parameter in early prostatic cancer. Therefore it should be added to the accepted staging modalities prior to a planned radical prostatectomy.

References

Bonney WW, Chiu LC, Culp DA (1978) Computed tomography of the pelvis. J Urol 120:457

Cerny JC, Farad R, Rian R, Weckstein ML (1975) An evaluation of lymphangiography in staging carcinoma of the prostate. J Urol 113:367

Haaga J, Reich NE (1978) Computed tomography of abdominal abnormalities. Mosby, St. Louis, pp 240, 393

Redman HC (1977) Computed tomography of the pelvis. Radiol Clin North Am 15:3, 441

Seidelmann FE, Reich NE, Cohen WN, Haaga JR, Bryan PJ, Havrilla TR (1977) Computed tomography of seminal vesicles and the seminal vesicles angle. Comput Axial Tomogr 1:281

Sukov RJ, Scardino PT, Sample WF, Winter J, Confer DJ (1977) Computed tomography and transabdominal ultrasound in the evaluation of the prostate. J Comput Assist Tomogr 1: 281

Van Engelshoven JMA, Kreel L (1979) Computed tomography of the prostate. J Comput Assist Tomogr 3:45

Nuclear Medicine in Diagnostic Urology

General Review

P. H. O'Reilly

In 1958, Taplin and Winter produced an activity-time curve on a chart recorder of the renal scintillations following an intravenous injection of ^{131}I-labelled diodrast and thereby established the first practicable isotope renogram. Two years later McAfee and Wagner (1960), using ^{203}Hg-labelled neohydrin and a rectilinear scanner, obtained the first detailed isotope images of the kidney. These events were hailed at the time as a major breakthrough in renal investigations, and when diodrast gave way to the superior hippuran (Tubis et al. 1960) and ^{203}Hg to the less radiotoxic ^{197}Hg (Sodee 1964), the new speciality of nuclear medicine was welcome as a significant advance in investigative urology. Unfortunately, the ambitions and aspirations of nuclear medicine specialists and urologists were not to be immediately matched by the efficiency of the available radiopharmaceuticals and detection equipment and, although renography became established as a useful qualitative test of individual renal function and the slow rectilinear scan provided a means of complementing the far superior images of the excretion urogram, enthusiasm for the techniques slowed down in the late 1960s to the extent that nuclear medicine failed to become generally accepted as an established mode of investigation. This had to wait for the following decade when the almost inevitable advances in science and technology made available a new generation of radionuclides such as iodine 123 and technetium 99m, and the gamma camera-computer system to replace the old

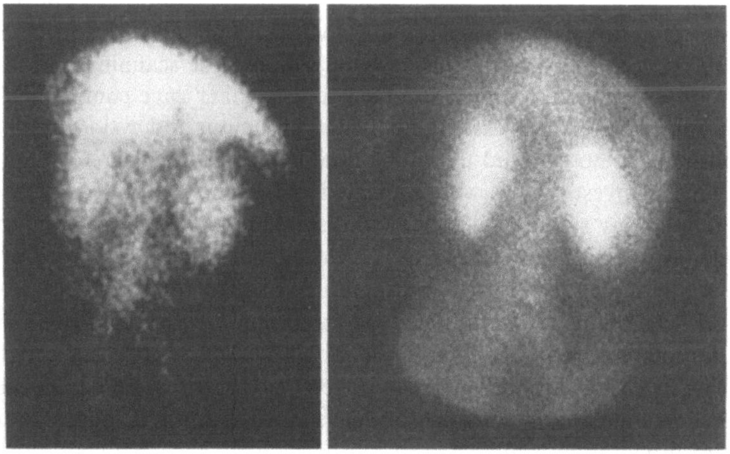

Fig. 1. **a** Normal vascular renal scan using ^{99m}Tc-gluconate. **b** Normal parenchymal renal scan using ^{99m}Tc-gluconate.

rectilinear scanner (Fig. 1). The result is that nuclear medicine has at last begun to achieve the potential it showed 20 years ago, and to establish itself as one of the most important and valuable investigative methods available to the clinical urologist.

The current spheres of importance of nuclear medicine to urology can be divided into three groups – radionuclide imaging, differential function and urodynamics.

Radionuclide Imaging

Excretion urography remains the standby for the initial radiological examination of the urological patient. The anatomical detail it provides, particularly when combined with nephrotomography, justifies its pre-eminence. There are, nevertheless, certain situations where standard radiology requires some complementary procedures to clarify urographic abnormalities.

Space-Occupying Lesions (Figs. 2, 3)

The true nature of renal space-occupying lesions detected by urography will be certain in only a minority of cases. Ultrasound is often called upon at this stage to distinguish between solid and cystic lesions; its accuracy varies 71%–98% (Barnett and Morley 1971) while Sherwood has achieved figures of 98% accuracy in cysts and 86% in tumours (Sherwood 1975). Radionuclide gamma camera imaging also has a place here: Using a gamma camera, it is possible to acquire dynamic 1-s pictures of the passage of ^{99m}Tc-gluconate through the aorta, renal arteries and intra-renal vasculature following intravenous injection. Fifty such frames are usually collected, and followed by parenchymal images at 2, 5 and 10 min or longer. The parenchymal images give further definition of the space-occupying lesion while the isotope angiogram permits assessment of the vascular characteristics of the suspect area. Thus, the vascular or avascular qualities can be assessed after urography by a simple, non-invasive 10-min procedure. Using this technique in a series of 62 consecutive patients, our diagnostic accuracy rate was 80% in hypernephroma and 96% in cysts (O'Reilly et al. 1979 a). In a further trial using both radionuclide scanning and ultrasound, the procedures showed similar accuracy, and together gave complementary accurate information in 82% of cases (28 patients) of tumour and cyst (O'Reilly et al., to be published). In no case did the two procedures mistakenly agree; where they disagreed, further investigations were indicated. While the urologist may not be prepared to rely on any single test, such as ultrasound or radionuclide scan, to make a decision regarding surgery, the combination of the two carries more diagnostic weight and reduces the need for arteriography. In cases remaining equivocal after these, CT scanning is now available for further non-invasive confirmation and we have so far found it impressively accurate in this context. Using such a plan (a protocol appears in Fig. 4) arteriography can be reserved for cases still equivocal, patients in whom some idea of the anatomy of the renal vasculature is required, or those cases where embolisation is indicated. It can be avoided in benign conditions where it is unnecessary and carries an adverse risk/benefit ratio compared to the non-invasive alternatives.

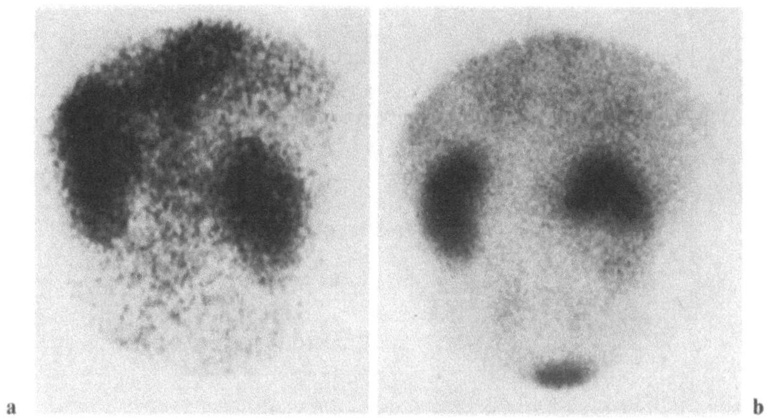

Fig. 2. **a** Vascular ^{99m}Tc-gluconate scan showing vascular right lower pole. **b** Parenchymal study showing right lower pole space-occupying lesion – vascular lesion.

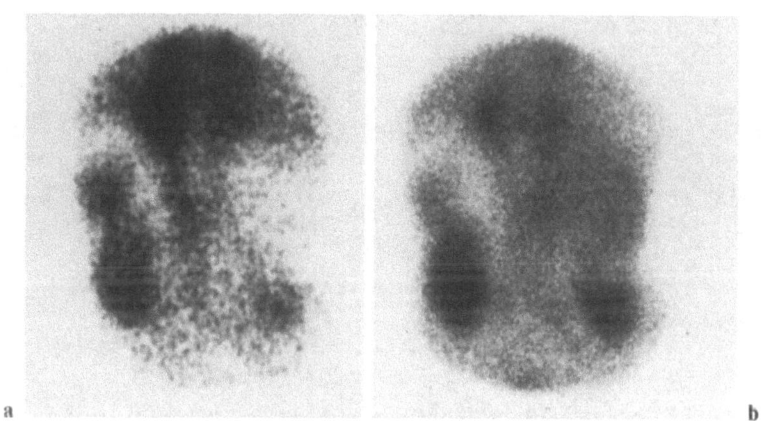

Fig. 3. **a** Vascular ^{99m}Tc-gluconate scan showing a vascular right upper pole. **b** Parenchymal study showing space-occupying right upper pole – avascular lesion.

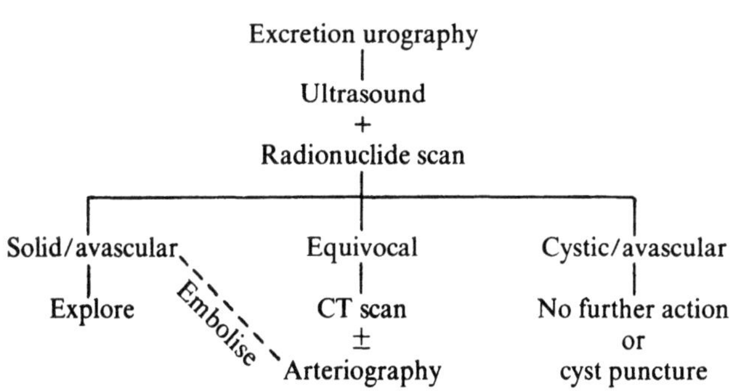

Fig. 4. Investigation of renal-space occupying lesions – the role of radionuclides.

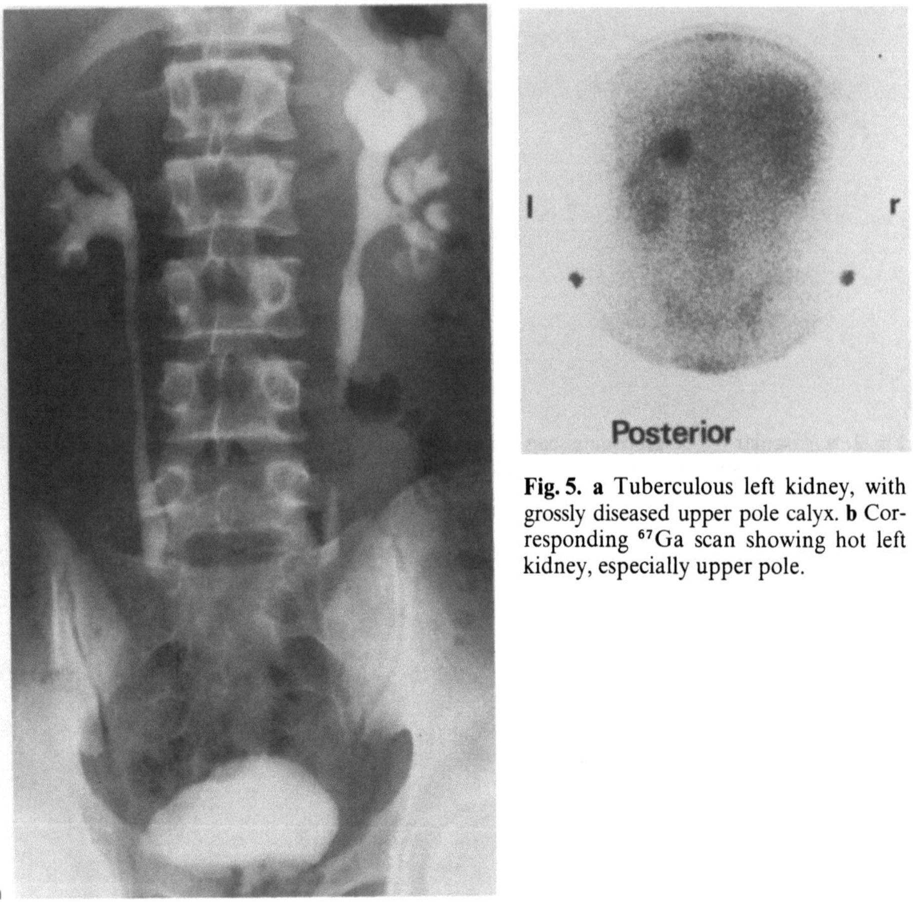

a b

Fig. 5. **a** Tuberculous left kidney, with grossly diseased upper pole calyx. **b** Corresponding ^{67}Ga scan showing hot left kidney, especially upper pole.

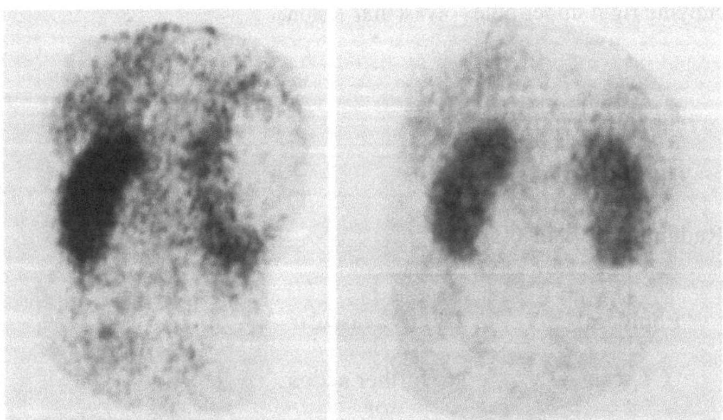

a b

Fig. 6. **a** Right renal abscess on ^{99m}Tc-gluconate parenchymal renal scan. **b** Corresponding ^{99m}Tc-gluconate parenchymal scan after treatment.

Parenchymal Disorders (Figs. 5, 6)

Cortical scarring and focal inflammatory disease are often seen on urography, although in obese or poorly prepared patients detail may be poor and nephrotomography needed. The standard urogram gives better collecting-system detail than cortical detail. Radiopharmaceuticals such as ^{99m}Tc-gluconate allow imaging by the fact that after injection they are actually retained in the cells of the proximal convoluted tubules, making parenchymal visualisation the outstanding characteristic of the radionuclide scan. In several situations where background makes renal visualisation difficult on the urogram, such gamma camera imaging can be of great value. Examples include localising ectopic kidneys, assessing the isthmus of horseshoe kidneys, locating renal tissue not seen on urography (e.g. pelvic organs) and evaluating grafts after renal transplantation. We have also found the technique useful in assessing parenchymal involvement in absecesses and particularly renal carbuncles (O'Reilly et al. 1980). Other agents such as DMSA are also available: It has a longer injection-to-scanning time, but a higher level of fixation than gluconate, 50% being retained in the kidneys after 1 h and as much as 70% at 2 h. Scanning at 2 h gives very sharp cortical images with little or no background or even renal pelvic activity: It is a useful agent for detailed assessment of functioning parenchymal mass and cortical scarring in pyelonephritis. A further agent worthy of mention in inflammatory renal disease is gallium −67. This radiopharmaceutical is well known for its ability to concentrate in lymphoid tissue, and is used clinically in conditions such as Hodgkin's disease; however, the lymphoid concentration and intestinal excretion have contributed to false-positive results during attempts at specific organ visualisation. Nevertheless, it has been shown to be useful in the assessment of perinephric abscess and pyelonephritis (Hurwitz et al. 1976) and we have been encouraged in pilot studies by its ability to demonstrate foci of genitourinary tuberculosis.

Skeletal Imaging

Little need be said regarding the value of isotope bone scanning using the ^{99m}Tc phosphate compounds. Its importance is indisputable and it is firmly established as a necessary part of the assessment of metastatic disease in carcinoma of the prostate.

Prostatic Lymphoscintigraphy (Fig. 7)

The importance of nodal metastases in carcinoma of the prostate is well-known but they are notoriously difficult to demonstrate, even by lymphography. Attempts to overcome this problem using radionuclides have recently been reported (Stone et al. 1979; Gardiner et al. 1979). The technique involves the injection of ^{99m}Tc-labelled antimony sulphide into the prostatic capsule transperineally or transrectally, followed by gamma camera imaging of the pelvis 3 h or more later (Fig. 8). Unfortunately the technique has run into several problems during early trials. As much as 85% of the activity lingers at the injection site, and there is a great deal of variation in the distribution of uptake in the regional nodes, even in normal patients. The injection must be accurately located in the capsule, rather than the parenchyma, of the gland. Furthermore, theoretical objections to the procedure, because of the

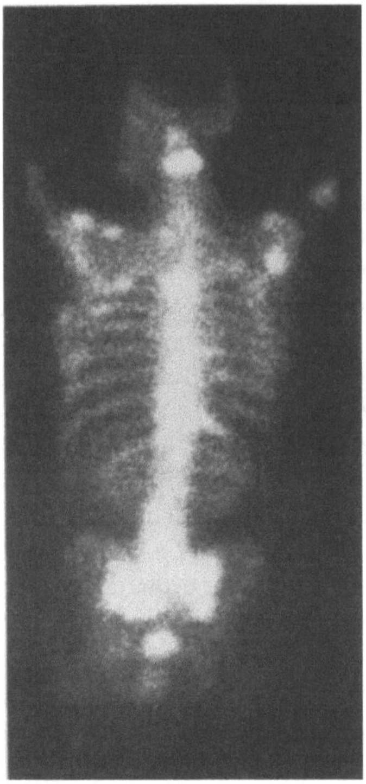

Fig. 7. ^{99m}Tc-MDP bone scan in case of skeletal prostatic metastases.

possibility of disseminating tumour cells, have been raised. Nevertheless, with increasing interest in radical-beam radiotherapy for the treatment of prostatic cancer and the knowledge that the presence of regional nodal metastases has an adverse effect on the prognosis after total prostatectomy and radiotherapy, the search for a reliable, reproducible and preferably quantifiable means of assessing prostatic regional lymphatics should be continued. The early radionuclide attempts are sufficiently encouraging to stimulate further studies.

Differential Renal Function

One of the most exciting advances in urological nuclear medicine in recent years has been the ability to accurately measure differential renal function without resorting to invasive ureteric catheterisation. Raynaud pioneered this role for radionuclides using ^{197}Hg-chloride (Raynaud 1975). This remains an accurate procedure but it is time-consuming, complex and nephrotoxic, delivering as much as several rads to the kidneys in children. The same workers have recently reported attempts to use same technique with less toxic agents such as ^{204}Bi and ^{99m}Tc-TMA (Raynaud et al. 1980). ^{99m}Tc-DMSA has been used in similar fashion as a test of renal fixation. Although it gives probably the best current scintigraphic images, it is formed of several complexes, the renal kinetics of which can differ: This instability gives a wide dispersion of normal values, and can make reproducibility difficult. Perhaps the simplest radionuclide differential renal function test is that which can be performed during ^{131}I-hippuran or preferably (because of its optimal physical qualities) ^{123}I-hippuran renography (Fig. 8). Following intravenous injection, 20-s frames of the passage of activity through the kidneys are collected for 20 min in the normal fashion. The renal areas and a suitable area of background are defined with a light pen on the display screen, and a series of subtracted counts for the renal areas alone can then be produced. The counts for 1–2 and 2–3 min for each kidney are summed, the average value calculated and the differential function expressed as the percentage contribution of each kidney to the total counts. This simple technique shows good correlation with constant hippurate infusion and individual renal urine collection techniques (Hayes et al. 1974) and with the aforementioned ^{99m}Tc-DMSA method (Holter and Storm 1979). While hippuran gives an estimate of individual renal plasma flow, an alternative agent is available to measure glomerular filtration rate – ^{99m}Tc-DTPA. Although this agent is purely filtered and not retained in the cortex like gluconate, it is in the kidneys long enough and in sufficient concentration to give good renal images. It is thus a truly functional renal imaging agent (Neilson et al. 1977). A recent report of its use in 101 children with various uropathies demonstrated good correlation with total and separate clearance, the Raynaud Hg-Cl_2 test and maximal urinary concentration. The authors rightly emphasised the par-

a

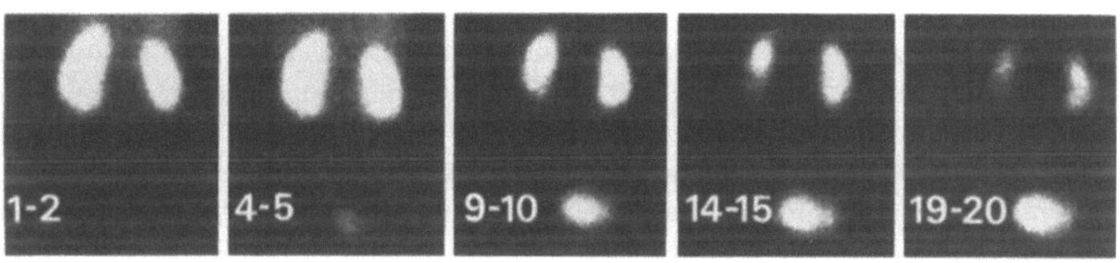

b

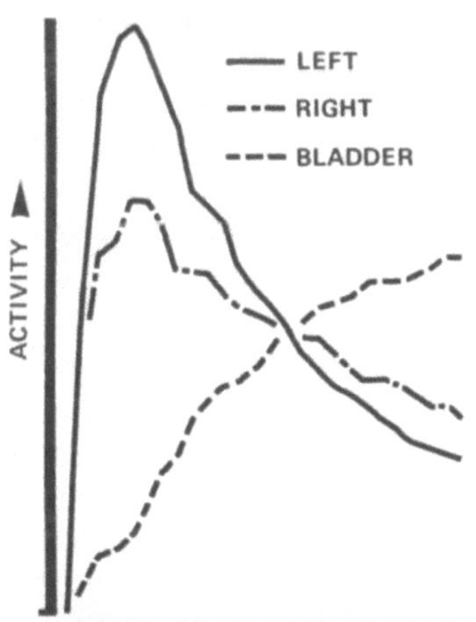

Fig. 8. a Series of ^{123}I-hippuran gamma camera images. b Computer-derived renograms.

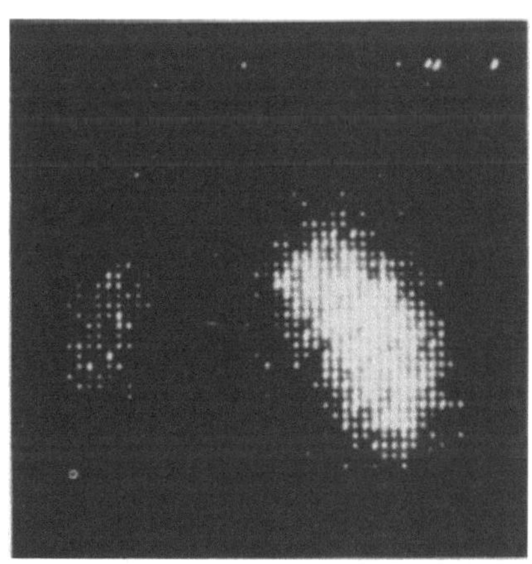

Fig. 9. ^{131}I-hippuran gamma camera images in left hypoplastic kidney for divided-function calculation.

ticular suitability of such radionuclide scanning to paediatric practice because of its simplicity, atraumatism and low radiation dose (Piepz et al. 1978). Many situations exist where an index of differential function is vital to correct patient management – obstructive uropathy, chronic pyelonephritis, glomerulonephritis, hypertension, vesico-ureteric reflux, primary megaureter and renal hypoplasia or dysplasia to mention but a few. The urologists must know the functional status of the kidneys to make appropriate decisions regarding nephrectomy or kidney preservation, or to assess progress after surgery or during conservative treatment. Radionuclide methods make such information readily available and accurately quantifiable (Fig. 9). Nor need such measurements be confined to individual kidneys: Modern gamma camera-computer systems make it possible to estimate function in separate moieties of duplex systems and even in intrarenal areas of interest.

Urodynamics

Obstructive Uropathy

Few subjects have undergone such thorough reappraisal in recent years as the diagnosis and management of urinary obstruction, and particularly equivocal states of obstruction and dilatation of the upper urinary tracts. It has been appreciated that the static anatomical images of the excretion urogram cannot give an accurate measure of the degree of obstruction or underlying renal function. The distinction between obstructive and non-obstructive dilatation is particularly crucial in situations such as idiopathic hydroephrosis, post-pyeloplasty dilatation, primary megaureter, ureters remaining dilated after reimplantation or ureterolithotomy and ureters which become dilated after urinary diversion. Radionuclides have found an important role in the assessment of these problems. Dilatation from any cause will result in retention of tracer in the renal areas or ureters during renography. However, when retention is found at 20 min, increasing the urine flow rate by an intravenous injection of 0.5 mg/kg of the diuretic Frusemide will help to make the distinction between genuine and hypotonic non-obstructive dilatation. The truly obstructed tract remains obstructed at low- and high-flow rates, whereas the capacious, floppy non-obstructive tract does not impede the increased flow. Rather, the state of stasis allowing the initial, *apparently* obstructive pattern is unmasked and the renogram curve shows a prompt, rapid and complete elimination from the upper tract in response to the Frusemide. The details of such diuresis renography have been reported elsewhere (O'Reilly et al. 1979a, b) and it is gaining widespread acceptance as a useful method of assessing the dilated urinary tract (Koff et al. 1979). It has the advantage that the 2-min hippuran-uptake method of measuring individual renal function is inherent in the technique, and so the procedure gives a simultaneous assessment of differential function and urodynamics. Another radionuclide method of detecting obstructive nephropathy in these patients is the technique of measuring parenchymal transit times reported by Whitfield and his colleagues (Whitfield et al. 1977). This provides yet another non-invasive means of assessing this difficult group of patients and such methods represent a significant step foreward in understanding and managing the dilated urinary tract.

Urinary Reflux

Conventional radiological micturating cystourethrography remains the initial investigation for the assessment of vesicoureteric reflux. If conservative management is decided upon, however, repeated radiological examinations to monitor progress will entail a large radiation dose to the patient, particularly children and adolescent females. Direct radionuclide cystography, instilling a small amount of ^{99m}Tc-pertechnetate or sulphur colloid into the bladder and continuously monitoring bladder and renal activity on the gamma camera during filling, straining and voiding is a well-established alternative (Conway et al. 1972; Rothwell et al. 1977). The radiation dose to the patient is very low, 30 min exposure to 1 mCi of ^{99m}Tc delivering about 30 mrad to the bladder and 2.3 mrad to the gonads (Blaufox et al. 1974). More recently a further advance has been reported which does away with the need for urethral catheterisation (Merrick et al. 1979; Meller et al. 1980). Here the isotope is introduced into the bladder by injecting it intravenously and allowing it to pass through the kidneys into the bladder as during standard renography. ^{123}I-hippuran or ^{99m}Tc-DTPA may be used for such indirect radionuclide cystography. Using a computer-optimized display so that small numbers of frames may be inspected in detail and analysed, even small degrees of reflux can be detected. Thus, catheterisation is not required, the radiation dose is small, the overall cost is less than conventional radiological methods and the method is at least as sensitive. It can be repeated at frequent intervals. This technique is ideally suited to follow up children and adults undergoing medical treatment for established reflux, to assess patients after ureteric reimplantation and as a screening test in children and adults found to have scarred kidneys. Clearly, where anatomical detail is required, and for initial examination after urography, the conventional method of radiology is preferable.

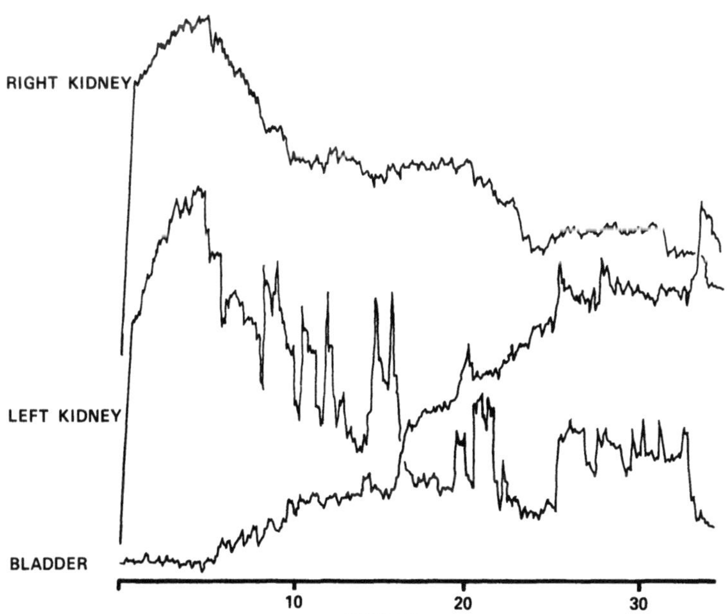

Fig. 10. Renogram pattern of uretero-ureteric reflux showing characteristic saw-tooth waves.

A further form of reflux in which gamma camera assessment is valuable is uretero-ureteric reflux between the moieties of duplex upper urinary tracts (Fig. 10). Duplication is the commonest congenital urological abnormality, and the incomplete form is twice as common as the complete. However, the incidence of urodynamic abnormalities in this condition is not clear, and the search for them up to now has required attempts to catheterise both ureters above the common stem, or radiotoxic fluoroscopy. By performing ^{123}I-hippuran renography, deriving images and renograms over both moieties, ureters and the ureteric confluence, and analysing the fluctuations in activity over all these areas, it is possible to detect the presence of ureteroureteric reflux, to distinguish between the up-and-down and see-saw varieties and to measure differential function in the two moieties (O'Reilly et al. 1978). To date, we have examined 23 consecutive patients with incomplete duplication by this method and detected gross urodynamic abnormalities in seven (30%). These patients often give a long history of loin pain but have entirely normal urological investigations other than the presence of the duplication, which is often regarded as a normal variant of little clinical significance. Radionuclide studies should help to establish the true incidence of urodynamic abnormalities and select patients in whom surgery is indicated.

Lower Tract Radionuclide Studies

Scrotal Scanning

The application of radionuclides to the lower urinary tract has not received widespread attention. One exception is scrotal imaging. The main application is to distinguish between inflammatory processes such as epididymo-orchitis and avascular conditions such as torsion of the testis. The technique is simple, requiring one intravenous injection of ^{99m}Tc-pertechnetate followed by serial 3-s ir 5-s pictures on the gamma camera, the scrotum lying on a lead or tape bridge. The pictures show the passage of the isotope trough the vessels and tissues of the testes, and a vascular or hypervascular pattern is indicative of normal or inflamed tissues while avascularity indicates torsion. Although academically attreactive, many urologists would prefer to opt for immediate surgical exploration if acute torsion of the testis is suspected rather than accept even the short delay inherent in performing any diagnostic studies. Even one false-negative result in such a situation is a tragedy, and reactive hyperaemia, sub-total torsion and spontaneous de-torsion all represent potential events which will give a vascular scan where fixation is indicated. Unless the facilities for the performance of the technique are immediately available and the results are interpreted in the most critical fashion, it is difficult to recommend the procedure in children and young adults. It must be added, however, that several reports exist giving excellent results from such procedures (Datta and Mishkin 1975; Riley et al. 1976).

Lower Tract Urodynamics

There are only two current ways in which radionuclide studies can help in the assessment of lower tract urodynamics – the measurement of urinary flow rate and the estimation of residual urine. Following renography using ^{123}I-hippuran or ^{99m}Tc-DTPA, the bladder contains a volume of highly active urine in quantification terms. Gamma camera imaging during voiding will monitor the rate at which this activity leaves the bladder allowing a curve to be derived to give the flow rate. In our experience, the technique does not give an instantaneous and accurate reflection of rapid, small changes in flow such as can be obtained using other apparatus such as the rotating drum (DISA) mictiometer, and such fluctuations and intermittency can be of clinical significance. Furthermore, the smoothing of the data necessary to obtain the curves from the computer tend to slightly underestimate maximum flow rate. Nevertheless it is useful for average flow rate where conventional urodynamic apparatus is not available.

The measurement of residual urine by radionuclides is well established. The pre- and post-voiding counts in the bladder are recorded, the volume of urine passed is measured and the residual urine is calculated by the following formula:

$$\text{residual volume} = \frac{\text{voided volume} \times \text{full bladder counts}}{\text{initial bladder counts} - \text{final bladder counts}}.$$

In patients with suspected lower tract obstruction, the ^{123}I-hippuran study is useful since it gives an estimate of individual renal function, a renogram curve, renal and ureteric visualisation, an average flow rate and an estimate of residual volume. Where such information is likely to be of value, the renogram should be complemented by the lower tract study which takes only a few extra minutes.

In conclusion, this brief review reflects the development and current role of nuclear medicine in urological practice. Its major achievement has been to complement existing methods of urinary tract visualisation with alternative imaging techniques, objective quantifiable renal functional data and urodynamics. Further improvements are certain to evolve with sophisticated detection and computer hardwarde. The inherent qualities of non-invasiveness, low radiotoxicity and computer quantification make such procedures indispensible to the practice of modern clinical urology, and establish nuclear medicine as one of the most exciting current developments for the practical urologist since the introduction of the excretion urogram.

Acknowledgements. Much of the work reported in this review forms part of a continuing study based at the Manchester Royal Infirmary into the role of radionuclides in nephrourology. Credit is due to all the clinicians and scientists involved, but particularly to Dr. H. J. Testa, Consultant in Nuclear Medicine; Mr. R. A. Shields, Principal Physicist; Dr. R. S. Lawson, Senior Physicist; and Mr. Eric Charlton Edwards, Senior Consultant Urologist.

References

Barnett E, Morley P (1971) Ultrasound and the investigation of space-occupying lesions of the kidney. Br J Radiol 44:733–742

Blaufox MD, Gruskin A, Sandler P (1971) Radionuclide cystography in the detection of vesicoureteric reflux in children. J Pediatr 79:239–245

Constable AR, Joekes AM (1972) Scintiscans and renography applied to duplex kidneys. In: Blaufox MD, Funck Brentano JL (eds) Radionuclides in nephrology. Grune & Stratton, New York

Conway JJ, King LR, Belman AB, Thompson T Jr (1972) The detection of vesicoureteric reflux with radionuclide cystography. AJR 115:720–725

Datta NS, Mishkin FS (1975) Radionuclide imaging in intrascrotal lesions. JAMA 231:1060 to 1062

Gardiner RA, Fitzpatrick JM, Constable AR, Cranage RW, O'Donaghue EPN, Wickham JEA (1979) Improved techniques in radionuclide imaging of prostatic lymph nodes. Br J Urol 51:561–564

Hayes M, Brosnan S, Taplin GV (1974) Determination of differential renal function by sequential scintigraphy. J Urol 3:556–559

Holten I, Storm HH (1979) Kidney scintigraphy with ^{99m}Tc-DMSA and ^{131}I-Hippuran. Scand J Urol Nephrol 13:275–283

Hurwitz SR, Kessler WD, Alazaku P, Ashburn WK (1976) ^{67}Ga imaging to localise urinary tract infection. Br J Radiol 49:156–160

Koff SA, Thrall HA, Kempes JR (1979) Diuretic radionuclide urography. Non-invasive method for evaluating nephroureteral dilatation. J Urol 122:451–455

McAfee JG, Wagner HN Jr (1960) Visualisation of renal parenchyma. Scintiscanning with ^{203}Hg-neohydrin. Radiology 75:820

Neilson SP, Lehd-Moller M, Trap Jensen J (1977) ^{99m}Tc-DTPA scintillation camera renography. A new method for estimation of single kidney function. J Nucl Med 18:112–117

O'Reilly PH, Lawson RS, Shields RA, Testa HJ, Charlton Edwards E, Carroll RNP (1978) A radioisotope method of assessing ureteroureteric reflux. Br J Urol 50:164–168

O'Reilly PH, Shields RA, Testa HJ (eds) (1979a) Nuclear medicine in urology and nephrology. Butterworths, London

O'Reilly PH, Lawson RS, Shields RA, Testa HJ (1979b) Idiopathic hydronephrosis. J Urol 121:153–155

O'Reilly PH, Lupton EW, Shields RA, Testa HJ, Charlton Edwards E (1980) Diagnosing renal carbuncles – the role of radionuclides. Br J Radiol 53:504–507

O'Reilly PH, Osborne DE, Shields RA, Testa HJ, Asbury DL, Best JJK, Barnard RJB (to be published) Renal imaging; a comparison of radionuclide ultrasound and CT scanning in the investigation of renal space-occupying lesions

Piepz A, Denis R, Ham HR, Dobbeleir A, Schulman CC (1978) A simple method for measuring separate glomerular filtration rate using a single injection of ^{99m}Tc-DTPA and the scintillation camera. J Pediatr 93:769–774

Raynaud C, Verhas M, Ricard S, Bardy A, Goret F (1980) ^{206}Bi, ^{99m}Tc-DMSA and ^{99m}Tc-TMA in measuring renal uptake. In: Hollenberg, Lange (eds) Radionuclides in nephrology. Thieme, Stuttgart

Raynaud EC (1975) The renal uptake of radioactive mercury. Thomas, Springfield

Rothwell D, Constable AR, Albrecht M (1977) Radionuclide cystography in the management of vesicoureteric reflux. Br J Urol 49:628–632

Sherwood T (1975) Renal masses and ultrasound. Br Med J 11:682–683

Sodee DB (1964) A new scanning isotope, ^{197}Hg-neohydrin. J Nucl Med 51:74

Stone AR, Merrick MV, Chisholm GD (1979) Prostatic lymphoscintigraphy. Br J Urol 51:556–560

Taplin GV, Meredith OM, Kade H, Winter CC (1956) The radioisotope renogram. J Lab Clin Med 48:886

Tubis M, Posnick M, Nordyke RA (1960) The preparation and use of ^{131}I-labelled sodium ortho-iodohippurate in kidney function test. Proc Soc Exp Biol Med 103:498

Measurement of Separate Renal Function with 197 $HgCl_2$

A. Schoutens and M. Verhas

After intravenous injection of radiomercury bichloride, renal activity rises slowly to reach 75% of its maximum at 6 h and a constant activity or plateau at 24 h. Urinary excretion of activity is negligible.

The uptake of radiomercury is limited to the cortex and is dependent on the tubular function. It is correlated with inulin and PAH clearances and Tm of PAH.

The very nature of the uptake process makes it independent of the circumstances of the injection, vasovagal reflex for example, and allows repeted measurements if some technical bias is suspected. The measure of the uptake by each kidney takes place routinely 2 days after injection with a gamma camera equipped with some unsophisticated processing unit. Renal activity is corrected for kidney depth and for the small liver interference.

In normal adults, 19% and 19.5% of the injected radioactive dose are found in each kidney and the results are expressed as a percentage of this normal mean (normality: 100% ± 13% of normal mean for each kidney and 100% ± 11% for uptake of both kidneys).

In the child, uptake rises from 5% of I.D. at 2 months to values observed in adults at 3 years. The radiation dose absorbed by the kidneys being rather high in very young children (up to 10 rads), we avoid use of this technique before 6 months of age.

Reproducibility of results is fair. Repeated measurements in 15 patients with time intervals of several months and even years went along with a variation coefficient just less than 5%.

A one-sided renal disease goes along with an increase of the renal mass of the controlateral kidney. This process of compensatory hypertrophy develops slowly so that 1 to 3 years are needed after uninephrectomy for the radiomercury uptake by the kidney left in place to near 200% of the normal mean for one kidney. If no renal compensatory hypertrophy develops, integrity of the residual kidney must be questioned.

Demonstration of the absence of renal compensatory hypertrophy in supposed unilateral chronic disease will incite the clinician to reconsider his diagnosis.

However, it will be noticed that the diseased kidney could hinder the development of a controlateral compensatory hypertrophy in certain circumstances. Indeed, in some patients with diminished global radiomercury uptake, uninephrectomy was followed by a dramatic increase in the uptake of the kidney left in place. As the functional parameter was initially low, it was suppossed that some incitement to renal hypertrophy existed but was ineffectual not because of the renal status of the less-diseased kidney (function increased after surgery on the other kidney) but because of some inhibition.

The interpretation of results will also take advantage of the observation of a transient decrease in renal uptake of mercury just after acute ureteral obstruction (stone with nephritic colic). If controlled one month later, function will be found normalized.

Radiomercury uptake by the kidneys taken as a measure of renal tubular function was assayed in different diseases and situations related to nephrology and urology. It appears today that the urologist is the most liable to use a technique giving a reproducible measure of the functional state of each kidney. In obstructive uropathies, the technique helps him to choose between conservative surgery and nephrectomy and to choose the kidney to be first operated upon; it also helps him to appreciate the efficiency of the chosen therapy. In vesicoureteric refluxes the measure will point to some unexpected functional damage or objectivate functional deterioration in the course of therapy.

To sum up, measurement of renal uptake of mercury is a simple, highly reliable, and reproducible technique which informs us about the evolution of the separate renal function in obstructive uropathies and vesicoureteric refluxes.

References

Raynaud C (ed) (1973) La fixation rénale du mercure radioactif. Masson, Paris

Raynaud C (ed) (1976) The renal uptake of radioactive mercury. Method for testing the functional value of each kidney; technical results and clinical application in urology and nephrology. Thomas, Springfield, Ill.

The ^{99m}Tc-DTPA Functional Study in the Child and the Adult

A. Piepsz, H. R. Ham, M. Hall, and C. C. Schulman

The renogram, introduced by Taplin in 1956, has been used widely in child and adult urology. Although useful clinical information can be obtained on this basis, the interpretation of the renographic curves remains empirical. This is due to the interference of three components simultaneously influencing the entire time–activity renal curve, namely, the blood background or the uptake and the removal component.

Since the introduction of the sophisticated gamma camera connected to computer system, it is now possible to extract more physiologic parameters from the renogram. In our department, the separate glomerular filtration rate (SGFR), the intrarenal transit times, and the renal response to a frusemide injection are routinely obtained by means of one test of short duration, necessitating only the intravenous injection of a single radiotracer and providing a minimal irradiation to the patient.

The patient is well hydrated before the examination and is asked to empty his bladder. He is positioned on a scintillation camera connected to a minicomputer. A dose of 0.50 mCi/kg Tc-DTPA is injected intravenously, and all the information is stored at 20-s intervals for the first 20-min period. Polaroid images are regularly taken and a frusemide injection is decided in function of the renal emptying at 15 min. At 20 min a blood sample is taken and the frusemide is injected if necessary at a dose of 2 mg/kg followed by a second 15-min recording period. The test ends with two lateral views of 1 min each, allowing the correction for the renal depth.

Separate Glomerular Filtration Rate

The method has been described in previous papers (Piepsz et al. 1977, 1978a). By definition, the amount of radioactivity that accumulates in the kidney per unit time, divided by the corresponding plasma concentration, yields the separate clearance value in so far as no significant amount of the tracer escapes from the kidney.

$$\mathrm{SGFR\ (miC/min)} = \frac{1}{\mathrm{p\,(t)}} \cdot \frac{\mathrm{dR\,(t)}}{\mathrm{dt}} \quad \text{if} \quad t < 3\ \mathrm{min},$$

where t = time in minutes, dR(t)/dt = slope of corrected renal curve at time t, P(t) = plasma concentration at time t.

Renal, background, and cardiac curves are determined from regions of interest, and the cardiac curve is calibrated by means of the blood sample taken at 20 min. Correction factors have been introduced for kidney depth and body surface area.

Normal values have been established and are in the range of normal inulin clearance (60 ml/min).

The SGFR is correlated well with separate creatinine clearance carried out in postoperative patients by urine diversion. The sum of left and right SGFR is also well correlated with the total creatinine clearance. A fairly good correlation was observed between the SGFR and $HgCl_2$ uptake test. A comparison with intravenous pyelography has shown in one-third of the cases a significant discrepancy, which confirms that renal function can only grossly be estimated by X-ray methods. A recent preliminary follow-up study on vesicoureteric reflux patients (Piepsz et al. 1978 b) did not show any significant SGFR change, whatever the grade of reflux, the degree of initial SGFR alteration, the type of treatment (medical or surgical), and the age of the patient.

Intrarenal Transit Times

The descending part of the clinical renogram provides some information on intrarenal transport of the tracer. It is, however, strongly dependent upon the variation of plasma concentration of the tracer with time. By a mathematical technique called deconvolution, a new function called the "retention function" can be obtained which represents the shape of the renogram that would be obtained if an injection could be given directly into the renal artery. The slope of this retention function is exclusively representative of the intrarenal transit times. An international joint project devoted to the clinical indications of this is still in progress.

The normal values of transit times were determined, and this parameter was shown to be helpful in the diagnosis of obstruction and in the follow-up of relieved acute obstructions.

Abnormal transit times were observed in vesicoureteric reflux, but the significance of these alterations is still a matter of study.

The Frusemide Test

Chronic obstruction is associated with dilatation of the collecting system which is not reversed by operative interference. Neither the classic renogram nor the transit times performed on the whole renal area can differentiate obstruction from simple dilatation of the renal cavities. This is the reason why the frusemide test, already described by several authors, completes successfully and in the function of the clinical circumstances the Tc-DTPA functional test.

In conclusion, the Tc-DTPA test appears as a very complete procedure, providing multiple information on the separate renal function, the intrarenal transport, and the renal emptying under frusemide.

References

Piepsz A et al. (1977) Eur J Nucl Med 2:173
Piepsz A et al. (1978 a) J Pediatr 93:769
Piepsz A et al. (1978 b) 2nd Congress of the European Society of Nuclear Medicine. London

Separate Renal Function Evaluation by I 131-Hippuran in Chronic Renal Obstruction

M. Mebel, P. Müller, B. Schönberger, D. Strangfeld, and H. Siewert

The estimation of the function of hydronephrosis due to the partial and intermittent pelviureteric junction obstruction is very difficult. Knowledge of divided renal function is helpful in the surgical management of patients with hydronephrosis. In 59 patients with pelviureteric junction obstruction we performed renal sequential scintigraphy by a standard technique using an Anger Camera (Dyna-Camera 3C/12 Fa. Picker with Krupp-Atlas Computer). After an injection of I 131-Hippuran in average 250 μCi the split renal function in percentage was estimated using the integral from zero to the 2nd minute and a background correction (Strangfeld et al. 1979). We found that the degree of impairment of drainage and the split renal function did not proceed parallel (Table 1).

Twenty-three patients were treated conservatively. Nine of them underwent pyeloplasty some years ago. But we had to decide if the second pyeloplasty was needed or not. Function and drainage were better in this group than in the group in which pyeloplasty was indicated. Thirty-two patients were treated by a pyeloplasty. Eighteen patients had an impaired drainage function but a normal parenchymal function of the obstructed kidney. Even advanced and "big" hydronephrosis in ten patients still showed a split parenchymal function of about 30%. On the strength of X-ray image and sequential renal scintigraphy the primary nephrectomy was performed in four patients. The function of obstructed kidney was below 20% of the global function.

Follow-up investigations of divided renal function were performed in two groups (operated and nonoperated patients). No difference was observed in com-

Table 1. Results of renal sequential scintigraphy in patients with pelviureteric junction obstruction.

Separate renal function of the obstructed kidney in percentage	Conservative treatment	Pyeloplasty	Primary nephrectomy
40%	15 (4)	18***	–
30% – 39%	5 (3)	10*	–
20% – 29%	1 (1)	–	–
20%	2** (1)	4*	4
	23 (9)	32	4

* Case(s) with bilateral pelviureteric junction obstruction.
() Patients underwent pyeloplasty some years ago but with unsatisfactory results.

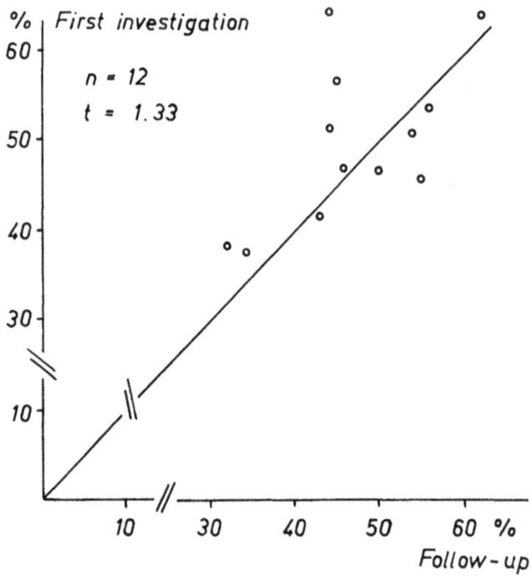

Fig. 1. Separate renal function of the obstructed kidneys which were treated conservatively. There is no difference between the two investigations during an observation period of 1 year.

parison of the first and the second investigation (after 12 months) in patients who were treated conservatively (Fig. 1).

The split parenchymal function also remained unchanged pre- and postoperatively during an observation period of 2 years in patients who underwent a pyeloplasty (Fig. 2).

There were only two exceptions. In one case of an asymmetric horseshoe kidney the "healthy" part showed a decreased parenchymal function, but the whole kidney, an unchanged global function. The second patient underwent an acute pyelonephritic episode on the day of preoperative investigation. The postoperative investigation demonstrated a much better split function. The shape of the radioisotope renography altered in only half the cases. The other patients had an unchanged renogram curve. A similar observation was reported by Bratt et al. (1977). We believe

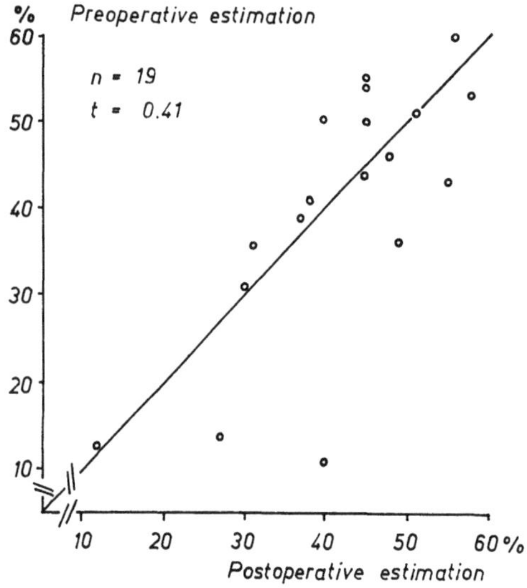

Fig. 2. Separate renal function of the obstructed kidneys which were treated surgically. There is no difference between the pre- and postoperative investigations.

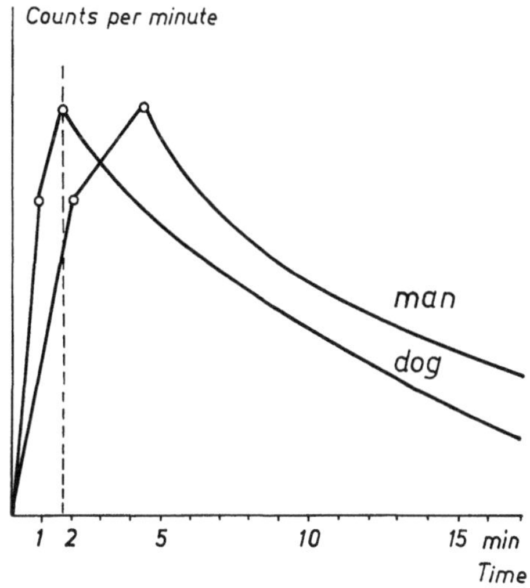

Fig. 3. Comparison of radioisotope renograms from humans and dogs. The time parameters of the dog curve are shortened significantly.

that improvement occurred more often when there was an interval of a year or more between surgery and the repeat renogram (Davis et al. 1969).

The moderately decreased renal function in sequential scintigraphy in some cases was contradictory to the X-ray and the intraoperative findings. Some authors (Doppelfeld et al. 1979, Creutzing et al. 1979) believe it can be proved that the divided renal function estimation included the possibility of overestimation of the obstructed kidney up to plus 10%. In their opinion a considerable part of the tracer passes the pyelon and the ureter in the estimating period up to the second min, whereas it remains in the obstructed kidney and does not leave the measuring device. This means that the obstructed kidney is overestimated and the normal one is underestimated. In an experimental study with dogs we investigated the transit time for I 131-Hippuran. Fifteen male and femal dogs weighing 20–25 kg each were

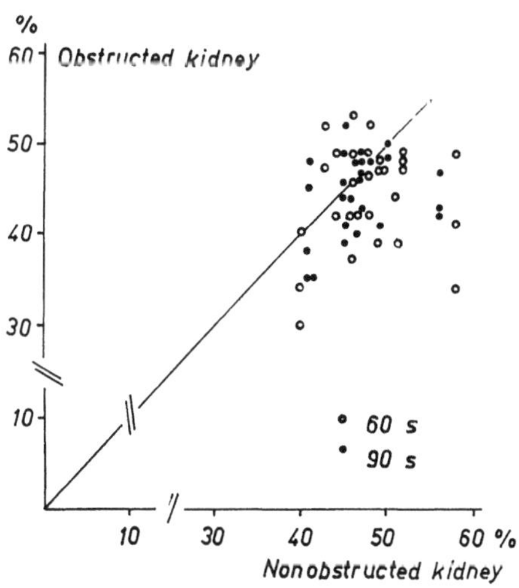

Fig. 4. Separate renal function of the nonobstructed and the obstructet kidneys in a experimental study. There is no difference using a calculation period up to the 60th and 90th s.

used. The urine was collected in 20-s periods through a catheter which was conducted from the pyelon through the ureter penetrating the skin. The count rates were measured in a well counter. We found a quick appearance of the radioactivity in urine, but the count rate until the peak of the renogram is reached is smaller than 5% in comparison to the amount of radioactivity up to the 25th min.

The comparison of the radioisotope renogram in man and in dogs illustrated the unfavorable conditions for our model (Fig. 3). The peak of the curve was reached between the 80th and 110th s. This means it was reached considerably earlier than in the human body. In our first study we examined the split renal function under normal conditions. Then the urine flow was blocked 30 s before tracer injection and released 5 or 6 min after injection. A comparison of the divided renal function in percentage of the same kidney – nonobstructed and obstructed – showed in the calculating period up to the 60th and 90th s no significant difference (Fig. 4). But by using for calculation a period after reaching the peak (for dogs up to the 120th s) the differences became significant. The calculation of the split renal function is only allowed in a period which lies before the peak of the renogram. We will report more about this study in a further publication.

Our conclusions are as follows:

1) Hydronephrosis is frequently functionally better than one would suppose from X-ray image.
2) The functional damage to the kidney with pelviureteric junction obstruction proceeds very slowly over a period of years.
3) After pyeloplasty one can evaluate an unchanged split renal function of the operated kidney as a success.
4) Overestimation of the obstructed kidney is not probable if the divided renal function is calculated in the first 2 min when the uptake of the kidney is lower than 80% of the maximal uptake.

References

Bratt C, Awell M, Nilsson S (1977) Renal function in hydronephrosis. Br J Urol 4:249–255

Creutzig H, Schindler E, Reuter ThD, Fröhlich D (1979) Abschätzung der seitengetrennten Nierenfunktion bei Harnabflußstörungen – ein Vergleich verschiedener nuklearmedizinischer Verfahren. Urologe [A] 18:316–320

Davis RJ, Jones DJ, Croft DN (1969) An assessment of Anderson-Hynes pyeloplasty by radioisotope renography. Proc R Soc Med 62:1123–1124

Doppelfeld E (1979) Untersuchungen zur I-131-Hippuran-Clearance bei der Stauungsniere. Die Extraktion von Para-Amino-Hippursäure und I-131-Hippuran in der akut gestauten Hundeniere. Nuklearmedizin 18:181–185

Doppelfeld E, Weissbach L (1979) Untersuchungen zum Einfluß von Harnabflußstörungen auf die Ergebnisse der katheterlosen seitengetrennten Bestimmung der renalen Hippuran-Clearance. Aktuel Urol 10:85–94

Doppelfeld E, Weissbach L, Hanisch K, Breuel HP, Wesener K, Winkler C (1978) Wird die Steigerung der gesamten Phase II des ING durch Harnabflußstörungen beeinflußt? Nuc Compact 9:6–7

Strangfeld D, Müller P, Schönberger B, Correns HJ (1979) Die Bedeutung der seitengetrennten Funktionsszintigraphie bei der Beurteilung urologisch-nephrologischer Erkrankungen. Dtsch Gesundheit-Wesen 34:97–101

Separate Renal Function Evaluation by DMSA

C. C. Abbou, J. L. Moretti, D. Chopin, E. Sanabria, M. Msallag, T. Nebout, and J. Auvert

Radioisotope exploration of the kidneys allows separate renal function determination without retrograde catheterization (Taylor and Nelson 1979). Dimercaptosuccinic acid (DMSA) is a chelate which was first used as a protective agent against irradiation, in the deintoxication of heavy metals, and in the treatment of schistomiasis (Cannava and Cugarra 1961; Fraga de Azevedo and Braganca 1966). DMSA labeled with technetium 99m (DMSA sn ^{99}Tc) was proposed to obtain images of renal parenchyma (Enlander et al. 1974; Lin et al. 1974; Arnold et al. 1975; Mandmaker et al. 1975; Vanlic Razumedic and Gorkic 1976; Daly et al. 1977); afterwards it was used as an index for separate renal function (Moretti et al. 1975; Raynaud et al. 1975; Dumery et al. 1977; Rapin et al. 1979).

The stability and stereochemical form of this complex is dependent on the pH in specific concentration ($1/3 < SnCl_2/DMSA < 1/2$). In an acid pH, the complex has shown very satisfactory renal fixation (Raynaud 1975). Our preliminary studies using two complexes (DMSA/Sn 2/1) have shown that the plasmatic transport takes place preferentially according to the non-specific linkage with an alphaglobulin and albumin.

Renal fixation primarily takes place in the cortex. The mechanism of fixation for this complex hexa- (Fraga de Azevedo and Braganca 1966), penta- (Krejcarer et al. 1976), or tetralinkage (Laroche and Travert 1979) is still controversial. The fixation requires the dissociation of the complex into separate molecules of DMSA ^{99}Tc; the liberated functional thiols then fix to the renal tubular proteins (Laroche and Travert 1979). The microsomes in the proximal renal tubules constituted the preferential fixation site (Raynaud 1975).

A study concerning 131 renal scintigraphies using DMSA Tc 99m was made in order to determine the place of DMSA in the evaluation of separate renal function and its value in an urologic work up. This DMSA Tc 99m has certain advantages over mercury bichloride: limited irradiation, better image quality, tracer availability, and the possibility of completing the examination in 24 h.

Material and Methods

The agent used was furnished by Saclay's C.E.N. The complex is obtained in a pH of 2 by the addition of Tc 99m pertechnetate (produced by a generator) to a lyophilic mixture of DMSA $SnCl_2$ of inositol and an antioxidator preservative (ascorbic acid).

The DMSA is injected intravenously. Renal scanning is performed at the 3rd and 6th h using a posterior incidence. The count was corrected in function of the muscle and bone background activity. Kidney depth was estimated according to Raynaud formula (1975):

$$D(\text{cm}) = -1.017 + 0.049\,P\,(\text{kg}) + 2.198\,T\,(\text{m})$$

where D = renal depth, P = weight, T = height.

Percentage of fixation was thus obtained by the following formula:

$$\text{Fix R} = \frac{T_R - T_f}{T_0} \cdot \frac{A_0}{A_i} \times 100\,,$$

where T_R = kidney area count, T_f = background count, T_0 = count from the renal depth control, A_i = injected radioactive dose, and A_0 = radioactive dose of the control.

This formula was also used by Tauxe and Burfe (1968) for adults more than 19 years old.

The blood and urinary cinetic evaluations were obtained in 12 patients by sequential blood samples connected to a scintigraphic recorder at the 3rd and 6th h. One hundred and thirty-one renal scans were performed; five groups of patients were studied:

1) A control group of 16 patients,
2) A group of 36 patients with a solitary kidney,
3) A group of 31 patients with a unilateral nephropathy,
4) A group of 37 patients with bilateral nephropathy. (We have separated in this group the patients presenting symmetrical renal lesions from those presenting obviously asymmetrical lesions.)
5) A group of 11 patients with normal renal function presenting obstructive uropathy without prior surgical treatment.

The following biologic tests were performed: creatinemia, creatinuria, BUN and urine urea, beta 2 microglobulin, and alphaglobulin. All patients were satisfactorily hydrated (diuresis > 1500 ml/24 h). Medications that could eventually modify the percentage of fixation by competition with specific protein carriers such as Lipavlon, phenylbutazone, sulfamids, and Dihydan were discontinued. The delivered dose to the kidneys varied from 0.6 to 0.76 mCi^{-1}.

Results

The urinary activity collected over 6 h was 12% of the injected dose. The plasmatic activity decreased according to a multiexponential mode. Thus there probably exists a complex compartmental model (> 2 compartments).

In the control group the average percentage of fixation is from 25.7% ± 2.48% for the right kidney and 24.4% ± 2.86% for the left kidney (Fig. 1). In the group of

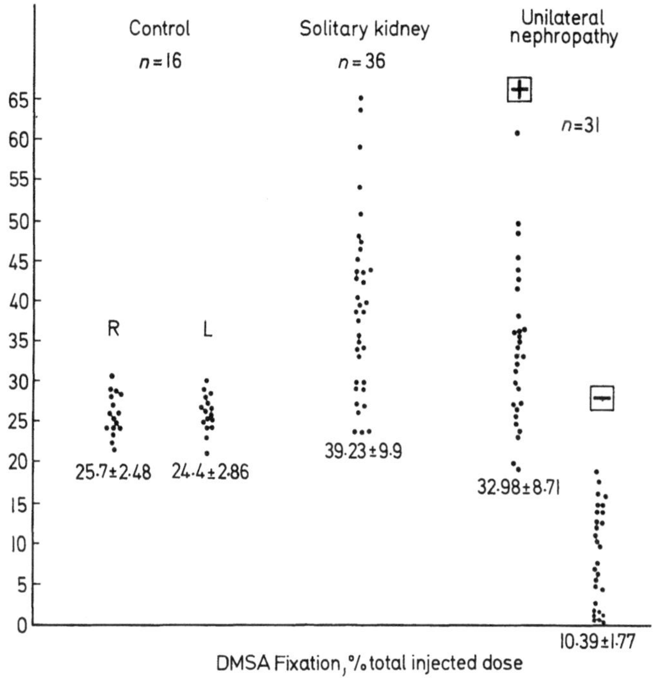

Fig. 1. Average value of DMSA fixation in control group, in solitary kidneys, and in unilateral uropathy group.

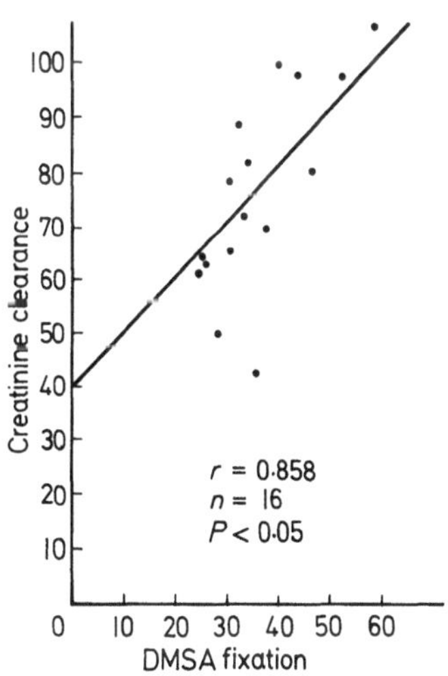

Fig. 2. The correlation between the renal fixation of DMSA and urinary clearance of creatinin in the group of solitary kidneys.

36 patients with a single kidney the indications of nephrectomy are shown in the Table 1. The average value of fixation is from 39.23% ± 9.9% (Fig. 1). This elevated percentage expresses the phenomenon of compensating hypertrophy existing in certain patients.

Table 1. Solitary kidneys after surgery. Disease of the kidney removed.

Hydronephrosis	12
Renal hypoplasia and HBP	5
Lumbar contusion	3
Renal lithiasis	4
Pyonephrosis	2
Renal artery stenosis	1
Renal tuberculosis	4
Renal haemorrhage	2
Retroperitoneal fibrosis	2
Bladder tumor	1
Total	36

Table 2. Unilateral nephropathy and renal disease.

Junction syndrome	4
Renal hypoplasia and HBP	3
Renal aplasia	2
Pyonephrosis	2
Pyelonephritis	1
Vesicorenal reflux	1
Renal lithiasis	2
Total	15

In 16 patients there was a correlation between the value of fixation and the clearance of creatinine ($r = 0.858$, $P < 0.05$) (Fig. 2). In the group with unilateral nephropathy, the average fixation is from 10.39% ± 1.77% for pathologic kidneys and 32.98% ± 8.71% for healthy kidneys. These quantitative findings clearly suggest that the healthy kidney compensates for the pathologic kidney. After renal scanning 15 patients underwent nephrectomies; the other patients either had conservative surgery or no surgery. The fixation value for the removed kidneys ranged from 0.4% to 9% with an average of 4.33% ± 4.04%. The causes resulting in nephrectomy are shown in Table 2.

In the group of patients having bilateral nephopathy 19 patients had a symmetrical bilateral nephropathy with an average fixation of 9.67% ± 5.51% for the right kidneys and 8.46% ± 6.2% for the left kidneys. The creatinemia ranged from 15 to 50 mg with an average of 24.73% ± 9.24% (Fig. 3).

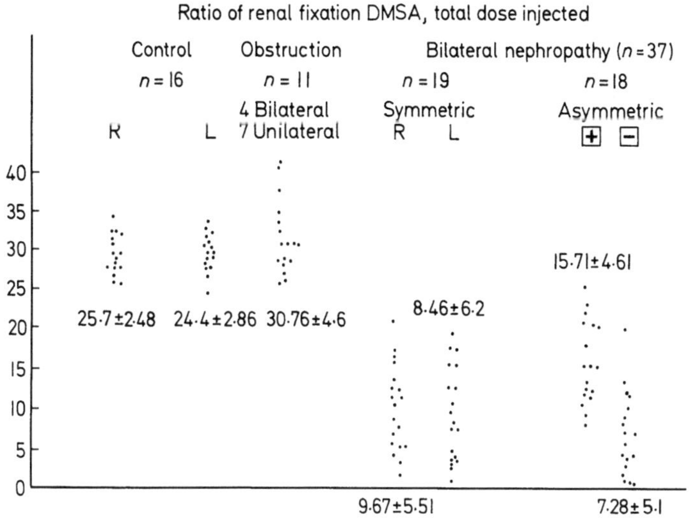

Fig. 3. The average values of DMSA fixation in the control group, in obstructive uropathy, and in the group with bilateral nephropathy.

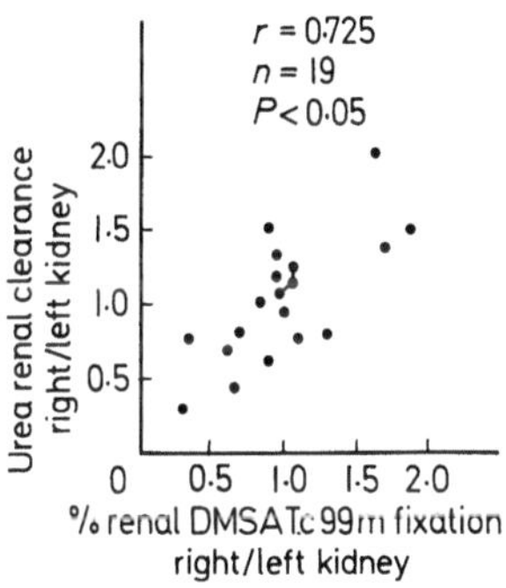

Fig. 4. Correlation between separate urea renal clearance and renal DMSA Tc 99 m fixation.

Eighteen patients had an asymmetrical nephropathy. The average fixations is 7.28% ± 5.1% in the most severely diseased kidneys and 15.71% ± 4.61% in the other kidney, with creatinemia ranging from 150 to 1500 μmol/liter and the average being 354.3 ± 448.8.

Between groups 3 and 4 19 patients had separate urine collections after surgical treatment of an uni- or bilateral uropathy. A correlation existed when we compared the ratio of separate kidney urea clearance and separate kidney fixation of DMSA ($r = 0.725$, $P < 0.05$) (Fig. 4). However, the group of patients having an obstructive uropathy and maintaining normal renal function present an elevated renal fixation when comparing the average fixation value to the control group (m = 30.75% ± 4.6%).

Discussion

Renal scanning has been proposed as a useful complementary exploration in the radiologic and biologic work-up that attempts to more precisely substantiate therapeutic indications and provide continued control of the functional value of a kidney after conservative surgery. DMSA has been selected because of its numerous advantages over others tracers. The renal scanner using mercury bichloride introduced by Raynaud remains the most precise and consistently reproducible quantitative functional means of kidney exploration (Raynaud 1975). However, the practical use of mercury bichloride is limited because of its radiotoxicity and the complexity of the methodology.

The isotopic renogram obtained by Hippuran 131 studies the function of renal excretion (Taplin et al. 1963). Xenon 133 is a satisfactory index of renal perfusion and thus has a specific indication in patients with renal artery disease (Cosgrove and Raphael 1968). DMSA Tc 99m is both an index of renal perfusion and renal excretion; however, its most important test is qualitative analysis.

As with mercury bichloride, DMSA evaluates the function of renal fixation (capacity of renal tubules to fix heavy metals). Therefore, it is an index of the functional cortical mass which differs from the tubular renal function studied by renal clearances. This explains why until recently in renal pathology there has been no direct comparison made between fixation and renal clearance.

The first results presented by different authors (Raynaud 1975; Kawamura et al. 1978) suggested a certain number of errors when using DMSA: firstly, the loss of precision in early measurement, which is the consequence of the excreted fraction which exaggerates the fixation rate in renal obstruction, and secondly, the instability of the complex after being labeled with technetium.

The average results obtained in our controlled studies are similar to those reported by other authors (Table 3). Moreover, our result variations were reduced by 50% when compared to equivalent result variations reported by other authors. This may be explained by the greater stability of the DMSA furnished by Saclay's C.E.N.

The results obtained in obstructive uropathy demonstrated an overestimation of renal function which was probably related to a stagnation of the product in the renal cavities (Bin Gham and Maisey 1978). Certain authors proposed to measure the re-

Table 3. DMSA fixation – control values. Review of literature.

	Number of patients	Right kidney	Left kidney	Total	Product
Study presented	16	25.7±2.5	24.4±2.9	50.1±4	DMSA (CEN)
Kawamura et al. (1978)	65	27.8±5.5	26.2±6.5	54 ±8.8	DMSA (Mediphysics)
Raynaud (1975)	11	27.2±6	27.2±4.8	54.4±8	DMSA (Mediphysics) 57 Patients DMSA (CEN) 27 Patients

Table 4. DMSA fixation – values obtained in renal pathology. Review of literature.

	Unilateral nephropathy		Solitary kidney	Symmetric bilateral nephropathy		Asymmetric bilateral nephropathy	
	Safe kidney	Pathologic kidney		Left kidney	Right kidney	Pathologic kidney	More pathologic kidney
Study presented	$n=31$ 33±8.7	8.7±6.2	$n=36$ 39.2± 9.9	$n=19$ 6.4±6.2	9.7±5.5	$n=18$ 15.7±6.6	7.3±5.1
	Total: 41.7±10			Total: 18.1±8.3		Total: 23±8	
Kawamura et al. (1978)	$n=77$ 29.1±7.2	9.1±5	$n=29$ 38.0±10.6	$n=19$ 10.1±5.7	12.1±5.8	$n=13$ 14.6±4.4	4.0±2.8
	Total: 38.0±8.3			Total: 22.2±11.2		Total: 18.5±5.2	

nal fixation after the 24th h in order to permit maximum elimination of the product. In the different pathologic groups, our results confirmed those found by Kawamura et al. (1978) (Table 4). In the group with a solitary kidney or unilateral nephropathy, scanning clearly demonstrates the evidence of compensatory hypertrophy of the healthy kidney. In the case of either uni- or bilateral kidney disease, renal scanning allows one to both objectively recognize and quantify renal disease.

There exist a satisfactory correlation in the group of patients with solitary kidneys between creatinine clearance and the percentage of fixation of DMSA. Moreover, in the group of patients in which urine was collected separately, there was a significant correlation between the ratio of urea excretion over 24 h and the ratio of fixation between both kidneys. The awareness of the advantages and the disadvantages of the DMSA with respect to the other tracer clearly indicates the place of DMSA renal scanning in a urologic work-up:

1) As an objective appreciation of the value of separate kidney function when discussing the possibility of conservative surgery or nephrectomy while understanding the limits of this method in the case of obstructive uropathy;
2) the appreciation of the benefit of conservative surgery and long-term follow-up;
3) the determination of the quantitative value of compensating hypertrophy in patients with unilateral disease or after nephrectomy.

Summary

Renal uptake of DMSA Tc 99m was studied to evaluate divided renal function. One hundred and thirty-one patients were distributed in five groups: normal (16), patients with a single kidney (36), unilateral (31) or bilateral (37) renal disease, or obstructive uropathy (11). Each patient received DMSA Tc 99m (C.E.N. Saclay) intravenously. A quantitative scintigraphic examination was performed 6 h afterwards.

In normal subjects, right renal uptake was 25.7% ± 2.5% and left renal uptake was 24.4% ± 2.9%. Correlation between the uptake and creatinine clearance was obtained in the 16 patients with compensatory hypertrophic kidneys ($r = 0.858$). In case of diseased kidneys, the ration of DMSA uptake between both kidneys correlated significantly with the ratio of urea output ($r = 0.725$).

These results are helpful in decisions affecting conservative surgery or nephrectomy and to appreciate compensatory hypertrophy. Quantitative renal scintigraphy with DMSA TC 99m does not appear to be useful in obstructive uropathy.

Acknowledgment. We would like to thank Dr. James Goldberg for his help in the edition and translation of this paper.

References

Arnold RW, Subramanian G, McAfee JG, Blair RJ, Thomas FD (1975) Comparison of 99m Tc complexes for renal imaging. J Nucl Med 16:357–367

Bin Gham JB, Maisey MN (1978) An evaluation of the use of 99m Tc dimercaptosuccinic acid (DMSA) as a static renal imaging agent. Br J Radiol 51:599–607

Cannava A, Cugurra F (1961) Pharmacologic activity and antitoxic properties of dimercaptosuccini acids. Arch Int Pharmacodyn Ther 131:283–300

Cosgrove E, Raphael J (1968) The use of xenon 133 to measure blood flow in patients. Br J Surg 55:245

Daly MJ, Jones WA, Rudd TG, Tremann JA (1977) Differential Tc 99m dimercaptosuccinic and renal localisation, correlation with renal function. J Nucl Med 18:594–595

Dumery JP, Reaulth, Rapin JR, Moretti JL, Galle P (1977) Study of the fixation of a complexe dimercaptosuccinic acid (DMSA) technitium. Comm. First European Congress on Nuclear Medecine, Lausanne

Enlander D, Weber PH, Dos Remedios LV (1974) Renal cortical imaging in 35 patients superior quality with 99m Tc DMSA. J Nucl Med 15:743–749

Evrin PE, Wibell (1973) Serum β_2 microglobulin in various disorder. Clin Chim Acta 43:183–187

Fraga de Azevedo J, Braganca G (1966) Absorption and elimination of Atisban labeled with 12n Sb. An Inst Med Trop (Lisbon) 23:191–198

Johannsen B, Spiles H, Syhre R (1979) Study on complexation of Tc 99m with dimercaptosuccinic acids with regards to organ specificity of Tc 99m radiopharmacocorticals. Eur J Nucl Med 2:148

Kawamura J, Mosokana S, Yoshida O (1978) Validity of 99m Tc dimercaptosuccinic acid renal uptake for an assessment of individual kidney function. J Urol 119:305–309

Krejcarer GE et al. (1976) The structures of stannous dimercaptosuccinic acid chelates. J Nucl Med 17:565

Laroche D, Travert G (1979) Etude physicochimique et biologique d'un agent scintigraphique rénal. J Fr Biophys Med Nucl 3, 4:181–198

Lin TH, Khentigan A, Winchell WS (1974) A 99m Tc chelate substitute for organomercurial renal agents. J Nucl Med 15:34–35

Mandmaker H, Young BW, Lowenstein LM (1975) Clinical experience with 99m Tc DMSA, a new renal imaging agent. J Nucl Med 16:28–32

Moretti JL, Meignan M, Dumery JP, Galle P, Auvert J, Lagrue G (1975) Le dimercaptosuccinate de Technetium en exploration rénale 99m Tc DMSA. Nouv Presse Méd 19:1430

O'Reilly PM et al. (1977) Dynamic scintigraphy in clinical urology. Br J Urol 49:575–582

Price RR, Born ML, Jones JP (1979) Comparison of differential renal function determination by Tc 99m DMSA, Tc 99m DTPA, I 131 Hippuran and ureteral catheterization. J Nucl Med 20:631

Rapin JR, Moretti JL, Compagnon M (1979) Fixation rénale du complexe doublement marqué Acide Dimercapto-2-3-succinique 14C,2,3 Sn 99m Tc. Comm. XX Coll. Med. Nucl. Bordeaux, 20–22 Sept., I, 21–22

Raynaud C (1975) La fixation rénale du mercure et du DMSA. In: Raynaud C (ed) Compte-rendu du 11ème Colloque International sur la Fixation Rénale. Svce Doc. C.E.N.-Saclay, Paris, 24–25 Oct.

Taplin GV, Dore EK, Johnson DE (1963) The quantitative radiorenogram for total and differential renal blood flow measurement. J Nucl Med 4:404

Taylor A, Nelson M (1979) Current status of quantitative differential renal scanning. Applied Radiology, May, pp 111–114

Taylor A, Hollenbeck J, Hagan PL (1979) DMSA scanning: an index of relative renal plasma flow. J Nucl Med 20:630–631

Tauxe WN, Burfe EC (1968) Kidney depth and isotope renography. J Nucl Med 9:225

Vanlic Razumedic NM, Gorkic DA (1976) Studies of chemical and biological properties of 99m Tc DMS renal imaging agent. Eur J Nucl Med 1:232–242

Wibell L, Evrin PE, Berggard I (1973) Serum β_2 microglobulin in renal disease. Nephron 10:320–331

Catheter-Free Isotope Reflux Studies

P. Alken, G. Hutschenreiter, and K. Hahn

Three different techniques to establish the diagnosis of reflux are currently available: conventional X-ray micturition cystography, direct radionuclide cystography (Winter 1959; Rothwell and Constable 1977), and indirect radionuclide cystography (Dodge 1963; Rothwell and Constable 1977). The latter technique offers the special advantage of simultaneous determination of kidney morphology, split renal function, and reflux. The radiation dose is low (Hedmann et al. 1978) and catheterization of the bladder with the hazard of introducing infection is avoided.

Methods and Patients

After intravenous injection of 1–2 μCi of 123-Iodine-Hippuran, gamma camera scintigraphy is performed and split renal function calculated with computerized background substraction. When scintiscanning shows the kidney collecting system to be free of isotope material – usually within 20 min – low pressure reflux is simulated by manual bladder compression in a supine position. High pressure reflux is recorded during voiding, the patient in a sitting position. Reflux is determined either by visual monitoring of the scintiscanning photographs that are taken in 5-s intervals or by the time–activity curve registered over the kidney region.

Sixty-two patients with recurrent urinary tract infection in 48 cases, recurrent pyelonephritis in 30, and previous positive reflux studies in 15 were subjected to indirect radionuclide cystography with 123-Iodine-Hippuran, conventional micturition cystoureterogram and IVP, usually within 1 month.

Results

There were identical findings with both investigations, showing reflux in 16 patients and no reflux in 24 (Table 1). Radionuclide cystography missed four refluxes that had been radiologically documented. In 18 patients reflux was only detected during the isotope investigation.

The IVPs of group 1 and 2 patients showed a high rate of pyelonephritic changes. This was a rare finding in group 4 patients, who showed no reflux in either examination.

Table 1. Incidence of reflux and pyelonephritis in 62 patients.

Group		Reflux	Pyelonephritis
1	Isotope + X-ray +	16	13 of 16 = 81%
2	Isotope + X-ray −	18	14 of 18 = 78%
3	Isotope − X-ray −	4	1 of 4 = 25%
4	Isotope − X-ray −	24	2 of 24 = 8%

Discussion

Discrepancies between X-ray and isotope reflux studies are explained by three factors:

1) Continuous monitoring on the gamma camera during isotope studies detects intermittent phases of reflux that are missed during X-ray examination with spot films.
2) The viscosity of the contrast medium used during the X-ray examination may impede free reflux.
3) Reflux is not a constant finding in the same patient.

In this patient series, however, an additional factor is of interest: most urologists would agree that reflux is the cause of the pyelonephritic changes in group 1 patients with positive X-ray findings. The nearly identical rate of pyelonephritic changes in group 2 patients with positive findings only during the isotope studies seems to indicate that this technique is even able to detect an earlier reflux that had been the cause of pyelonephritis but can no longer be detected during radiologic investigation. This situation is often described as "reflux maturation."

The findings in two patients will serve to illustrate the value of the isotope technique.

Case 1. The IVP (Fig. 1 a) of a 9-year-old child with recurrent urinary tract infection and fever shows pyelonephritic scarring of the lower part of the duplicated collecting system. Reflux in these cases is a frequent finding. Micturition cystography showed no reflux (Fig. 1 b). Isotope studies done on the same day revealed a high pressure reflux in the lower left collecting system (Fig. 2). In this case, the isotope study confirmed the reflux that had to be expected because of the anatomic situation. One might argue that a second radiologic investigation could equally have detected reflux, but this would only be at the risk of another exposure to radiation.

Case 2. The higher sensitivity of the radioisotope method is demonstrated in this case. A 38-year-old woman was first investigated for recurrent urinary tract infection at the age of 5. Reflux on the left side was documented, but for unknown reasons, no antireflux operation had been performed. Since the age of 29 she again had recurrent bouts of urinary infection. Reflux studies from 1974, 1976, and 1978 (Fig. 3) never showed more than reflux in the lower left ureter. Not the low-grade reflux documented between 1974 and 1978 but probably a high-grade reflux in

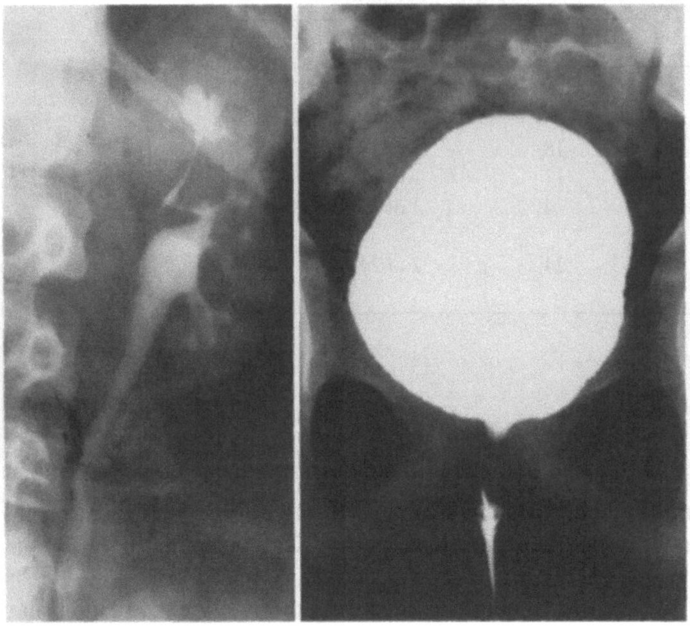

Fig. 1. a IVP of 9-year-old child with recurrent urinary tract infection and fever. b Absence of reflux on micturition cystography.

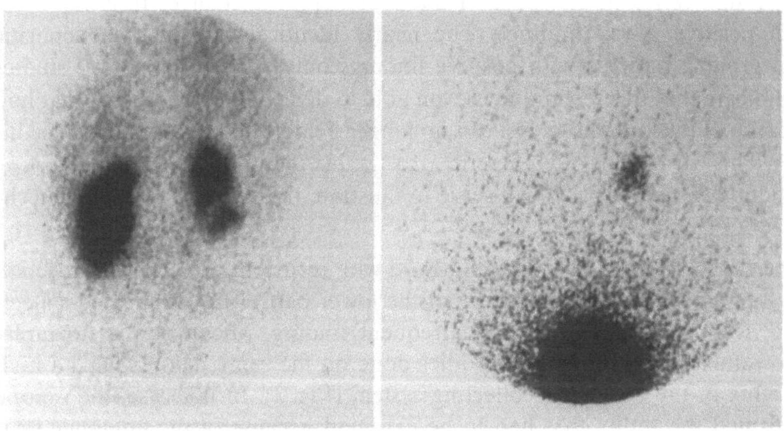

Fig. 2. a Kidney scintiscanning shows reduced accumulation of tracer in the lower part of the left kidney. b After tracer excretion into the bladder. Reflux into the lower part of the left kidney is shown during the "low pressure" study.

childhood was the cause for the pyelonephritic scarring of both kidneys (Fig. 4). The reflux isotope studies done in 1978 clearly documented a still-existing vesicorenal reflux on both sides (Fig. 5).

In the series of patients we investigated, the mean age was 29 years. Isotope studies showed a high sensitivity in a retrospective manner, detecting reflux as the

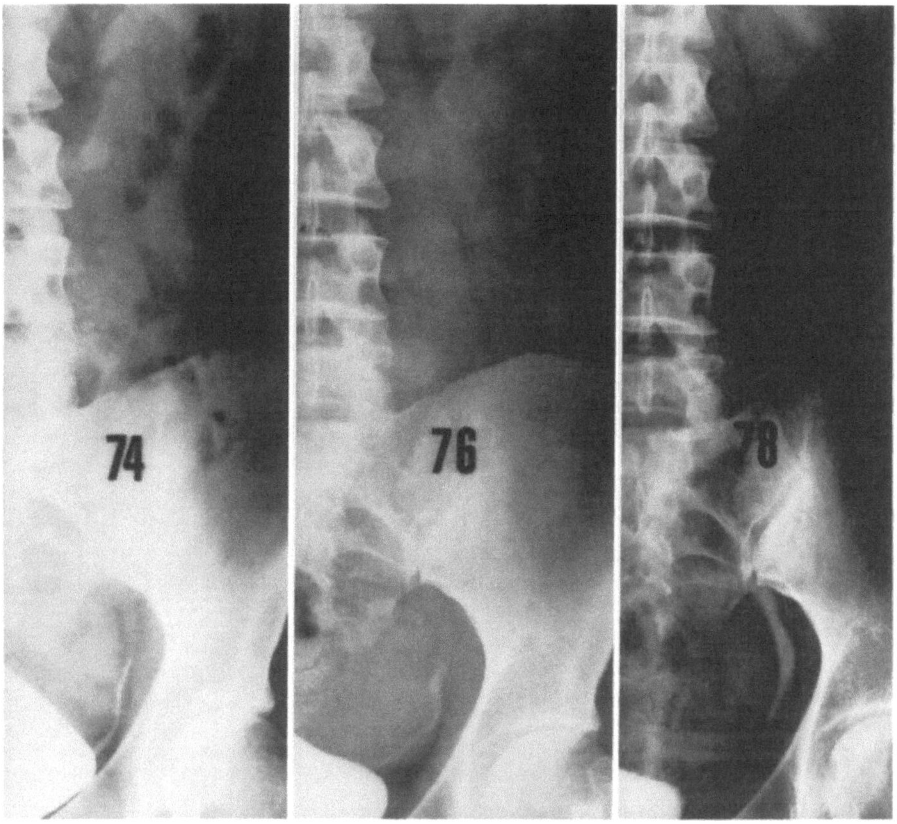

Fig. 3. Studies from 1974, 1976, and 1978 showing low-grade reflux in case 2.

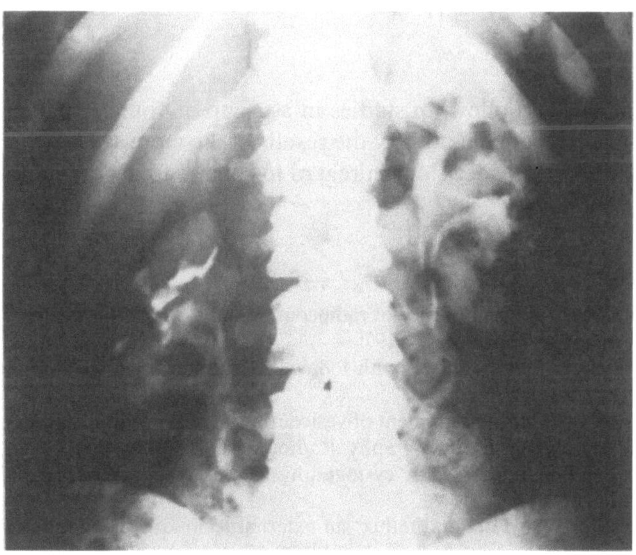

Fig. 4. Pyelonephritic scarring of both kidneys (case 2).

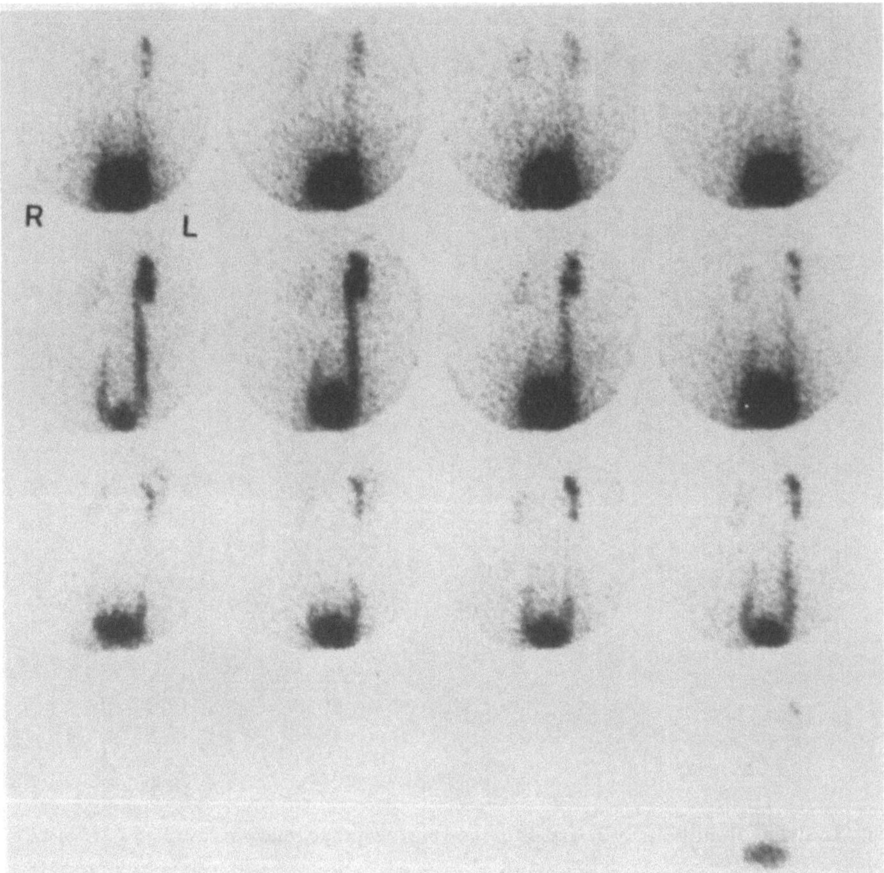

Fig. 5. Bilateral vesicorenal reflux during low-pressure and high-pressure conditions (figures must be read from right to left).

possible cause of pyelonephritis. Follow-up studies in a group of younger patients are currently underway to determine if and how the results of the more sensitive isotope study will influence therapeutic decisions in regard to conservative or operative treatment.

References

Baker GA, Lum DJ, Smith EM (1974) Significance of radiocontaminants in ^{123}J for dosimetry and scintillation camera imaging. J Nucl Med 4: 197

Dodge EA (1963) Vesicoureteric reflux: diagnosis with iodine-131 sodium ortho-iodohippurate. Lancet 1:303

Hedmann JK, Kempi V, Voss H (1978) Measurement of vesicoureteral reflux with intravenous 99mTc-DTPA compared to radiographic cystography. Radiology 126:205

Rothwell DL, Constable AR (1977) Radionuclide cystography in the management of vesico ureteric reflux. BJU 49:621

Winter CC (1959) A new test for vesico-ureteral reflux: an external technique using radioisotopes. J Urol 81: 105

Quantitative Bone Scanning and the Supervision of Bone Metastases in Prostatic Cancer

C. Bollack, G. Methlin, A. Oliveux, J. C. Grob, and I. Carloz

Bone scanning, the isotopic exploration of the skeleton, holds at the present time a privileged place among the techniques for assessing the extension of osteophilic cancers, especially prostatic cancers. In 1976 and 1979, we reported on the use of this simple test for the early detection and localization of bone metastases from prostatic carcinoma. In addition to the diagnostic use of bone scanning, we investigated the possibility of using quantitative techniques to evaluate the evolution of the metastatic process discovered at the first examination.

Methods

Physiopathologic Basis

When a metastasis occurs in bone, the replacement of healty tissue by neoplastic tissue causes an increase in calcium turnover which is dependent on the type of metastasis (lytic or condensing). Using a radioactive tracer whose behaviour resembles that of calcium bone salts, the local increase in calcium metabolism results in a hyperfixation of the tracer which causes an increase in radioactivity measurable by the scintillation camera.

Examination Technique

The tracer is Tc 99m methylene diphosphonate. A dose of approximately 10 mCi is administered intravenously. Two types of documents are made 2–3 h after administration:

1) First, a total body scan is done using a Picker Dynacamera and an "Omni-View" whole-body system. The information gathered during a period of 400 s is stored and processed by computer.
2) Next, static views are taken of pathologic and suspicious areas.

Once the information is stored, we determine by means of a program of selection by zones the ratio of activities between the pathologic zones and a normal zone chosen as reference (usually the humerus and occasionally the head).

We also tried to establish other criteria of fixation by using either a section of soft tissue as reference or the total activity detected during the examination.

Results

Ten patients studied with our initial protocol were retained for serial studies. After the initial quantitative bone scan we performed another 2 to 3 months after the beginning of hormone therapy. We specifically used high doses of estrogen (starting with 150 mg/day estradiol and decreasing over 6 weeks to 5 mg/day).

The results were expressed as ratios of activity between the pathologic zone and the reference zone which varied for each patient, but remained identical for the same patient. The results were then compared with the clinical course of the patient. This comparison allowed us to distinguish three groups of patients. The first group of patients corresponds to a favorable clinical course (Table 1). At the second quantitative bone scan 2–3 months after the beginning of therapy, five patients showed a regression of metastases indicated by a decrease in the fixation ratios of the pathologic zones discovered at the first scan. The degree of regression varied with each patient. Moreover, the degree of regression varied from one pathologic zone to another for the same patient, representing a different response to therapy of the different secondary localizations (Fig. 1).

Two points should be emphasized. A good correlation exists between the clinical course and the results of quantitative bone scanning. Hence, in three of the five patients the clinical examination showed a marked amelioration as a decrease in functional problems, good estrogenic impreganation, and decrease in pain when present. On the other hand, the comparison of the two total body scans showed no differences in at least three patients. The lack of change in total body scans does not allow an assessment of the course of the disease with treatment.

The second group of patients corresponds to an unfavorable clinical course (Table 2). In three of these patients quantitative bone scanning showed a deterioration of the lesions i.e., evolution of the metastases, indicated by an increase in the fixation ratios of the pathologic zones, even when the aspect of the total body scan did not permit prediction of the clinical courses (Fig. 2). The pathologic zones do not appear qualitatively to be more avid for the tracer on the second film than on the first. The increase is variable but generally parallel for all the zones, indicating a resistance or lack of response to therapy. At the same time, the clinical examination showed a clear-cut deterioration evidenced by the increase of bone pain and a worsening of the patient's general condition.

The third group (Table 3) was composed of two patients whose serial quantitative bone scans showed no significant differences. The results in these cases are difficult to interpret but seem to indicate the lack of metastatic growth and, thus, partial response to therapy which was confirmed by the clinical examination. One of the patients died of another disease.

Table 1. Group 1: Decrease in fixation ratios.

Patient	Detection	After therapy	Standard scan	Clinical course
1	EPG 3.3	2	Moderate activity	Improvement
	CD 5.2	2.7		
2	CD 8	4.4	Identical	Improvement
	CL 9.4	5.1		
3	FG 16.8	11.6	Moderate activity	Stable
	CD 23	19.5		
	CC 15.9	14.7		
4	CD 19	13.9	Identical	Stable
	SID 12.9	11.4		
	FD 14	11.6		
	EPG 12	5.4		
5	CC 5.4	4.1	Identical	Improvement
	CD 13.9	8.9		
	CC 9.4	5.6		

Table 2. Group 2: Increase in fixation ratios.

Patient	Detection	After therapy	Standard scan	Clinical course
1	AIG 4	8	Identical	Pain
	CL 9	10.5		
	ÉPD 5.6	9.4		
	CÔTE 6	9.4		
2	AIG 23	31.5	Moderate activity	Pain
	AID 5.3	5.8		
	CD 6.9	6.1		
3	AID 5.2	13.1	Identical	Poor clinical condition
	CD 8	19.4		
	CR 3.2	10.4		

Table 3. Group 3: Unmodified fixation ratios.

Patient	Detection	After therapy	Standard scan	Clinical course
1	C 1.2	1.5	Identical	Deceased
	SIG 5.5	4.8		
	SID 6.5	5.8		
	CD 3.6	4.4		
2	AI 5.7	6.4	Identical	Good condition
	CC 7.2	4.8		
	C 3	2.1		

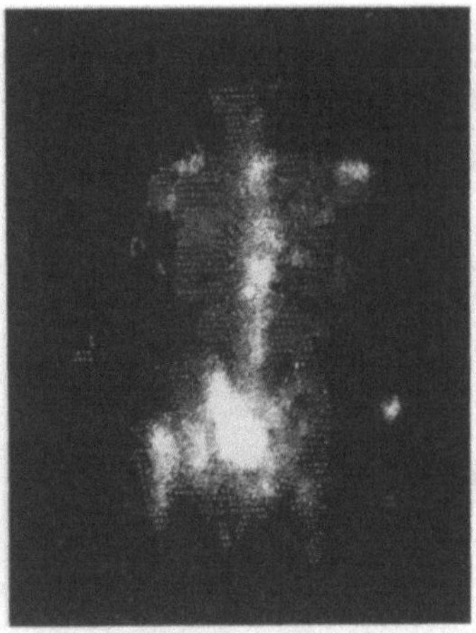

	Ratio Path. bone / Norm. bone
Left femur	16.8
Dorsal spine	22.9
Right shoulder	11.3

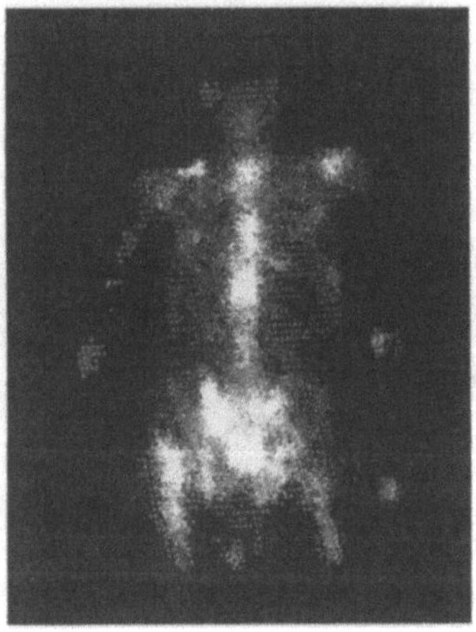

	Ratio Path. bone / Norm. bone
Left femur	11.6
Dorsal spine	19.5
Right shoulder	11.4

Fig. 1 a, b. Example of favorable response: decrease of the fixation ratio in several metastatic areas. **a** Before treatment; **b** during treatment (3 months).

L 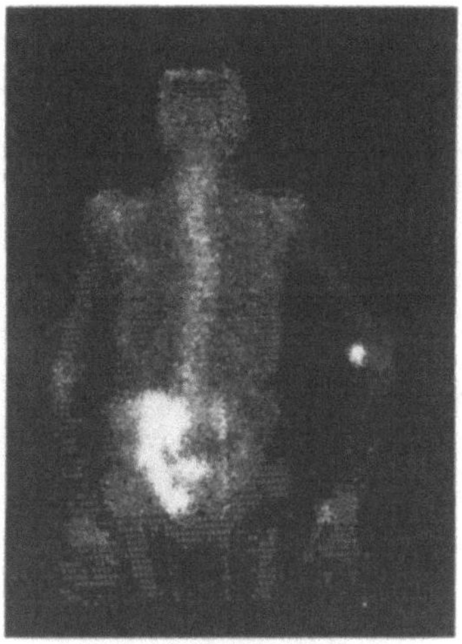 R

a

	Ratio Path. bone Norm. bone
Left ilium	23
Right ilium	5.3
Dorsal spine	6.9

L 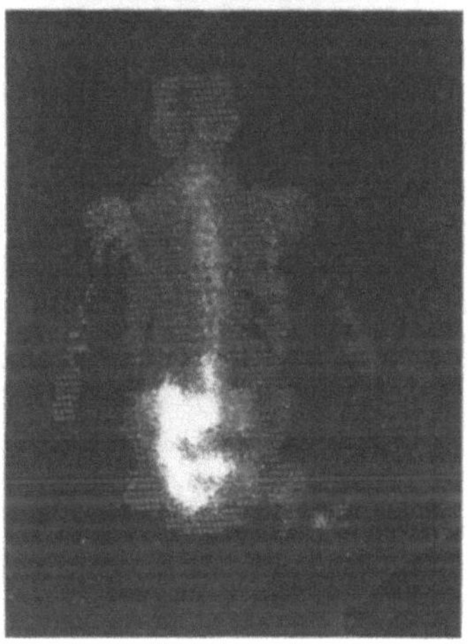 R

b

	Ratio Path. bone Norm. bone
Left ilium	31.5
Right ilium	5.8
Dorsal spine	6.1

Fig. 2a, b. Example of unfavorable evolution: increase in the fixation ratio in metastatic zones. **a** Before treatment; **b** during treatment (3 months).

Discussion

We wish to emphasize three points.

The Criteria Retained. We initially considered three possible criteria for quantifying the scan, but we were forced by our experience to discard two of the three. The ratio of activities to pathologic zone total activity was discarded since the total activity is directly linked to the quality of the patient's urinary function. Thus, this ratio changes with any patient presenting a renal insufficiency or difficulty in urine, excretion.

The ratio of activities to pathologic zone soft tissue also gave an unduly large statistical dispersion most certainly caused by the difficulty in choosing a zone of soft tissue reproducible from one examination to another. Moreover, soft-tissue activity is dependent on urinary excretion of the tracer.

Finally, we found the only valid criterion to be the ratio of activities between pathologic zone and reference zone. We discussed how we obtain this ratio in the preceding section on methodology. The only phenomenon capable of modifying this ratio would be the appearance of a metastasis in the zone of reference which was found to be normal during the first test. We never confronted such a case in our study.

The Interpretation and Validity of the Results. As stated earlier, the detection of a hyperactive zone indicates a change in the calcium turnover and must be confronted with the clinical and radiologic findings. However, we must point out that even if in most cases a hyperactive zone corresponds to a metastasis, relative hyperactive zones exist even in normal individuals, e.g., at the level of the sacroiliac joints. Moreover, certain benign osteoarticular lesions can produce a variable increase in activity. Certainly, a significant increase in the ratio indicates a metastasis but only confirms what is already obvious with the total body scan. In doubtful cases the real problem appears, since there is only a moderate increase in activity. Does this increase correspond to a metastasis? The real advantage of comparing the serial ratios is precisely in these doubtful cases.

The Advantages of Quantitative Bone Scanning. Aside from its diagnostic use in doubtful cases, quantitative bone scanning appears to be a valuable method to evaluate the evolution and the response to therapy of an osteophilic tumor. The analysis of our results clearly shows that this technique allows an objective approach to the clinical stage of a metastatic lesion undetected by other, more classical methods. The correlation of our results confirms the parallelism that exists between the clinical course and the results of quantitative bone scanning.

Conclusion

Total body scanning appears to be the best technique for detecting bone metastases in prostatic cancer. However, this technique does not allow an evaluation of the progression of the tumor. Serial studies with quantitative bone scanning, a relatively easy technique, allows an objective evaluation of the clinical course. We feel that this method should be used in the supervision of patients presenting a prostatic cancer and as an aid in conducting the therapy.

References

Adams FG, Horton PW (1978) Rectilinear bone scanning: Differentiation between metastases and degenerative spinal disease. Br J Radiol 51:281–285

Bollack C, Oliveux A, Methlin G, Vanegas M (1976) Notre expérience de la scintigraphie osseuse aux pyrophosphates technétiés dans le bilan d'extension du cancer de la prostate. J Urol Nephrol (Paris) 82:885–893

Charkes ND (1979) Mechanisms of skeletal tracer uptake. J Nucl Med 20:794–795

Citrin DL, Tuohy JB, Bessent RG, Greig WR, Blumgart IH (1974) Quantitative bone scanning. A method for assessing response of bone metastases to treatment. Lancet 1974:1132

Langhammer H, Sinterman R, Hor G, Pabst W (1978) Serial bone scintigraphy for assessing the effectiveness of treatment of osseous metastases from prostatic cancer. Nuklearmedizin 17:87–91

Lurye DR, Castronovo FP, Potsaid MS (1977) An improved method for quantitative bone scanning. J Nucl Med 18:1069–1073

Oliveux A, Grob JC, Moyses B, Methlin G, Bollack C (1979) Mise au point sur les explorations isotopiques du squelette dans les cancers de la prostate. Ann Urol 13:167–171

Piard JN, Moreau R, Vailland F, Souaille C, Minher JF, Larra F (1978) Scintigraphie numérique du squelette: intérêt dans la surveillance des cancers ostéophiles. Nouv Presse Med 7:1216

Robillard J, Couette JE, Lemouel J, Lyvanho A, Vernhes JC, Chedeville R (1976) Exploration quantitative et qualitative des métastases osseuses par scintigraphie corporelle totale à l'aide du 99m Tc pyrophosphate. J Radiol Electrol Med Nucl 57:424–433

Rudd TG, Allen DR, Hartnett DE (1977) Tc-99m Methylene Diphosphonate versus Tc-99m Pyrophosphate: Biologic and clinical comparison. J Nucl Med 18:872–876

Prostatic Lymphoscintigraphy

J. M. Fitzpatrick, A. R. Constable, and R. W. Cranage

Introduction

There is not much doubt that reliable imaging of prostatic lymph nodes could play a significant role in the staging and clinical management of prostatic cancer. Neither radiographic (lymphography) nor radionuclide (lymphoscintigraphy) methods have yet been developed sufficiently to be accepted as viable diagnostic procedures. The former technique relies on a passively introduced contrast medium while the latter depends primarily on the functional activity of phagocytes and macrophages for the removal of a radioactive colloid from the injection site into the lymphatic system. It would seem logical then that lymphoscintigraphy, with its more functional mode of operation, could be expected to yield more relevant clinical information when fully developed.

Lymphoscintigraphy has been used with some success in the assessment of lymph nodes in breast cancer (Boak and Agwunobi 1978; Ege 1978; Ege et al. 1979) but it has not yet gained widespread acceptance as a routine diagnostic procedure. There is little doubt, however, that in breast cancer the techniques of lymphoscintigraphy are sufficiently advanced to provide helpful additional means for assessing nodal involvement. Patterns of normality are fairly well-established and experienced workers (Ege et al. 1979) are able to interpret departures from normality with some confidence.

For any diagnostic procedure to become a successful routine investigation, it must acquire a high degree of reproducibility and achieve a large measure of simplification both to execute and to interpret. However, the very large range of variations that exist between normal patients and between those with some degree of abnormality have made these aims difficult to achieve for lymphoscintigraphy and have presented experienced workers with considerable problems in conveying satisfactory assessment criteria.

Internal mammary lymphoscintigraphy involves a small injection of a suitable colloid material labelled with ^{99m}Tc. Injections are normally made into the posterior rectus sheath and inaccurate injections must be avoided. Variations in the final images due to minor variations in depth of subcutaneous injection will add to the already wide range of variations of normal nodal anatomy as well as to the large variety of abnormal nodal patterns.

Despite the intrinsic difficulties of interpretation in breast lymphoscintigraphy the technique has achieved a measure of success and continues to be explored with some enthusiasm demonstrating the important role of nodal assessment in breast carcinoma.

Nodal assessment is, in principle, of equal importance in prostatic carcinoma but the pursuit of prostatic lymphoscintigraphy is fraught with difficulties which have denied workers in this field anything more than fleeting indications of success. But the subject continues to be of interest particularly as there is now evidence that under some circumstances the internal iliac nodes can be clearly visualised.

Lymphatic Drainage of the Prostate

Until fairly recently, it was thought that there was no lymphatic drainage of the prostate. This idea was strongly suggested by early investigations by O'Conor and Ladd (1937) and later Rounds and Evans (1956) who found that colloidal suspensions of radioactive compounds were not removed from the prostate. Further weight was added to this theory by Smith (1966), who was unable to demonstrate drainage of Patent Blue V dye to the lymph nodes after intraprostatic injection. Similarly, Rodin et al. (1967), Gittes and McCullough (1974) and McCullough (1975) failed to demonstrate the regional nodes after intraprostatic injection of contrast medium or vital dye.

This strong body of opinion suggested that lymphatic plexuses associated with prostatic alveoli were quite rare. It was felt that metastases to regional nodes occurred only after there was spread into or through the prostatic capsule. Two further ideas were put forward. Firstly, it seemed that carcinoma of the prostate spread in the perineural spaces both through the prostate and extraprostatically. Secondly, it was suggested by Gittes and McCullough (1974) that in view of the lack of demonstrable lymphatics, the prostate is an "immunologically privileged site."

However, Menon et al. (1977) injected ^{198}Au colloid through the open bladder into the dog's prostate, and demonstrated uptake by the regional lymph nodes. Most recently, Shridhar (1979), in an elegant experimental study in dogs, successfully demonstrated intraprostatic lymphatics following the injection of india ink into the

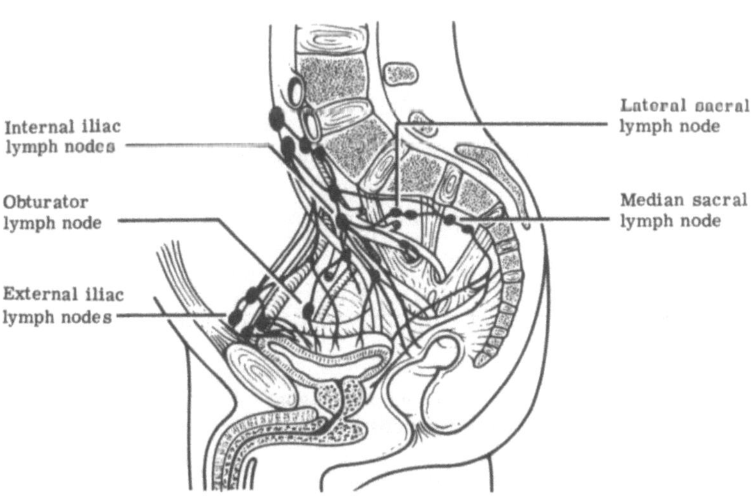

Fig. 1. Side view of pelvis showing prostatic regional lymph nodes.

prostatic parenchyma. He based the identification of intraprostatic lymphatics on the presence of an endothelial lining with no red blood cells in the lumen, but evidence of coagulated lymph. The continuity of these channels was traceable in serial sections, and they were also seen to have india ink particles in them as well as in the regional nodes. It seems, therefore, that there is no validity to the concept of the prostate as an "immunologically privileged site", and that it has a well-developed system of lymph channals.

Lymph drains to the regional lymph nodes, mainly to the internal iliac and obturator nodes and to the median and lateral sacral nodes. There may be some drainage to the external iliac nodes directly from the prostate. From these groups, lymph draws to the juxta-regional nodes, that is, the common iliac and paraaortic lymph nodes (Fig. 1).

Technique and Dosimetry

In the experimental work described above, ^{198}Au was the radionuclide used in an attempt to show the prostatic lymph nodes, because of its small particle size. The authors selected ^{99m}Tc-labelled antimony sulphide colloid for their study, because of its lower radiation dose and better imaging characteristics, and its particle size (4–12 mm) is still small enough to be transported by macrophages to the regional lymph nodes.

At the beginning of the study described by Gardiner et al. (1979a, b) the best site of injection was uncertain, and several were tried (Table 1). Using a fine-bore needle transperineally, it was difficult to site the tip accurately in the prostate, and there was no drainage to the lymph nodes. Menon et al. (1977) successfully demonstrated nodal uptake by injecting radionuclide transvesically in dogs, so in 15 patients an endoscopic method was used. Injections were made through a 21-gauge needle attached to the end of a 6FG ureteric catheter introduced and directed through the cystoscope.

Injections were made by this technique transurethrally into the prostatic parenchyma, both superficially and deeply into the trigone, into the anterior and posterior vesical walls and by multiple injections around both ureteric orifices. In only one of these, a transurethral intraprostatic injection, was any nodal uptake demonstrated on the scintigram and it was unsatisfactory because of the difficulty in accurately defining separate groups of nodes.

Table 1. Sites of injection of radionuclide.

Group I	Transperineal	
Group II	Intraprostatic	
	Intravesical	– Superficial and deep trigone
		– Anterior and posterior walls
		– Periureteric
Group III	Transabdominal (into retropubic space)	
Group IV	Transrectal (into prostatic capsule)	

Finally a transrectal approach was attempted. Using a Franzen needle, 0.1 ml was injected into the prostatic capsule. The colloid was either given in two separate injections of 0.05 ml into the postero-inferior capsule on either side of the midline, or as a single injection into the prostatic capsule in the midline. This has now been performed in 40 patients, all of whom were volunteers undergoing cysto-urethroscopy in the follow-up for their superficial bladder tumours. The injections were mostly given while the patients were under general anaesthetic, but could be given with the patient awake.

The complication of bacteraemia following transrectal needle biopsy of the prostate is well documented (Thompson et al. 1980), so patients undergoing transrectal injection were covered in a 5-day course of cortimoxazole (two tablets twice daily). There have been no side effects, apart from urinary tract infections in three, asymptomatic bacteriuria in one and proctalgia in one.

A similar investigation was carried out by Stone et al. (1979) in which both ^{99m}Tc-phytate and ^{99m}Tc-antimony sulphide colloid were used. The best injection site in this work was perianally using ^{99m}Tc-antimone sulphide colloid, although only four patients were investigated by this method. In three of these patients some nodal uptake was observed from which some anatomical location was possible. Poor visualisation resulted when ^{99m}Tc-phytate was used. The other injection sites used by these authors were transurethrally into the prostatic parenchyma and transperineally into the posterior prostatic capsule. The transrectal route into the prostatic capsule or parenchyma as described by Gardiner et al. (1979a, b) was not attempted by these authors.

Both of these studies (Gardiner et al. 1979a, b; Stone et al. 1979) used small injection volumes of less than 0.2 ml containing 250 μCi or less. Small volumes like this should present fewer drainage problems than larger volumes and have also been found more satisfactory for breast lymphoscintigraphy (Ege 1976, 1978). The radiation dose to patients undergoing this investigation will of course depend on how well the activity is removed from the injection site. In the event of it all remaining at the injection site and concentrated in a tissue volume of 1 cm^3, the dose to this region would be 2.5 rad for an administered dose of 250 μCi ^{99m}Tc-antimony sulphide colloid.

Results

Of the results so far reported, the most successful route for administering activity was the transrectal injection of radionuclide using the Franzen needle (Gardiner et al. 1979a, b). In all but six, imaging of at least one group of nodes was possible, nearly always the internal iliac nodes. Examples can be seen in Figs. 2 and 3. In some of the early patients radionuclide could be seen in the urethra (Fig. 4). This was almost certainly due to spillage of radioisotope into the prostatic ducts, which then drained into the urethra.

In order to know better the anatomical location of the lymph nodes, some recent improvements have been made by the authors. When markers were placed on the umbilicus, pubic symphysis and both anterior superior iliac spines, the pelvis could be mapped out and a "pelvic grid" superimposed on the scintigram (Figs. 5, 6). In-

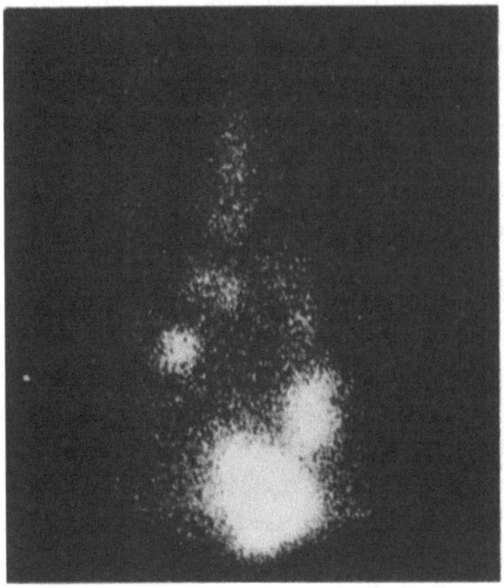

Fig. 2

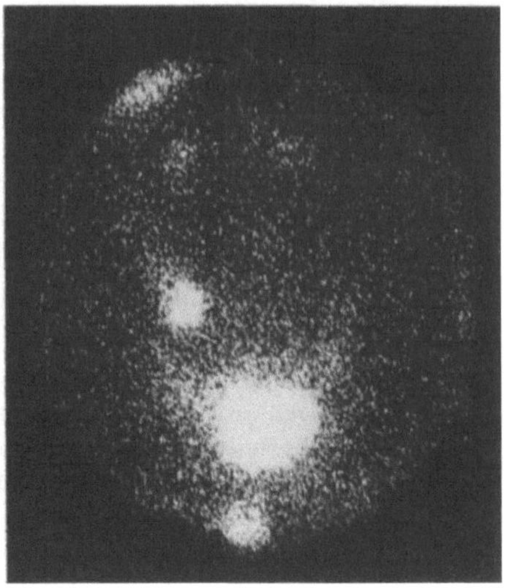

Fig. 3

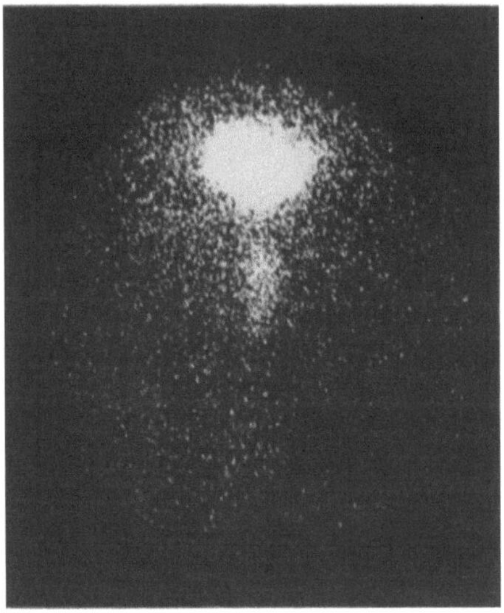

Fig. 4

Fig. 2. Demonstration of lymph nodes following transurethral injection of ^{99m}Tc-antimony sulphide colloid using the Franzen needle.

Fig. 3. Further demonstration of nodal uptake.

Fig. 4. Drainage of radionuclide into the urethra.

itially scintigrams were performed at 3 h and 6 h, but it was found that a better image was not obtained in the later pictures, so the 6 h examination was discontinued. There was an advantage in obtaining three views of the patient's pelvis: antero-posterior (AP), postero-anterior (PA) and lateral. If a group of nodes was nearer the back than the front of the patient it appeared more intense on the PA view and less so on the AP view (Fig. 7).

Although imaging of lymph nodes was possible in all but a few, accurate localisation of these nodes proved to be a difficulty at the beginning, although the improvements in technique described above made this significantly easier. What has

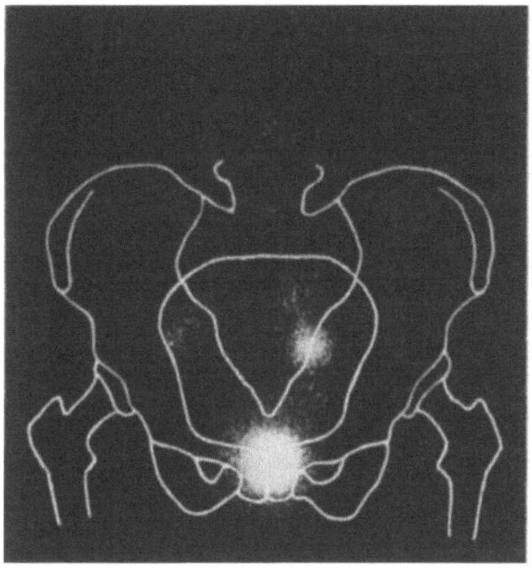

Fig. 5

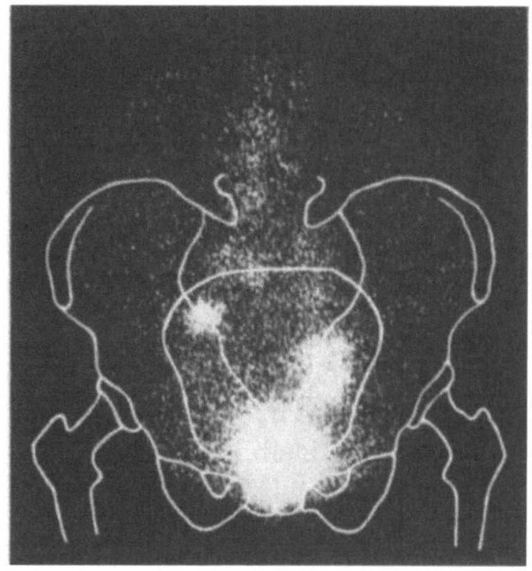

Fig. 6

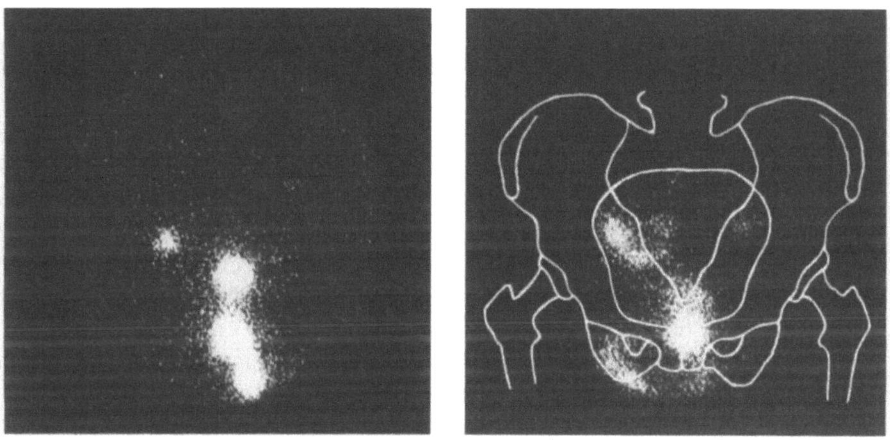

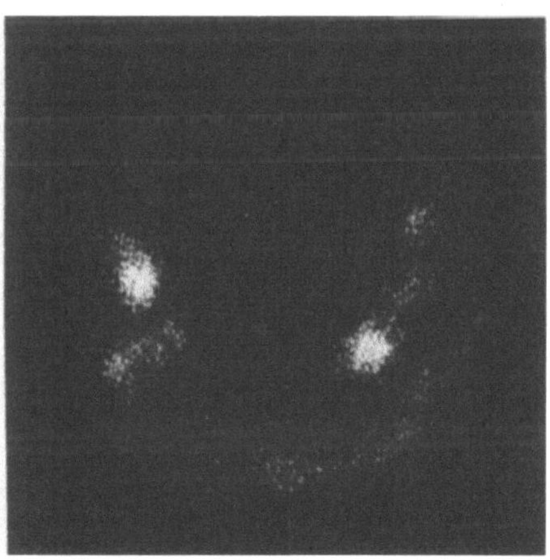

Fig. 7 a–c

Fig. 5. Superimposition of "pelvic grid", easing nodal localisation. It can be seen that drainage to one side is favoured.

Fig. 6. AP pelvic view showing a clear pattern of lymph drainage.

Fig. 7. **a** PA, **b** AP and **c** lateral views.

continued to prove difficult, however, is the fact that there has been inconsistent filling of the obturator node and the median sacral nodes. A recognisable pattern of normality was not established.

Another difficulty has arisen from the fact that about 85% of the radioactivity remains at the injection site, with drainage of only a small amount to the nodes. The authors have found that prostatic massage does not improve drainage, and hyaluronidase has not been of help in previous studies with ^{198}Au (Flocks et al. 1959). No satisfactory method has yet been devised for dispersing the large collection of radioisotope at the injection site.

Similarly, drainage was always greater on one side than the other, in spite of bilateral injections. The reasons for this are uncertain, but it has obvious drawbacks in relation to reproducibility.

In summary, this method of injection with ^{99m}Tc-labelled antimony sulphide colloid is nearly always successful in imaging at least one group of nodes, most commonly the internal iliac, although a high percentage of the radioactivity remains at the injection site, and drainage to nodes on one side is always greater than the other.

Discussion

There are many limitations in the accurate staging of prostatic carcinoma, but several new techniques have now been introduced. Ultrasound (Resnick et al. 1978; Peeling et al. 1979), vesoseminal vesiculography (Beck et al. 1978) and computerised axial tomography (Stewart et al. 1978) are being developed in order to assess local spread. Distant metastases in bone are accurately localised by a combination of serum phosphatases, bone scanning (Fitzpatrick et al. 1978; O'Donoghue et al. 1978) and urinary hydroxoproline (Bishop and Fellows 1977).

Involvement of lymph nodes by prostatic carcinoma may be an early event in the natural history of disease (Arduino and Glucksman 1962) and precede the spread to bones. It is also likely that unsuspected lymphatic metastases occur more frequently than previously thought (McLaughlin et al. 1976). Table 2 shows the incidence of nodal metastases related to tumour states in several reports. It has been found that the obturator nodes are most commonly affected, being involved in most cases in which nodal spread has occurred (Withmore and McKenzie 1959). It has also been shown that nodal metastases often occur without evidence of concomitant bone metastases (McLaughlin et al. 1976).

Table 2. Incidence of lymph node metastases in MO disease.

Author	T1 B_1	T2 B_2	T3 C	T4 D_1
Whitmore et al. (1972)	25%	25%	55%	–
McCullough et al. (1974)	21%	21%	40%	–
Paxton et al. (1975)	25%	46%	60%	92%
McLaughlin et al. (1976)	21%	30%	50%	–
Wilson et al. (1977)	14%	45%	53%	–

The importance of accurate staging of lymph node involvement is remarked on by Flocks (1973) and Spaulding and Whitmore (1978) who found that the survival after total prostatectomy with positive nodes is significantly worse than when nodes are not involved. Bagshaw et al. (1975) have shown that the same applies to patients treated by external beam radiotherapy.

Several methods for demonstrating nodal metastases have been devised, with varying degrees of success and invasiveness. Pedal lymphography is not always accurate, even in the most experienced hands, and only demonstrates the juxta-regional lymph nodes. Computerised axial tomography (Steward et al. 1978) is only of limited value in assessing lymph node involvement in carcinoma of the prostate. Raghavaiah and Jordan (1979) have described their experience with prostatic lymphography, but this involves injection under anaesthesia of a large volume of contrast medium (6–8 ml into each lobe). One of the more accurate of the relatively non-invasive methods of assessing nodal metastases is fine-needle aspiration of suspicious nodes after pedal lymphography (Pollen and Schmidt 1979; Eisenberger 1980, personal communication), but this method does not sample the obturator or internal iliac nodes.

Flock (1973) and McLaughlin et al. (1976) recommended pelvic lymphadenectomy as a vital part of the management of prostatic cancer. Golimbu et al. (1979) also suggested that extended pelvic lymphadenectomy should be performed to include the obturator nodes. Although all of these authors found the procedure safe, they list a large number of complications, and this was also found in a study by O'Donoghue et al. (1976).

A less invasive and equally accurate method for node staging is required, and the attempts to produce such a technique are described here. The attractions of this investigation are that it is easily and safely repeated, can be performed in the outpatients and when further developed should allow for quantitation by computerised gamma camera techniques. Several problems still remain and, before extending it to a trial of patients with prostatic carcinoma, these must be excluded and an easily recognisable pattern of normality established.

Acknowledgements. We wish to thank Mr. P. Shridhar, FRCS, for helpful discussion during the preparation of this chapter. We are grateful to the Editor of the British Journal of Urology for his kind permission to reproduce illustrations (Figs. 2–7).

References

Arduino LJ, Glucksman MA (1962) Lymph node metastases in early carcinoma of the prostate. J Urol 88:91–93

Bagshaw MA, Ray GR, Pistenma DA, Castellino RA, Meares EM Jr (1975) External beam radiation therapy of primary carcinoma of the prostate. Cancer 36:723–728

Beck PH, McAninch JW, Levinsky B, Whitlock NW, Stutzman RE, Goebel JL (1978) Vasoseminal vesiculography in staging adenocarcinoma of prostate. Urology 11:239–242

Bishop MC, Fellows GJ (1977) Urine hydroxyproline excretion – a marker of bone metastases in prostatic carcinoma. Urol 49:711–716

Boak JL, Agwunobi TC (1978) Study of technetium-labelled sulphide colloid uptake by regional lymph nodes draining tumour-bearing area. Br J Surg 65:374–378

Ege GN (1976) Internal mammary lymphoscintigraphy. Radiology 118:101–107

Ege GN (1978) Internal mammary lymphoscintigraphy: a rational adjunct to the staging and management of breast carcinoma. Clin Radiol 29:453–456

Ege GN, Warbick-Cerone A, Bronskill MJ (1979) Radiocolloid internal mammary lymphoscintigraphy. Monograph. Published by Nuclear Medicine Department, Princess Margaret Hospital, Toronto

Eisenberger F (1980, personal communication) Fine needle aspiration of lymph nodes in carcinoma of the prostate

Fitzpatrick JM, Constable AR, Sherwood T, Stephenson JJ, Chisholm GD, O'Donoghue EPN (1978) Serial bone scanning: the assessment of treatment response in carcinoma of the prostate. Br J Urol 50:555–561

Flocks RH (1973) The treatment of stage C prostatic cancer with special reference to combined surgical and radiation therapy. J Urol 109:461–463

Flocks RH, Culp D, Porto R (1959) Lymphatic spread from prostatic cancer. J Urol 81:194–196

Gardiner RA, Fitzpatrick JM, Constable AR, Cranage RW, O'Donoghue EPN, Wickham JEA (1979a) Human prostatic lymphoscintigraphy. A preliminary report. Br J Urol 51:300–303

Gardiner RA, Fitzpatrick JM, Constable AR, Cranage RW, O'Donoghue EPN, Wickham JEA (1979b) Improved techniques in radionuclide imaging of prostatic lymph nodes. Br J Urol 51:561–564

Gittes RF, McCullough DL (1974) Occult carcinoma of the prostate: an oversight of immune surveillance – a working hypothesis. J Urol 112:241–244

Golimbu M, Morales P, Al-Askari S, Brown J (1979) Extended pelvic lymphadenectomy for prostatic cancer. J Urol 121:617–620

McCullough DL (1975) Experimental lymphangiography: experience with direct medium injection into the parenchyma of the rat testis and prostate. Invest Urol 13:211–219

McCullough DL, Prout GR Jr, Daly JJ (1974) Carcinoma of the prostate and lymphatic metastases. J Urol 111:65–71

McLaughlin AP, Saltzstein SL, McCullough DL, Gittes RF (1976) Prostatic carcinoma: incidence and location of unsuspected lymphatic metastases. J Urol 115:89–94

Menon M, Menon S, Strauss HW, Catalone WJ (1977) Demonstration of the existence of canine prostatic lymphatics by radioisotopic techniques. J Urol 118:274–277

O'Conor VJ, Ladd RL (1973) Intraprostatic injection. J Urol 37:557–568

O'Donoghue EPN, Shridhar P, Sherwood T, Williams JP, Chisholm GD (1976) Lymphography and pelvic lymphadenectomy in carcinoma of the prostate. Br J Urol 48:689–696

O'Donoghue EPN, Constable AR, Sherwood T, Stevenson JJ, Chisholm GD (1978) Bone scanning and plasma phosphatases in carcinoma of the prostate. Br J Urol 50:172–177

Paxton RM, Williams G, MacDonald JS (1975) Role of lymphography in carcinoma of the prostate. Br Med J 1:120–122

Peeling WB, Griffiths GJ, Evans KT, Roberts EE (1979) Diagnosis and staging of prostatic cancer by transrectal ultrasonography. A preliminary study. Br J Urol 51:565–570

Pollen JJ, Schmidt JD (1979) Diagnostic fine needle aspiration of soft tissue metastases from cancer of the prostate. J Urol 121:59–61

Raghavaiah NV, Jordan WP Jr (1979) Prostatic lymphography. J Urol 121:178–181

Resnick MI, Willard JW, Boyce WH (1978) Ultrasonic evaluation of the prostatic nodule. J Urol 120:86–89

Rodin AE, Carson DL, Roberts DK (1967) Nature of the perineural space invaded by prostatic carcinoma. Cancer 20:1772–1779

Rounds WM, Evans TC (1956) Recording of radioactivity in the blood, liver and prostate following interstitial administration of ^{198}Au. A J R 75:1132–1138

Shridhar P (1979) The lymphatics of the prostate gland and their role in the spread of prostatic carcinoma. Ann R Coll Surg Engl 61:114–122

Smith MJV (1966) The lymphatics of the prostate. Invest Urol 3:439–444

Spaulding JT, Whitmore WF Jr (1978) Extended total excision of prostatic adenocarcinoma. J Urol 120:188–190

Steward BH, James R, Haaga J, Alfidi RJ (1978) Urological applications of computerised axial tomography: a preliminary report. J Urol 120:198–204

Stone AR, Merrick MV, Chisholm GD (1979) Prostatic lymphoscintigraphy. Br J Urol 51:556–560
Thompson PM, Talbot RW, Packham DA, Dulake C (1980) Transrectal biopsy of the prostate and bacteraemia. Br J Surg 67:127–128
Whitmore WF Jr, McKenzie AR (1959) Experiences with various operative procedures for the total excision of prostatic cancer. Cancer 12:396–405
Whitmore WF Jr, Hilaris B, Grabstald H (1972) Retropubic implantation of iodine 125 in the treatment of prostatic cancer. J Urol 108:918–920
Wilson CS, Dahl DS, Middleton RG (1977) Pelvic lymphadenectomy for the staging of apparently localized prostatic cancer. J Urol 117:197–198

The Diuresis Renogram in Obstructive Uropathy

P. H. O'Reilly, R. A. Shields, H. J. Testa, and E. Charlton Edwards

Obstruction of the upper urinary tract is not always unequivocal: Where it is, it is usually easy to evaluate. The ureteric stone with proximal dilatation and hydronephrosis will be clearly seen on the excretion urogram. Standard isotope renography may be useful to demonstrate the degree of functional impairment and obstruction, but the decision to operate is not usually difficult to make. There are many situations, however, where the urogram demonstrates dilatation of the upper urinary tracts, but an obstructing lesion is not apparent and the question is raised as to whether the dilatation is truly obstructive or not (Fig. 1). In this situation, the decision to operate is often as difficult as it is straightforward in the unequivocal case. Renal pelvic dilatation, post-pyeloplasty dilatation, ureters dilated after reimplantation or ureterolithotomy, vesicoureteric reflux and post-diversion ureteric dilatation all provide examples where it might be difficult to be certain of the true explanation for the distension. The urogram gives only a still, instantaneous ana-

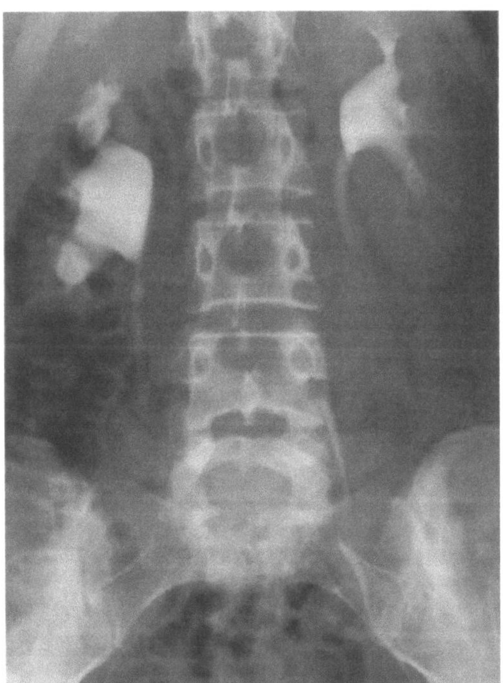

Fig. 1. Urogram demonstrating dilatation of the upper urinary tract.

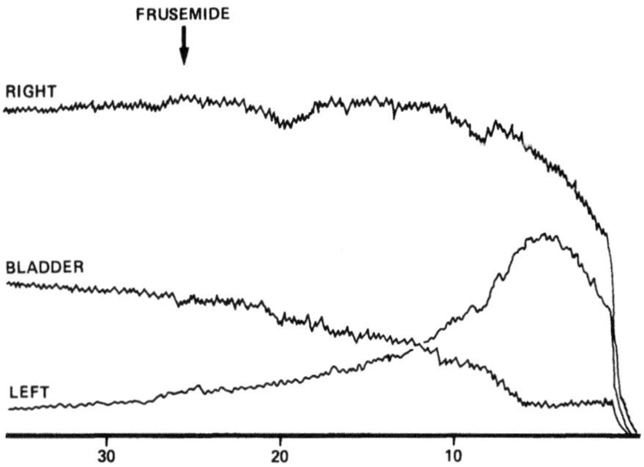

Fig. 2. Diuresis renogram of dilated, obstructed tract.

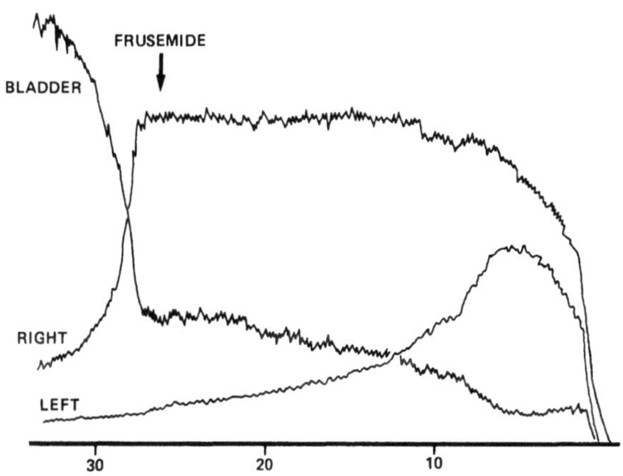

Fig. 3. Diuresis renogram of dilated, non-obstructed tract.

tomical picture; it says nothing about underlying function or upper tract urodynamics. The standard renogram will give a rising, *apparently* obstructive curve in any situation where there is retention of activity in the kidneys or ureters. Thus, stasis in non-obstructive dilatation *and* the truly impeded upper tract will give the same pattern.

It was against this background that we investigated and developed the diuresis renogram. The practical details have been reported before (O'Reilly et al. 1979a, b). Briefly, a gamma camera renogram is performed using either ^{131}I-hippuran, or preferably (because of its superior physical qualities) ^{123}I-hippuran. It is then repeated 3 min after the intravenous injection of 0.5 mg/kg of the diuretic frusemide. If the initial renogram shows a rising curve with retention of tracer at 20 min, the frusemide is given in continuity to observe its effect on the curve. Under diuresis, the rising or steady curve in the dilated, obstructed tract remains the same, reflecting obstruction at low and high flow rates (Fig. 2). Conversely, in the dilated, non-obstructed tract, increasing the urine flow rate by diuresis allows prompt unimpeded elimination of tracer from the pelvis or ureter (Fig. 3). This procedure has been performed in over 350 adults and children to date without complication. Using a butterfly (Abbott) cannula, only one intravenous injection is required. The study is carried out with the patient sitting, except infants, who are lain on top of the gamma camera. Some mild sedation is usually given to infants to discourage unwanted movement. A satisfactory state of hydration is demanded in all renogram work, and to this end, a glass of cola or orange juice is given before the test; this also helps relaxation in children.

Early studies using this technique showed good correlation with urography, clinical progress and operative findings (O'Reilly et al. 1978). Corroborative studies were required, however, to substantiate these impressions. These have shown equally encouraging results (Lupton 1980, personal communication).

Correlation with Perfusion Studies. Fifteen patients with idiopathic hydronephrosis have had diuresis renography and perfusion studies according to the technique of Whitaker (1973). In 11 patients, the correlation was exact. In one case the Whitaker test failed through extravasation. In one test, the renogram showed function to be so poor that no comment on elimination features could be made. The remaining two tests disagreed. Figures from other centres suggest even better correlation (Koff et al. 1979; Koff 1979, personal communication).

Correlation with Parenchymal Transit Times. Forty-six patients with idiopathic hydronephrosis and ureteric obstruction have had diuresis renography and transit time studies according to the technique of Whitfield (Whitfield et al. 1977). The correlation rate was 80%.

Correlation with Morphological Studies. Thirty-two patients with idiopathic hydronephrosis have had diuresis renography and objective morphological examination of the renal pelvis removed at Anderson-Hynes pyeloplasty. The specimens were examined according to the technique of Gosling and Dixon, whose description of the histological and electron microscopy features of the normal and hydronephrotic renal pelvis have recently been reported (Gosling and Dixon 1978). In a blind study, where the specimens were examined by these workers, the correlation rate was 88%.

It is now our policy where diuresis renography suggests the absence of obstruction to treat the patient conservatively. In a series of 28 consecutive patients with non-obstructive dilatation followed up for 5 years, only one required operation for continuing symptoms and renographic deterioration. One developed two asymptomatic renal pelvic calculi and one showed a slight deterioration in renal function without any evidence of developing obstruction. The remaining 25 patients became symptom-free and their renograms showed no evidence of deterioration in renal function or development of obstruction (O'Reilly et al. 1980).

The diuresis renogram has its critics. It does not directly measure pressure in the renal pelvis or ureter, and it is often emphasised that it is the increased pressure (or infection) which leads to renal damage in the patients. But it is debatable if a direct measure of pressure is an absolute requirement. We believe that synchronous assessment of differential function and urodynamics gives equally valuable information, and particularly in view of the good correlation of the technique with perfusion studies, transit times and especially objective morphological changes. The 2-min hippuran uptake test gives an index of differential function which correlates well with constant hippurate infusion and individual renal urine collection techniques (Hayes et al. 1974) and with other radionuclide procedures (Holten and Storm 1979). In addition, the excretion part of the study accurately demonstrates quantitative urodynamics under standard and provocative high flow rates. Since none of the other available techniques is able to give such a simultaneous index of both function and urodynamics, the diuresis renogram is our first choice for screening patients after excretion urography. Parenchymal transit studies and perfusion studies are reserved for those cases which remain equivocal thereafter. We do not think we have missed even minor degrees of obstruction with this policy. The gamma camera is a very sensitive indicator of obstruction. We would concede that in *grossly* dilated ureters the diuretic stimulus might be insufficient to fill the ureters and provoke the system. However, the normal protocol gives flow rates of 16–26 ml/min and this is sufficient to give a result in the overwhelming majority of cases. Arguments that the technique may be of value in pelvic dilatation but not in ureteric dilatation are no longer tenable. Probe detectors in this work have given way to gamma camera computer systems. Using these, ureteric visualisation is excellent if short half-life isotopes such as ^{123}- or ^{99m}Tc are used, in preference to the traditional ^{131}I.

Few subject in urology have undergone such a careful and detailed reappraisal in recent years as the dilated upper urinary tract and obstructive uropathy. The clinician now has a number of different procedures at his disposal to clarify suspected upper tract obstruction. Excretion urography clearly remains the first requirement in the patient suspected of upper tract obstruction to demonstrate the anatomical integrity of the pelvis and ureters. When a dilated upper tract is encountered and no clear cause is apparent, such as stone or tumour, a dynamic functional evaluation is mandatory to complement the urogram information. Only in this way can appropriate decisions regarding surgical or conservative management be made. We prefer to use the diuresis renogram at this stage because of the quantitative functional and synchronous urodynamic information it furnishes. If necessary, we then proceed to more complex radionuclide or invasive perfusion procedures. In this respect, all the available techniques are to be regarded as complementary rather than competitive. Their evolution represents an important step forward in understanding the pathogenesis and management of pelvic and ureteric dilatation and obstruction. Their considered and, where necessary, combined use will benefit both clinician and patient in terms of diagnostic accuracy and low morbidity.

Acknowledgements. This work is the result of an ongoing collaborative study involving the urologists, nuclear medicine physicians and medical physicists in Manchester, and particularly the authors wish to acknowledge Richard Lawson, Joe Cohen, Robin Barnard, Raymund Carroll and especially Eric Lupton. The work was initiated under the auspices of the Manchester & North West Region Kidney Research Association and the Independent order of Odd Fellows.

References

Gosling JA, Dixon JS (1978) Functional obstruction of the ureter and renal pelvis. A histological and electron microscopy study. Br J Urol 50: 145–152

Hayes M, Brosnan S, Taplin GV (1974) Determination of differential renal function by sequential renal scintigraphy. J Urol 3:556–559

Holten I, Storm HH (1979) Kidney scintigraphy with ^{99m}Tc-DMSA and ^{131}I-hippuran. Scand J Urol Nephrol 13:275–283

Koff SA, Thrall HA, Keyes JW Jr (1979) Diuretic radionuclide urography. Non-invasive method for evaluating nephroureteral obstruction. J Urol 122:451–455

O'Reilly PH, Shields RA, Testa HJ (1979a) Nuclear medicine in urology and nephrology. Butterworths, London

O'Reilly PH, Lawson RS, Shields RA, Testa HJ (1979b) Idiopathic hydronephrosis. J Urol 121:153–155

Whitaker RH (1973) Diagnosis of obstruction in dilated ureters. Ann R Coll Surg Engl 53:153–166

Whitfield HN, Britton KE, Fry IK, Hendry WF, Nimmon CC, Travers P, Wickham JEA (1977) The obstructed kidney. Correlation between renal function and urodynamic assessment. Br J Urol 49:615–620

Distinction Between Obstructive Nephropathy and Obstructive Uropathy by Deconvolution Analysis of Radionuclide Transit Times

H. N. Whitfield, K. E. Britton, W. F. Hendry, C. C. Nimmon, and J. E. A. Wickham

Probe renography is recognised to be unreliable in the diagnosis of upper urinary tract obstruction since a rising third phase may be seen for a number of different reasons. Even the presence of diminished function and a rising third phase is not reliable evidence of obstruction: A system which has been irreversibly damaged by an obstruction which has been relieved may remain capacious and will have the same appearance as a truly obstructed kidney. Diuresis renography has helped to overcome this problem (O'Reilly et al. 1978).

Gamma camera studies bring a new dimension to renography. It is possible to separate isotope handling by the renal parenchyma from isotope handling in the collecting system. The accurate separation of the two depends on the conversion of the familiar count-distribution image into a time-distribution image. This highlights the late arrival of isotope in the collecting system and parenchymal isotope transit is derived by subtracting the activity/time curve of the pelvis from that of the whole

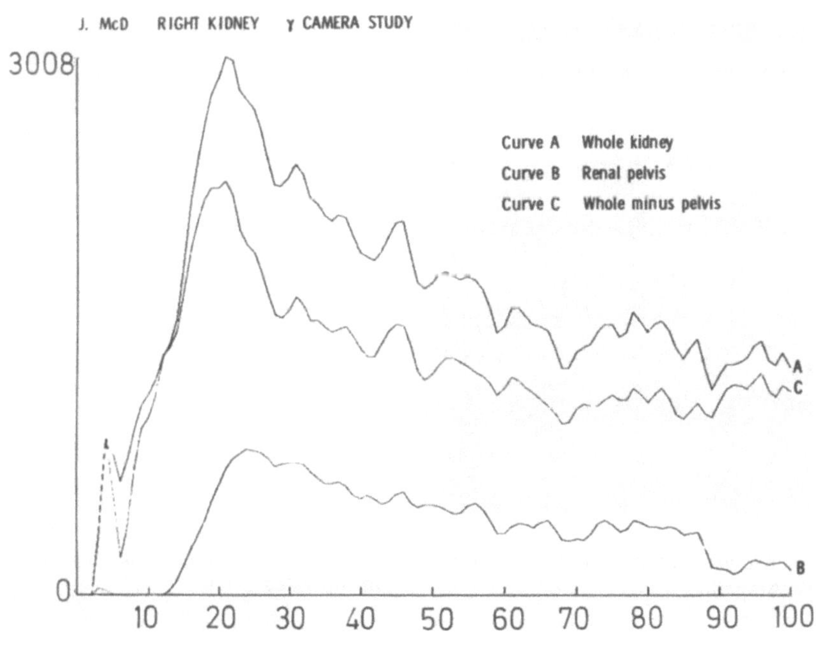

Fig. 1. Composite renogram of a normal kidney in which isotope handling of the parenchyma and renal pelvis have been separated.

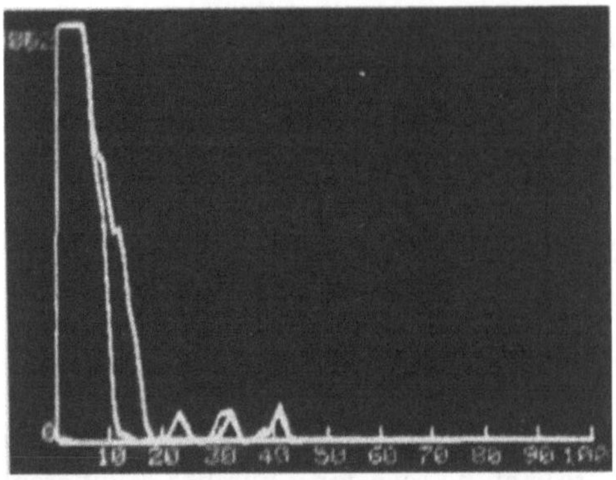

Fig. 2. Deconvoluted renogram of normal kidney.

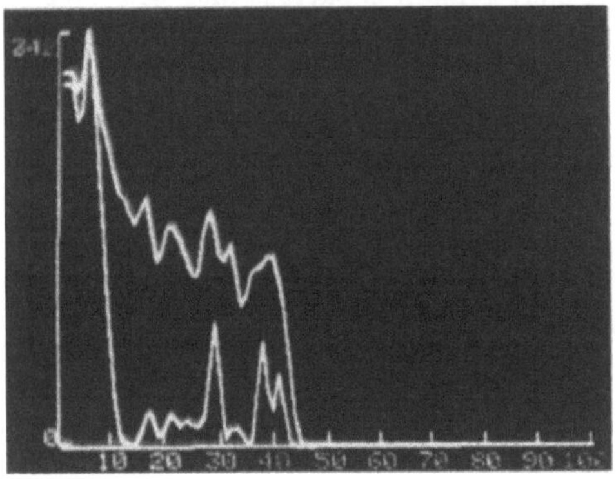

Fig. 3. Deconvoluted renogram of kidney with obstructive uropathy.

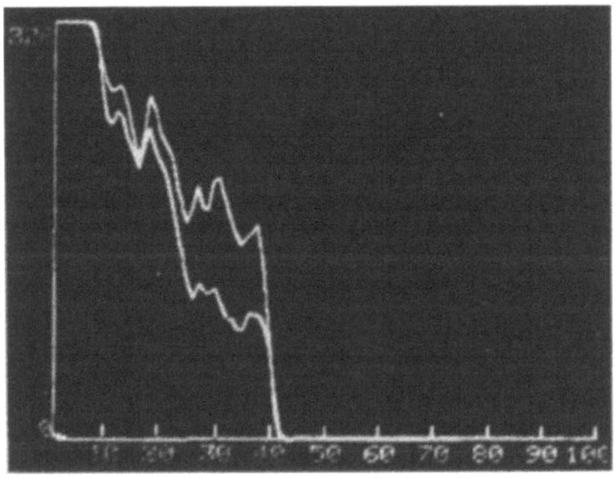

Fig. 4. Deconvoluted renogram of kidney with obstructed nephropathy.

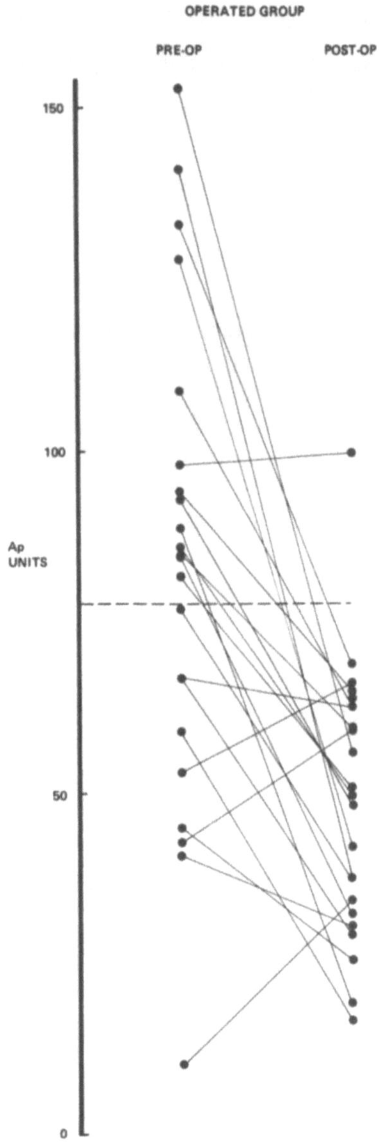

Fig. 5. Pre- and post-operative parenchymal isotope transit time results in the operated group.

kidney. Separate curves can then be drawn for the whole kidney, the collecting system and the parenchyma (Fig. 1).

Isotope transit times may be quantitated (Whitfield et al. 1978) by applying a standard mathematical technique, deconvolution analysis, that can be applied to any pair of input and output data. Essentially, this is the variation with time in the quantity of activity in selected regions which would be obtained after a theoretical spike injection into the renal artery.

After deconvolution analysis the curves obtained from a normal kidney show that parenchymal and whole kidney transit times are almost the same (Fig. 2). In a dilated but unobstructed system whole kidney isotope transit time is prolonged, but parenchymal isotope transit is normal (Fig. 3). In a kidney in which an obstructive process is affecting nephron function, not only will the whole kidney isotope transit time be prolonged but so will also the parenchymal isotope transit time (Fig. 4).

The distinction can thus be made between an obstructive uropathy in which the effect of an obstructing process on the outflow tract is apparent and an obstructive nephropathy, which monitors the effect of an obstructing process on nephron function.

Our hypothesis is that in the presence of a significant degree of obstruction at the pelvi-ureteric junction isotope transit time through the parenchyma will be prolonged since a rise in intratubular pressure relative to peri-tubular capillary pressure leads to increased proximal tubular reabsorption of salt and water and a delay in the tubular transport of a non-reabsorbable tracer such as technetium-DTPA.

We have validated this hypothesis in three ways. Experimental studies (Price et al. 1978) and clinical investigations (Piepsz et al. 1978) have shown that deconvolution of the renogram gives results which are very similar to actual intra-arterial bolus injection of isotope. In a study of 44 patients we have compared the diagnoses made after gamma camera studies with the diagnoses made on diuretic urography and pressure/flow studies, and the results correlate well (Tables 1 and 2). Thirdly, we have followed patients serially to see whether the outcome predicted on the results of gamma camera studies was fulfilled. Of the 30 patients who underwent surgery pre- and post-operative gamma camera information is available in 22 (Fig. 5). Thirteen of these operated cases were obstructed pre-operatively and 12 returned to normal post-operatively. The remaining patient remains symptomatic, has radiological evidence of obstruction and is awaiting surgery.

Of the nine cases who underwent surgery but were renographically unobstructed none have become renographically obstructed. Five patients, all of whom were radiologically or urodynamically unobstructed, were operated on for symptomatic indications and all five continue to have pain post-operatively. The remaining cases were all urodynamically or radiologically equivocal and closer to the level at which obstruction is diagnosed renographically and it would perhaps be more realistic to consider a range within which obstruction becomes increasingly likely rather than a rigid cut-off level.

Gamma camera studies have a number of advantages as an investigation for the diagnosis of obstruction. Differential renal function can be measured accurately, the test is non-invasive and parenchymal function is separated from that of the collecting system. Above all the small radiation dose makes it safe for serial investigations particularly in children.

Table 1. Comparison of diagnoses made on FIVU and deconvolution analysis of the gamma camera radionuclide study.

		FIVU		
		Obstructed	Unobstructed	Equivocal
Gamma camera study	Obstructed	6	1	1
	Unobstructed	2	4	2
	Equivocal	–	–	1
	Failed	3	–	–

Table 2. Comparison of diagnoses made on pressure/flow studies and deconvolution analysis of the gamma camera radionuclide study.

		Pressure/flow studies				
		Obstructed	Unobstructed	Equivocal	Failed	Not done
Gamma camera study	Obstructed	4	2	–	1	1
	Unobstructed	1	4	2	1	–
	Equivocal	–	–	–	1	–
	Failed	2	1	–	–	–

A number of questions still remain to be answered. There seems to be no direct relationship between the severity of obstruction and parenchymal isotope transit time. The relationship between the duration of obstruction and the appearance of delayed parenchymal transit time needs further investigation, since following relief of obstruction parenchymal transit time may take 3 months to return to normal. It seems that an obstruction may effect percentage renal function and parenchymal transit time in different ways and no direct relationship between the two exists. Papillary morphology may be as important in relation to obstruction as it is in vesico-ureteric reflux. The influence of pelvic wall compliance is poorly understood and although we have some experience of ureteric obstruction, in which the results seem to correlate well with those we have found in PUJ obstruction, longer term follow-up is needed.

Gamma camera renography with deconvolution analysis seems a very safe, reliable, non-invasive technique for the diagnosis of upper urinary tract obstruction at the level of the pelvi-ureteric junction.

References

O'Reilly RH, Testa HJ, Lawson RS, Farrar DJ, Charlton-Edwards E (1978) Diuresis renography in equivocal urinary tract obstruction. Br J Urol 50:76–80

Piepsz A, Denis R, Ham HR, Dobbeleir A, Schulman CC, Erbsmann F (1978) A simple method of measuring separate glomerular filtration rate using a single injection of ^{99m}Tc-DTPA and the scintillation camera. J Paediatr 93 (5):769–774

Price RR, Touya JJ, Branch R, Goddard J, Brill AB (1978) Validation of renal transit time calculation using compartmental models and direct measurements. A review of information processing in medical imaging. Oakridge National Laboratory Press, pp 536–554

Whitfield HN, Britton KE, Hendry WF, Nimmon CC, Wickham JEA (1978) The distinction between obstructive uropathy and nephropathy by radioisotope transit times. Br J Urol 50:433–436

Urodynamic Investigations in Urological Diagnostics
General Review

H. Melchior

The purpose of urodynamic investigations is to correlate morphology and function of the urinary tract. In the dynamical process, the morphological picture and the respective pathophysiological condition have to be coordinated.

At the present state of engineering, this task is best achieved by combined, simultaneous, roentgenological, and functional examinations. Since such combined techniques require, however, considerable expenditure on equipment; most urological departments and urologists have to content themselves with radiological and functional diagnostics being carried out in separate operations.

Various techniques of ureterometry and intraureteral pressure flow measurements for the evaluation of functional disturbances of the upper urinary tract have been clinically standardized and introduced into urological practice. Bladder dysfunctions, in particular neuromuscular dysfunctions, urinary incontinence, and functional bladder outlet obstructions are diagnosed by uroflowmetry and cystometry, possibly in combination with electromyography of the striated musculature of the pelvic floor. The clinical value of sphincterometry and urethral pressure profile has yet to be determined.

Retrograde Ureterometry

Retrograde transvesical ureterometry was introduced into clinical diagnostics by Kiil in 1953 (Kiil 1953, 1957). Electromanometry by means of retrograde catheterization is employed for the evaluation of ureteral dilatations, especially segmental dilatations. A peristalsis against resistance with high basic pressure and increased peristaltic frequency is found in cases of obstruction or functional stenosis, while ureteral hypoperistalsis caused by myogenic insufficiency is characterized by low basic pressure and irregular contractions with small pressure amplitudes.

An example of the use of ureterometry is shown in Fig. 1. After resection of a functionally obstructed ureteral segment in a 27-year-old female, dilatation of the upper ureter occurred despite wide anastomosis (Fig. 1 b). Postoperative ureteral dilatation is due to myogenic insufficiency of the upper segment. There are neither peristaltic concentrations in the dilated segment nor a pressure difference between the proximal and the distal ureter (Fig. 1 c).

Although retrograde ureterometry is not a particularly intricate or costly procedure, it has not been widely adopted by urologists. Besides the risk of transmission of infections, the main problem of retrograde ureterometry and cause of possible misinterpretations is the mechanical excitation of physioligical peristalsis. Animal

a b c
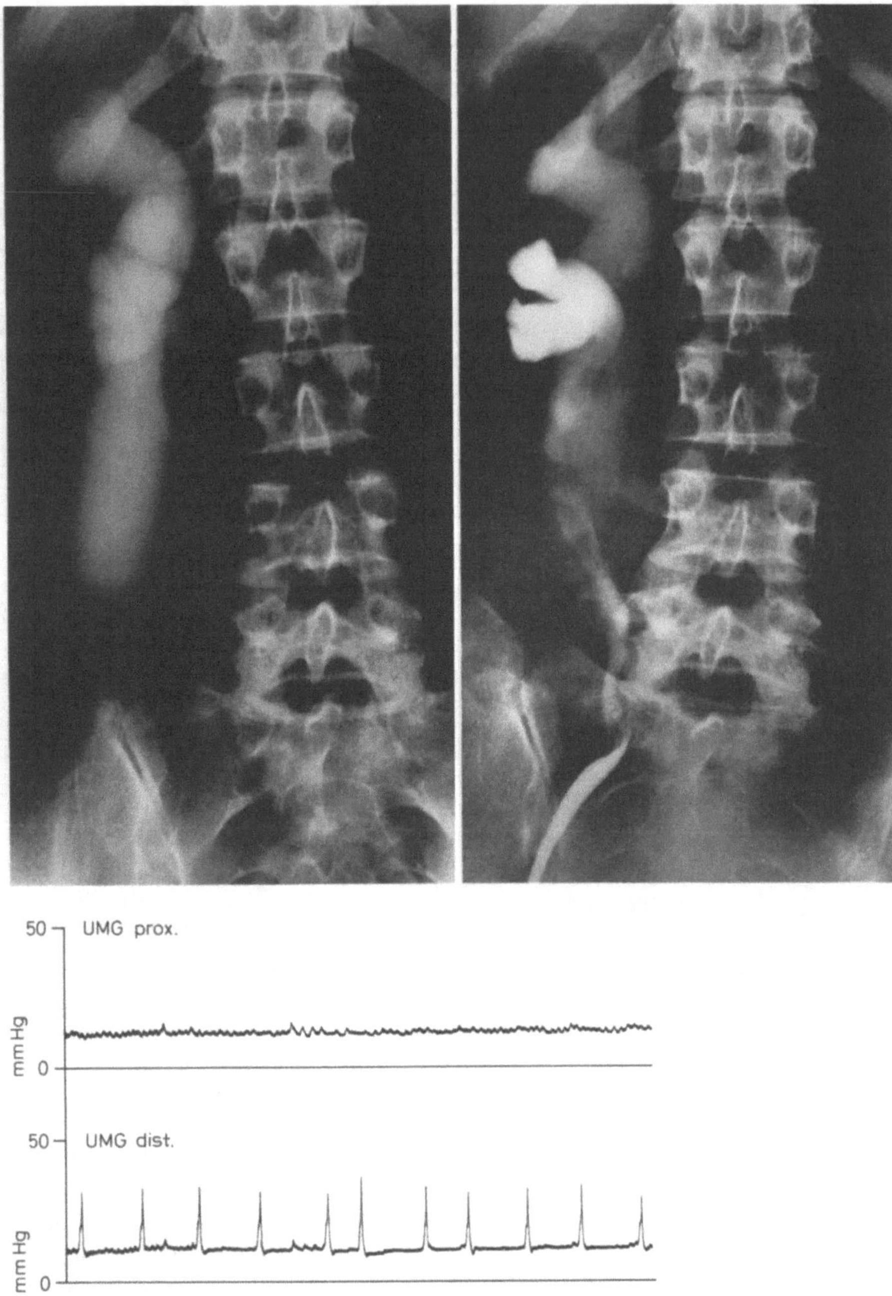

Fig. 1 a–c. Aperistaltic ureteral segment (ureterometry). **a** Preoperative excretory urography. **b** Postoperative retrograde ureterography. **c** Postoperative ureterometry: aperistaltic upper ureter (*UMG prox.*) and normal peristaltic contractions of the distal ureter (*UMG dist.*).

experiments and clinical studies showed that two thin catheters lying side by side cause less disturbance than a single catheter which is only slightly thicker.

Another argument against retrograde ureterometry is the fact that exact measurements of the static intraureteral pressure are nearly impossible. Between the measuring point and electromanometer there is always a difference in hydrostatic pressure up to a maximum of 5 mbar. This immanent inaccuracy can only be eliminated by the use of precisely calibrated tip manometers holding pressure receptors at the tip of the catheter. These tip manometers are, however, extremely expensive as well as prone to damage, so that the increase of information in comparison with standardized retrograde ureterometry does not justify the additional expenditure, still more so, because the dynamical pressure waves of ureteral peristalsis are of greater clinical relevancy than the absolute degree of the static basic pressure.

Urorheomanometry

The information on ureteral function derived from transvesical ureterometry will be even more useful if this examination is combined with intraureteral flow measurements. The velocity of urinary flow in the ureter is measured by urorheography. Urorheomanometry is simultaneous intraureteral pressure flow measurement, the combination of transvesical ureterometry and urorheography (Melchior et al. 1971 a, b; Melchior and Simhan 1971, 1973).

In clinical practice, the "two-catheter method" using separate pressure and flow receptors, is preferable to the technique which combines the two measuring units in one catheter. Combined pressure flow probes are equipped with an excellent dynamic sensitivity and accuracy of reproduction, but due to extreme thermic irritability of the strain gauges, they are affected by a relatively wide inconstancy of zero reference.

The procedure of intraureteral flow measurement is based on the physical principle of heat conduction, according to which a heated body radiates heat to its surroundings. In running fluid, heat conduction is – with some limitation – a function of the flow velocity. The interpretation of the data derived from urorheomanometry is founded on the hypotesis that pressure and flow velocity in the ureter are connected like dependent and independent variables of a mathematical equation and are modulated by external factors such as tension of the ureteral wall, diuresis, and flow resistance (Melchior 1980).

Examples of urorheomanometry can be seen in Figs. 2 and 3, which show two cases of segmental ureteral dilatation in which the X-ray photograph appeared to be identical; urodynamic examinations, however, revealed different disturbances:

1) A 20-year-old female (Fig. 2): Proximal to a stenosis in the dilated ureteral segment, a high basal pressure, low pressure amplitude, and irregular contractions [ureteromanogram (UMG)] were found, combined with a slow velocity of urinary flow [ureterorheogram (URG)]. These are the urodynamic characteristics of peristalsis against resistance. Distal to the stenosis in the normally configurated pelvic ureter, the peristalsis showed physiological data. The dilatation was caused by the functional stenosis.

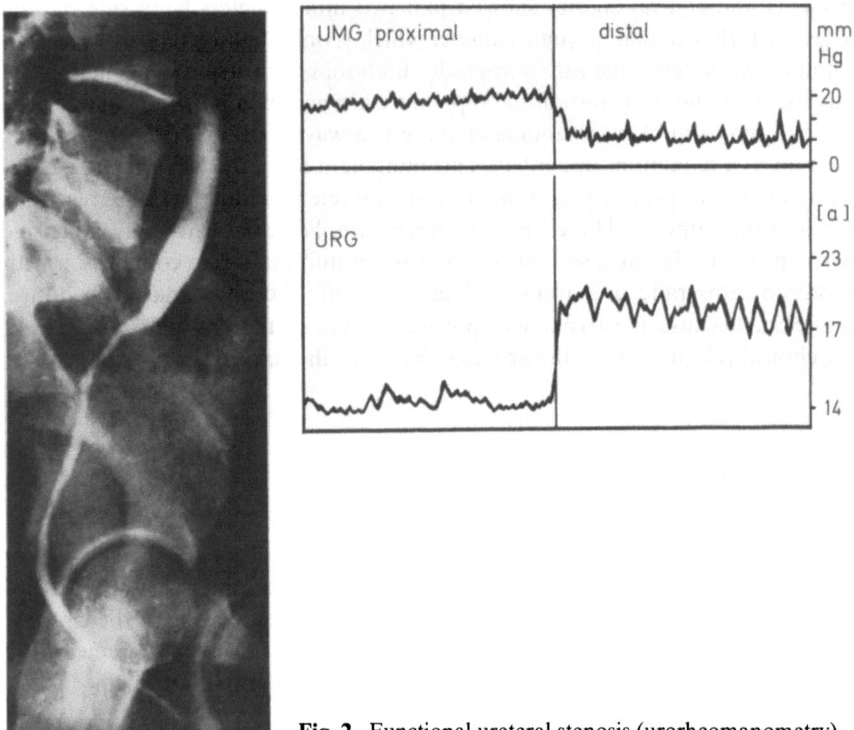

Fig. 2. Functional ureteral stenosis (urorheomanometry).

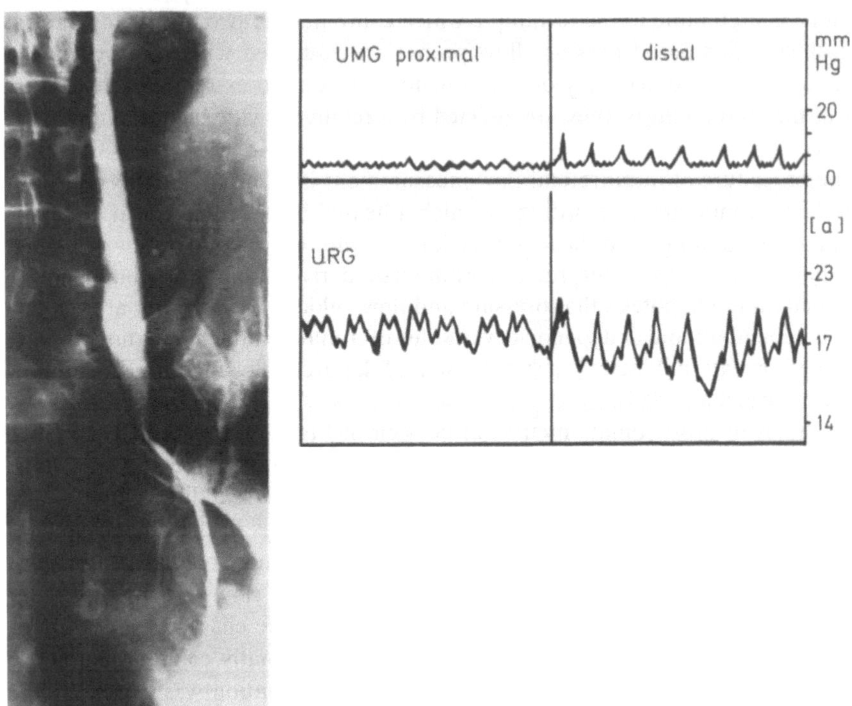

Fig. 3. Aperistaltic ureteral segment (urorheomanometry).

2) A 30-year-old female (Fig. 3): In the dilated ureteral segment, the basal pressure was normal, but there were only slight peristaltic concentrations with minimum amplitude (UMG) while the rheogram (URG) demonstrated an almost normal flow velocity with only a slight difference between systole and diastole. Below the dilated ureteral segment, peristalsis was normal with regular and efficient contractions; the basal pressure was the same as in the dilated segment. In this case, the dilatation was caused neither by functional stenosis nor by obstruction, but by segmental hypoperistalsis due to muscular insufficiency.

Antegrade Transrenal Pyeloureterometry

In contrast to retrograde transvesical ureterometry, Whitaker developed a technique of antegrade perfusion of the upper urinary tract for dynamical evaluation of obstructive or nonobstructive ureteral dilatation (Whitaker 1973, 1978). After percutaneous transrenal puncture of the pyelocaliceal system, pyelon and ureter are continuously perfused through a nephrostomy catheter, and the intrarenal pressure dependent on the perfusion volume is measured (Fig. 4). This procedure will gain in clinical relevance at the same time as percutaneous puncture of the kidney under sonographic control is standardized and adopted in clinical practice.

According to Whitaker, with a perfusion volume of 10 ml/min, normal perfusion pressure in the pyelon and ureter amounts to a maximum of 12 mbar. A perfusion pressure of more than 20 mbar is pathological and symptomatic of obstruction. The interpretation is critical in cases of medium pressure data within the range 15–18 mbar.

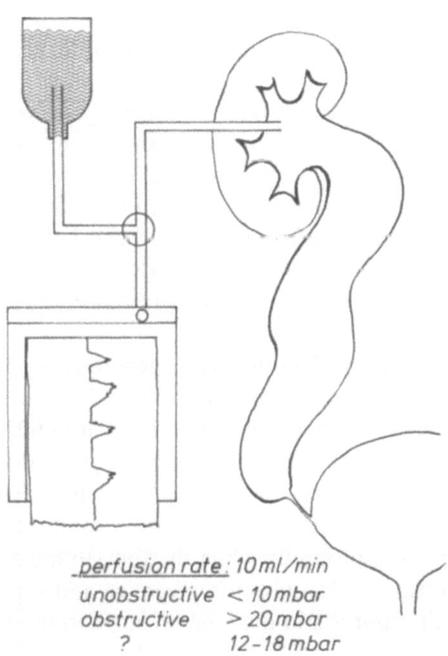

Fig. 4. Transrenal pyeloureterometry (schematic representation).

Videometry

Since retrograde transvesical and antegrade transrenal ureterometry have the disadvantage of being invasive methods, the development of noninvasive techniques would be a desirable object of urodynamics. For such demand, videometry may present a possible answer (Melchior 1980).

After recording individual peristaltic concentration waves on a tape recorder by X-ray video amplifier, the variations in ureteral diameter are measured by single scene analysis. According to hydrodynamic studies and their interpretation by Shapiro et al. (1969) and Simhan (1971), there is a purely bolar transport of urine if the quotient of the maximum ureteral diameter divided by its minimum diameter is more than 1.8. The clinical significance of this procedure has still to be established. At any rate, a basic requirement would be automatic recording and analysis in the manner of videodensitometry.

Analysis of the urine bolus as a time distance diagram is another possibility of noninvasive examination of ureteral peristalsis suggested by Durben et al. (1978), but so far only little clinical experience exists with regard to this method.

Uroflowmetry

In contrast to the functional evaluation of ureteral dynamics, diagnostics of lower urinary tract dysfunctions are a standardized part of urological routine examination. Uroflowmetry, in particular, proved useful after initial overestimation and subsequent disappointment (Melchior 1977).

The clinical significance of uroflowmetry depends on the conditions of micturition and the patients' readiness to cooperate. Therefore, a 'diagnostic toilet", which allows voiding in a physiological manner is just as important as a reliable uroflowmeter.

The interpretation of the flow curve is not only based on the statistical analysis of different parameters such as maximum flow, average flow, or voiding time, but on the complete diagram of micturition (Fig. 5). Initially, physiological uroflow rises quickly to a maximum ("time to maximum flow"), keeps a plateau of maximum flow for a short while, and decreases toward the end of voiding (Fig. 6). In healthy patients with medium voiding volumes, micturition time is relatively constant and amounts to approximately 20 s. Large voiding volumes, however, may cause a prolonged micturition time and a pseudoplateau.

Patients with functional or mechanical bladder outlet obstruction generally show an attenuated urinary stream with reduced maximum flow and prolonged micturition time. Furthermore, there are rather specific criteria which allow a differentiation between the various voiding disturbances by uroflowmetry (Fig. 6): A delayed start of micturition, prolonged time to maximum flow, and an early decrease of the flow curve are characteristic of a bladder outlet obstruction by prostate. In patients with urethral stenosis, micturition starts promptly while the time to maximum flow is short, so that the plateau of maximum flow is quickly reached and kept nearly constant for a relatively long time in proportion to the total micturition time. An irregular micturition without a plateau of maximum flow is typical of detrusor-

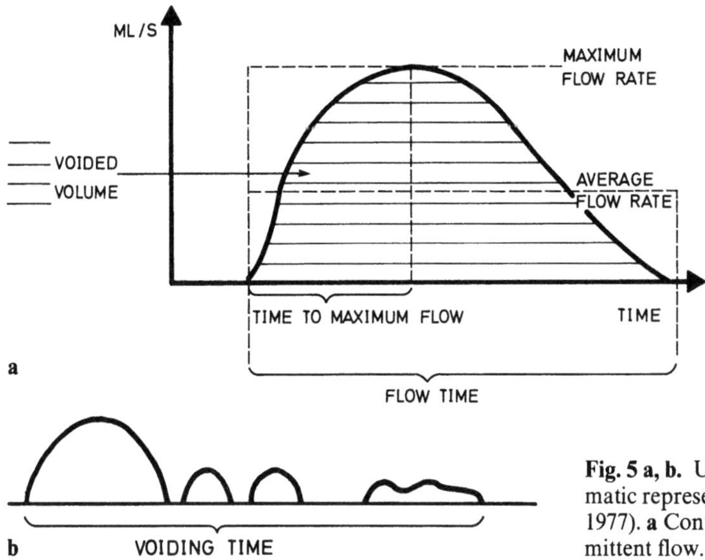

Fig. 5 a, b. Uroflowmetry (schematic representation; Bates et al. 1977). **a** Continuous flow. **b** Intermittent flow.

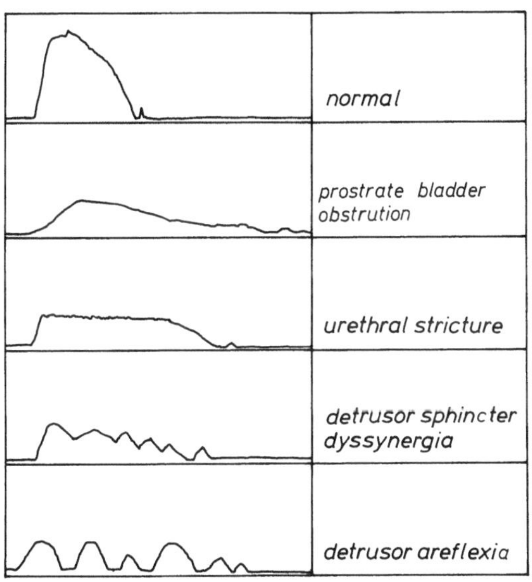

Fig. 6. Uroflowmetry (schematic representation): types of micturition.

sphincter dyssynergia. In the case of detrusor areflexia, the micturition pattern is characterized by intermittent voiding with complete interruption of the urinary flow (Frimodt-Møller 1977; Melchior 1977).

Since uroflowmetry is a very simple technique which causes no strain on the patient or the physician, it can always be carried out in urological practice. The greatest advantage of uroflowmetry is the avoidance of invasive instrumental manipulations of the urinary tract. Uroflowmetry is suited to check results of treatment and progression of disease, or as a screening procedure, if a functional or mechanical bladder outlet obstruction is suspected.

Cystometry

Cystometry is the technique by which the pressure–volume relationship of the bladder is measured (Bates et al. 1976). It is the most important diagnostic method for qualitative and quantitative evaluation of detrusor function. Cystometry reflects the viscoelastic properties of the bladder wall, the contraction power of the detrusor, the pathophysiology of bladder innervation, and micturition resistance. With respect to the filling medium, one distinguishes between liquid and gas cystometry.

Gas cystometry is the less complicated technique and therefore particularly suited for urological use (Bradley et al. 1968, 1975). The basic requirement for clinical employment of gas cystometers is secure reducing valves which reduce the high gas pressure in the supply cylinders of more than 600 mbar to physiological filling pressure. Furthermore, precise volumeters are necessary for determination of the pressure-dependent filling rate.

The most important advantages of gas cystometry are the possibility of rapid bladder filling using single-lumen catheters, and the independence of zero reference. Zero reference is not required because the specific gravities of bicarbonate and air are practically identical. Since the resistance against flow of bicarbonate is much smaller than that of fluid, up to a filling rate of 200 ml/min the pressure gradient along the tubing is negligible, so that single-lumen 8–12 French catheters may be used for bladder filling. Furthermore, with gas cystometry, the risk of bacterial contamination is extremely small. The interpretation of provocative tests, however, is difficult. Due to the compressibility of gas, the reproduction of sudden fluctuation is pressure – as caused by coughing – is delayed, moderated, and contorted. Therefore, it is often impossible to decide whether registered pressure wave from the provocative test itself, or from a reactive contraction of the detrusor. Moreover, with gas cystometry, the determination of micturition pressure – and consequently an analysis of voiding – is impossible. Because of hyperemic reaction of the bladder mucosa on bicarbonate, a cystoscopy following a gas cystometry mostly results in misinterpretation.

Fluid cystometry requires a much greater expenditure of time and equipement than gas cystometry. Regardless of the medium – water, NaCl solution, X-ray contrast medium – care has to be taken that:

1) The difference in hydrostatic pressure between the bladder and manometer is eliminated by precise zero adjustment, preferably at the level of the upper symphysial edge.
2) The perfusion pressure of the instilled liquid is not transmitted to the measured intravesical pressure and this is best prevented by employment of double-lumen catheters.
3) The results are not altered by the moderating effect of air bubbles in the tubing (Bates et al. 1976).

Besides, there is a certain risk of contamination, especially in the case of repeated use of the expensive tubing and double-lumen catheters.

The advantages of fluid cystometry are:

1) Exact reproducibility of the results, in particular those of the provocative tests;

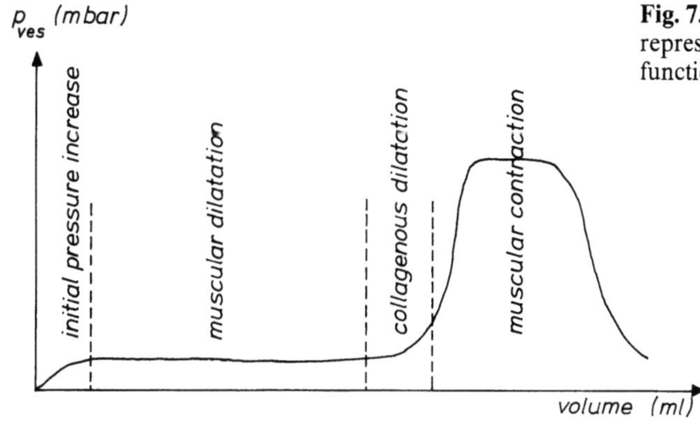

Fig. 7. Cystometry (schematic representation): phases of bladder function.

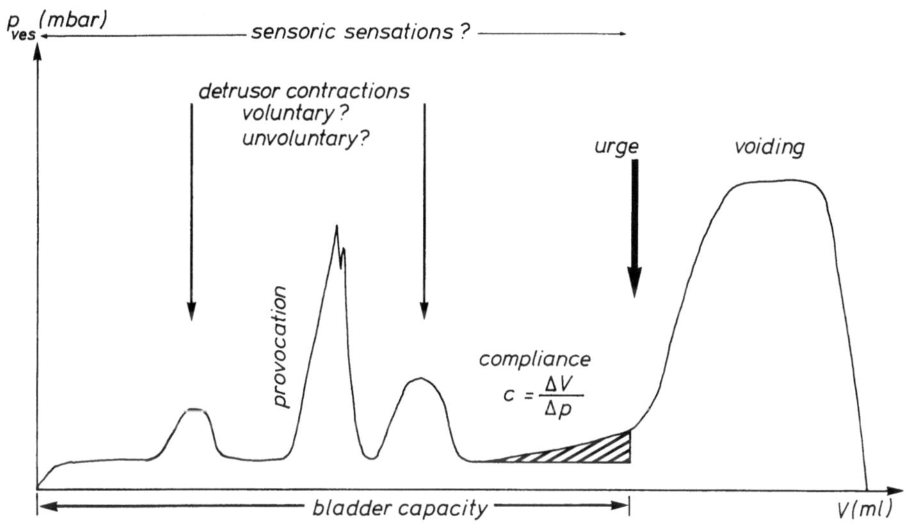

Fig. 8. Cystometry (schematic representation): findings. p_{ves}, Intravesical pressure.

2) determination of the micturition pressure, which enables an analysis of voiding with estimation of the resistance against voiding.

Furthermore, combined pressure flow measurements as well as extended diagnostics, such as videocystometry and simultaneous cine pressure flow measurements, are based on liquid cystometry. As a screening test, liquid cystometry and cystoscopy can even be carried out in the same operation.

Irrespective of the technique and the filling medium, because of the inhomogeneous structure of the bladder wall with viscous and contractile elements, three phases of bladder filling are distinguished from the fourth phase of muscular contration during micturition (Fig. 7):

1) Phase of initial rise in pressure,
2) phase of muscular dilatation,
3) phase of collagenous extension.

The phase of initial increase of pressure is clinically irrelevant and probably conditional on the method. During the phase of muscular dilatation, no voluntary musculatur contractions occur in a normal bladder; involuntary contractions are always pathological (Fig. 8). The absence of sensation and an urge to urinate during contractions of the detrusor indicates a disturbance of the bladder innervation. If involuntary detrusor contractions are perceived as an urge to urinate, this is symptomatic of a peripheral excitation of the micturition reflex.

The elasticity of the bladder wall is reflected in the coefficient of expansion, i.e., the "compliance". A compliance of less than 20 ml/mbar is characteristic of muscular hypertonus and inflammatory or degenerative defects of the elastic elements with development of a contracted bladder. Based on the studies of Coolsaet et al. (1973), a differentiation between muscular and collagenous hypertension is possible by incremental cystometry. Additional information is derived from the Pro-Banthine test.

In the case of undisturbed bladder innervation, the patient is generally able to induce and to suppress voluntarily the micturition reflex, and with it the muscular detrusor contraction. It has to be considered, however, that – due to inhibition – some people are unable to induce a micturition under laboratory conditions. In such cases the examination should be completed by uroflowmetry.

If the bladder outlet is unobstructed, the intravesical rise in pressure during micturition in the recumbent position amounts to less than 50 mbar in men and less than 30 mbar in women.

Sphincterometry

In many neurourological units, sphincterometry, i.e., the retrograde measurement of the urethral perfusion pressure (Fig. 9), is regarded as an important examination on which the indication of surgical or medicinal treatment of the urethral sphincter mechanism is based (Lapides et al. 1960). The indication of external sphincterotomy, in particular, is largely dependent upon the results or retrograde sphincterometry.

The significance of the information derived from sphincterometry is, however, limited since it is not the sphincter tone in the state of rest, but that during micturi-

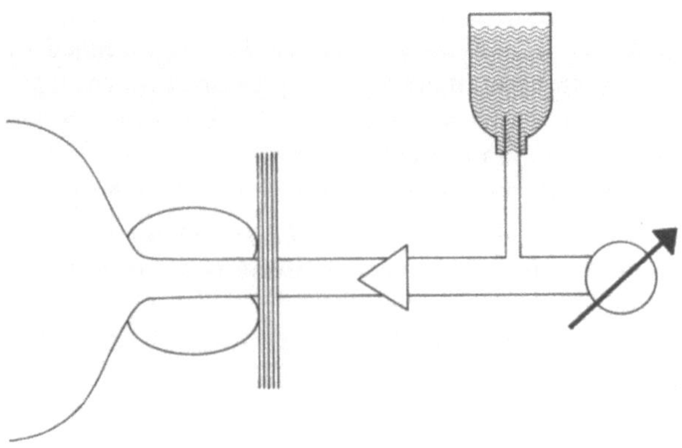

Fig. 9. Sphincterometry (schematic representation).

tion which is decisive of the resistance against voiding, especially in the case of neuromuscular bladder dysfunction. Detrusor-sphincter dyssynergia, the missing coordination of detrusor contraction and sphincter relaxation during micturition, is the main cause of the severe destructive effects that a neurogenic bladder has upon the kidneys and upper urinary tract. Therefore, the measurement of the intravesical pressure during voiding and the determination of the micturition pressure by cystometry should be given preference over retrograde sphincterometry.

Urethral Pressure Profile

The urethral pressure profile is a diagram of the intraluminal pressure along the urethra during the resting period of the bladder. Dependent upon the technique, it allows a segmental or a continuous analysis of the sphincter mechanism at the vesical outlet. The urethral pressure profile may be regarded as a measure of the closing pressure of the individual segments of the urethral sphincter mechanism. It proved to be useful for the evaluation of urinary incontinence. According to Enhörning (1961). A patient is continent if the intraurethral pressure exceeds the intravesical pressure.

The Standardization Committee of the International Continence Society recommend the following definitions (Bates et al. 1977; Fig. 10): *Maximum urethral pressure* is the maximum pressure of the measured profile. *Maximum urethral closure pressure* is the difference between the maximum urethral pressure and the intravesical pressure. *Functional profile length* is the length of the urethra along which the pressure exceeds the bladder pressure, i.e., the length of the urethral segment along which the closing pressure is positive. Generally, the morphological length of the urethra is clinically irrelevant.

Besides the perfusion method, according to Brown and Wickham (1969), the original measuring technique of Lapides et al. (1960) has been improved by Heidenreich and Beck (1971) as well as by Schreiter (1973): For the perfusion of the urethra, the measuring catheter has a central hole at its tip instead of a lateral open-

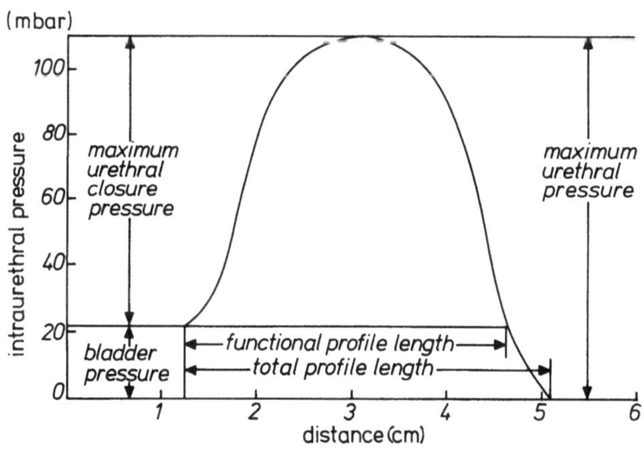

Fig. 10. Urethral pressure profile (schematic representation: Bates et al. 1977).

ing. There is no fundamental difference between these two techniques of perfusion as long as the perfusion rate is low in comparison with the withdrawal rate. In the procedure recommended by Heidenreich and Beck as well as by Schreiter, however, the perfusion rate of 5 ml/min is relatively high in comparison with the withdrawal rate of 1 cm/min; so that not the urethral closing pressure is measured point by point, but the perfusion resistance of the urethral segment proximal to the end of the catheter. Accordingly, the result is a profile of the perfusion resistance instead of a profile of the intraluminal closing pressure along the urethra, so that the findings of the two perfusion methods are not really comparable to each other. Normally, passive intraabdominal variations of pressure, as caused by coughing and straining, are not transmitted to the femal urethra if the sphincter mechanism at the bladder neck is closed. In the case of rapid perfusion of the urethra through a catheter with a central hole at its end, however, an open although only capillary communication is established between the vesical lumen and the measuring catheter, so that intraabdominal fluctuations in pressure are transmitted from the bladder through the intraurethral liquid column to the manometer.

The clinical value of the urethral pressure profile should not be overestimated. In the case of stress incontinence, it serves as an important supplementary test for quantitative evaluation of a sphincter insufficiency, but the diagnosis of stress incontinence itself can be neither confirmed nor disproved only by urethral pressure profile.

Electromyography of the Pelvic Floor

No information can be derived from electromyography (EMG) of the striated musculature of the pelvic floor as to activity and effectiveness of the sphincter mechanism. But if combined with cystometry, the interaction of detrusor and sphincter is demonstrated: Detrusor-sphincter dyssynergia is one of the severest functional disturbances of the lower urinary tract in the case of neuromuscular dysfunction (Allert and Jelasic 1969, 1974).

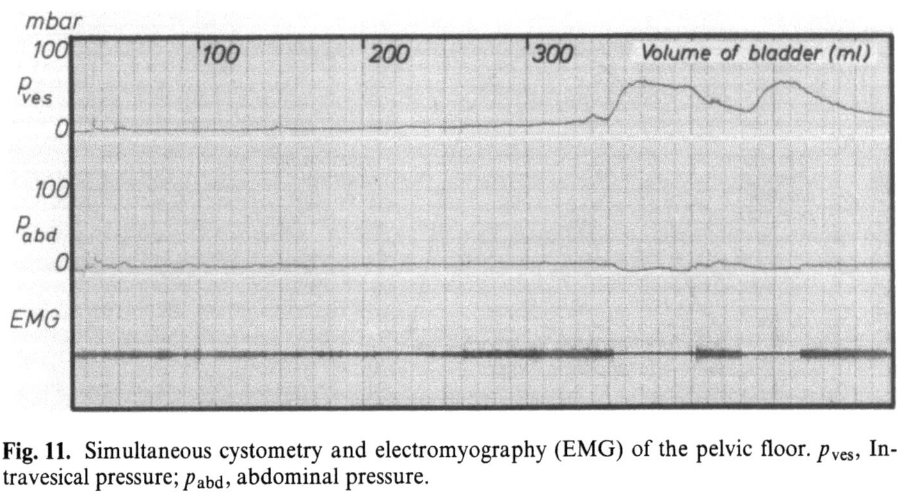

Fig. 11. Simultaneous cystometry and electromyography (EMG) of the pelvic floor. p_{ves}, Intravesical pressure; p_{abd}, abdominal pressure.

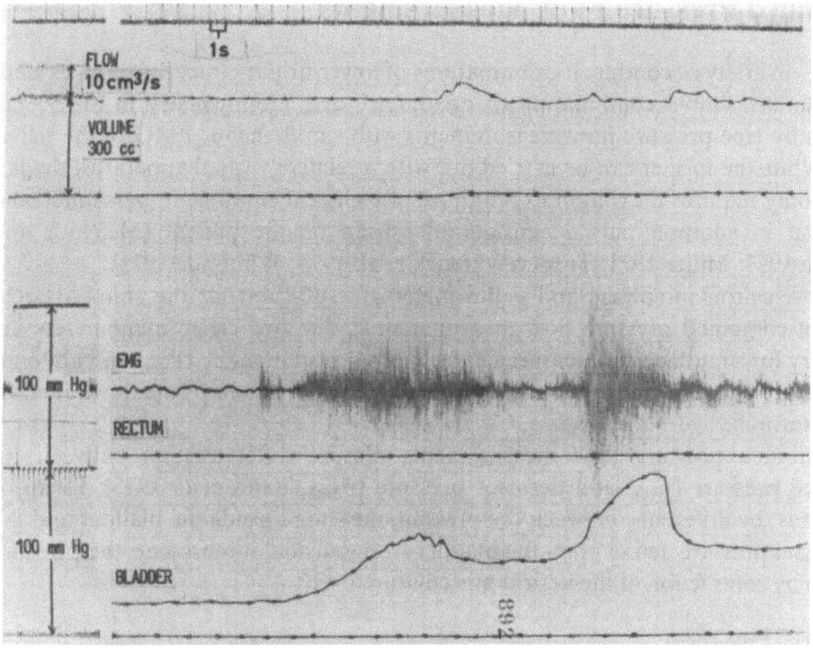

Fig. 12. Simultaneous pressure flow measurements and electromyography (EMG) in the case of neuropathic reflex bladder with detrusor-sphincter dyssynergia (Madersbacher 1976).

Since a selective conduction from the striated periurethral sphincter musculature is impractiacable, one has to content oneself with an accumulated conduction of the bioelectric potentials of the pelvic diaphragm.

If the bladder innervation is undisturbed, the motor activity of the striated sphincter musculature increase in parallel with the bladder filling (Fig. 11), reaches a maximum intensity near the limit of the bladder capacity, and stops abruptly at the beginning of the micturition phase: That EMG shows zero activity shortly before the detrusor contraction with increasing intravesical pressure is demonstrated by cystometry. If a patient with otherwise normal bladder innervation is psychically inhibited from inducing an active detrusor contraction, even during his attempt at voluntary micturition, the bioelectric activity of the striated sphincter musculature diminishes. At the end of voiding, there is maximum activity of the pelvic floor.

Nonexistent increase of the bioelectric activity of the striated sphincter musculature at the end of bladder filling as well as at the end of voiding suggests a reflex insufficiency of the sphincter (Madersbacher 1976; Fig. 12). More serious, however, is a missing activity decrease of the striated sphincter musculature during detrusor contractions, which is indicative of a bladder outlet obstruction by detrusor-sphincter dyssynergia.

Combined Pressure Flow Measurements

There is a variety of combined examinations of lower urinary tract function, extending from the simple combination of cystometry and uroflowmetry to an overall analysis by cine pressure flow measurements with simultaneous EMG of the pelvic floor. While the former can be carried out with a relatively small apparatus, the latter not only requires maximum expenditure of technical equipment, personnel, and time, but in addition puts a considerable strain on the patient (Melchior and Froelich 1977; Miller 1971; Turner-Warwick et al. 1973; Whiteside 1973).

Two electromanometers and a flowmeter are sufficient for the simplest technique of combined pressure flow measurements: The two electromanometers are necessary for simultaneous measurement of intravesical pressure (P_{ves}) and abdominal pressure (p_{abd}) during cystometry, while the flowmeter records the flow rate during micturition.

Combined pressure flow measurements require differentiation between intravesical pressure (p_{ves}) and detrusor pressure (p_{det}) (Bates et al. 1977). Detrusor pressure is the difference between the pressure measured inside the bladder and the abdominal pressure acting upon the bladder from outside; it represents the pressure built up by contraction of the vesical musculature itself:

$$p_{det} = p_{ves} - p_{abd}.$$

The intravesical pressure should preferably be measured suprapubic-percutaneously and the abdominal pressure transrectally.

Three phases of micturition are differentiated from one another (Fig. 13): (1) premicturation phase, (2) opening phase, and (3) voiding phase.

So far, all attempts have failed to determine from the correlation between micturition pressure and flow rate a factor "micturition resistance". Irrespective of the question whether the "micturition pressure" should mainly be related to the detrusor pressure, the abdominal, or the intravesical pressure, it is impossible to establish a mathematical correlation between micturition pressure and flow rate from which a clinically efficient measure for the micturition resistance would result. The lack of a generally applicable correlation between micturition pressure and flow rate is caused by the numerous variations of individual voiding characteristics as well as the biological properties of the urethra.

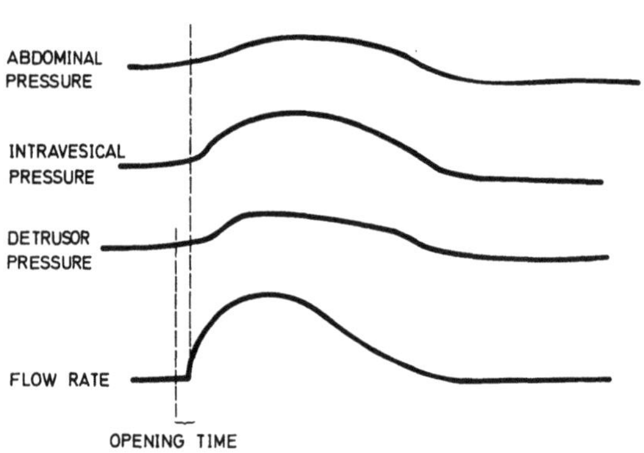

Fig. 13. Combined pressure flow measurements (schematic representation; Bates et al. 1977).

The spectrum of information derived from combined pressure flow measurements is substantially enlarged by simultaneous EMG of the pelvic floor. Depending on the mode of evaluation, two- to four-channel recorders of medium speed (5–10 mm/s) are required for the recording of the data.

The basic demand for correlation of morphology with function is best fulfilled by combined pressure flow measurements under X-ray amplifier video control. Such cine pressure flow measurements allow simultaneous study of the functional process and the morphological situation so that the recognition of pathophysiological disturbances may result in optimal therapeutic measures. Because of the extensive and costly apparatus required for cine pressure flow measurements, however, this technique is unlikely to become part of the routine diagnostics of urological practice, but will be reserved for some specially equipped urodynamic centres where patients with problematical disturbances are examined.

Summary

In recent years, a new line of thought and work known as urodynamics has matured in urology, which – conceived by urologists, bioengineers, physiologists, and morphologists – attempts to correlate morphology and function of the urinary tract. Detached from the traditional concept "a consistent morphology knows organs without function, a consistent physiology knows amorphous processes" new ideas of form and process have been developed. By improved diagnostics which enable direct functional evaluation in situ, pathophysiological correlations could be better revealed. From this resulted not only more accurate pathogenetic ideas of known dysfunctions of the urinary tract, but also the discovery of new syndromes. Furthermore, it has become possible to establish a standardized diagnostic program, and with it an equally clearly defined scheme of treatment for most functional disturbances of the urinary tract.

References

Allert ML, Jelasic F (1969) Elektromyografische Befunde am Blasen- und Analschließmuskel während der Miktion. In: Allert ML, Dressel M, Sökeland J (eds) Neurogene Blasenstörungen, Thieme, Stuttgart, pp 18–22

Allert ML, Jelasic F (1974) Diagnostik neurogener Blasenstörungen durch Elektromyographie. Thieme, Stuttgart

Bates P, Bradley WE, Glen E, Melchior H, Rowan D, Sterling A, Hald T (1976) The standardization of terminology of lower urinary tract function. Eur Urol 2:274–276

Bates P, Rowan D, Glen E, Sterling A, Griffiths D, Zinner N, Melchior H, Hald T (1977) Second report on the standardization of terminology of lower urinary tract function. Eur Urol 3:168–170

Bradley WE, Clarren SA, Shapiro R, Wolfson JR (1968) Air cystometry. J Urol 100:451–455

Bradley WE, Timm GW, Scott FB (1975) Cystometry. III. Cystometers. Urology 5:843–848

Brown M, Wickham JEA (1969) The urethral pressure profile. Br J Urol 41:211

Coolsaet BLRA, van Duyl WA, van Mastright R, van der Zwart A (1973) Step-wise cystometry of urinary bladder. Urology 2:255–257

Durben G, Gerlach R, Hannappel J (1978) Graphisch-radiologische Erfassung der unterschiedlichen Boluskonfiguration beim peristaltischen Harntransport. 4. Symposion Experimentelle Urologie, Kassel

Enhörning G (1961) Simultaneous recording of intravesical and intraurethral pressure. A study on urethral closure in normal and stress incontinent women. Acta Chir Scand [Suppl] 276:1
Frimodt-Møller C (1977) Die Aussagekraft der Uroflowmetrie. 1. Seminar Urologisch. Funktionsdiagnostik, Kassel
Heidenreich J, Beck L (1971) Simultane Druckmessung in Harnblase und Harnröhre zur Diagnostik der Harninkontinenz. Arch Gynaekol 211:325
Kiil F (1953) Pressure recordings in the upper urinary tract. Scand J Clin Lab Invest 5:383
Kiil F (1957) The function of the ureter and renal pelvis. Saunders, Philadelphia
Lapides J, Ajemian EP, Stewart BH, Breakly BA, Lichtwardt JR (1960) Further observations on the kinetics of the urethrovesical sphincter. J Urol 84:86
Madersbacher H (1976) Die neurogene gestörte Harnröhre: Urethrogramm und pathophysiologische Aspekte. Urologe [A] 15:1–12
Melchior H (1977) Harnröhrenobstruktionen: Der Wert urodynamischer Untersuchungsmethoden. Urol Int 32:413–427
Melchior H (1980) Urologische Funktionsdiagnostik. Thieme, Stuttgart
Melchior H, Froelich EJ (1977) Simultaneous cine-pressure-flow measurements by analogue video converter. 7th Annual Meeting International Continence Society, Portoroz (Yugoslavia)
Melchior H, Simhan KK (1971) Zur Problematik der Uro-Rheomanometrie. Biomed Tech (Berlin) 16:99–102
Melchior H, Simhan KK (1973) A new uro-rheomanometer. In: Lutzeyer W, Melchior H (eds) Urodynamics. Springer, Berlin Heidelberg New York, pp 30–34
Melchior H, Diemer KF, Simhan K, Lutzeyer K, Lutzeyer W (1971a) Ureterdynamik. I. Der Einfluß von Diurese und Stauung auf die Ureterdynamik. Z Urol Nephrol 64:81–91
Melchior H, Diemer KF, Simhan K, Lutzeyer K, Lutzeyer W (1971b) Ureterdynamik. II. Der Einfluß des autonomen Nervensystems auf die Ureterdynamik. Z Urol Nephrol 64:93–101
Miller ER (1971) Combined monitoring for the study of continence and voiding. In: Hinman F Jr (ed) Hydrodynamics of micturition. Thomas, Springfield, Ill., pp 5–17
Schreiter F (1973) Descending simultaneous measurement of the urinary bladder and sphincter pressure during continuous perfusion of the urethra after operations for incontinence. In: Lutzeyer W, Melchior H (eds) Urodynamics. Springer, Berlin Heidelberg New York, pp 42–45
Shapiro AH, Jaffrin MY, Weinberg SL (1969) Peristaltic pumping with long wave-lengths at low Reynolds number. J Fluid Mech 37:799
Simhan KK (1971) Über ein theoretisches Modell zur Erfassung des peristaltischen Transportvorganges. In: Lutzeyer W, Melchior H (eds) Ureterdynamik. Thieme, Stuttgart, pp 60–69
Turner-Warwick R, Whitside CG, Worth PHL, Milroy EJG, Bates CP (1973) A urodynamic view of the clinical problems associated with bladder neck dysfunction and its treatment by endoscopic incision and transtrigonal posterior prostatectomy. Br J Urol 45:44–59
Whitaker RH (1973) Diagnosis of obstruction in dilated ureters. Ann R Coll Surg Engl 53:153
Whitaker RH (1978) Clinical assessment of pelvic and ureteral function. Urology 12:146–150
Whiteside CG (1973) Technique of routine cine pressure flow cystography. In: Lutzeyer W, Melchior H (eds) Urodynamics. Springer, Berlin Heidelberg New York, pp 35–39

Diuresis Urography and Pelvi-Ureteric Obstruction

H. N. Whitfield, K. E. Britton, W. F. Hendry, and J. E. A. Wickham

The diagnosis of pelvi-ureteric junction (PUJ) obstruction may be straightforward but not infrequently there are cases which give rise to some doubt. With standard radiological techniques it is not always possible to be sure whether a significant degree of obstruction is present and this has led to the development of other methods of diagnosis. Urodynamic measurements (Whitaker 1973) provide accurate information about pressure/flow relationships but the test is open to criticism since it is invasive and carries a certain morbidity (Whitfield et al. 1976) and is not suitable for serial studies in an individual patient or for routine post-operative evaluation. Furthermore, the test is no guide to parenchymal renal function.

The importance of tailoring intravenous urography to answer specific questions in different circumstances has been stressed by many observers (Covington and Reeser 1950; Johnson and Robinson 1969; Davies et al. 1978). This study describes a simple method of diuretic intravenous urography for the diagnosis of PUJ obstruction.

Patients and Methods

Urography was performed in the hydrated patient and contrast medium was given in a dose of 650 mg iodine/kg body weight (Figs. 1, 2). Forty milligrams of frusemide was injected intravenously 20 min after the contrast. Five radiological features were examined:

1) Size of the renal pelvis before and after frusemide;
2) size of the calices before and after frusemide;
3) contrast dilution within the renal pelvis after frusemide;
4) presence of ureteric filling;
5) the occurrence of pain during the examination.

The only reliable and consistant feature was found to be the change in size of the renal pelvis. This was measured by outlining the pelvis on a tablet with a pressure-sensitive surface linked online to a computer. The surface area of the pelvis was measured in square centimetres and the change in size 20 min after contrast and 15 min after frusemide was expressed as a percentage.

On the results of these measurements we divided the patients into three groups:

1) Those in whom the increase in pelvic size after frusemide was greater than 20%.
2) Those in whom the increase in pelvic size after frusemide was 10–20%.
3) Those in whom the increase in pelvic size after frusemide was less than 10%.

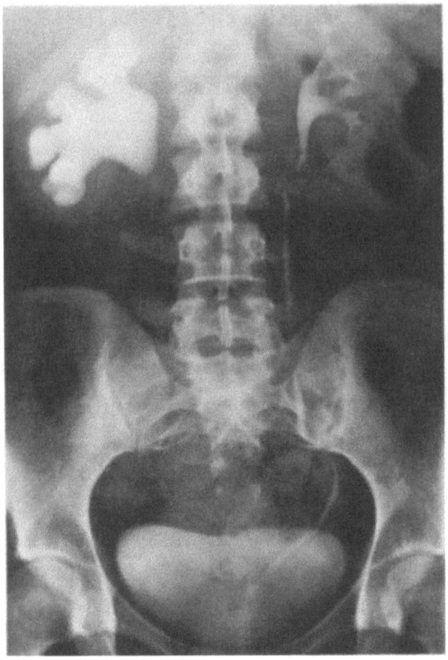

Fig. 1. Patient with equivocal PUJ obstruction, 20 min after contrast.

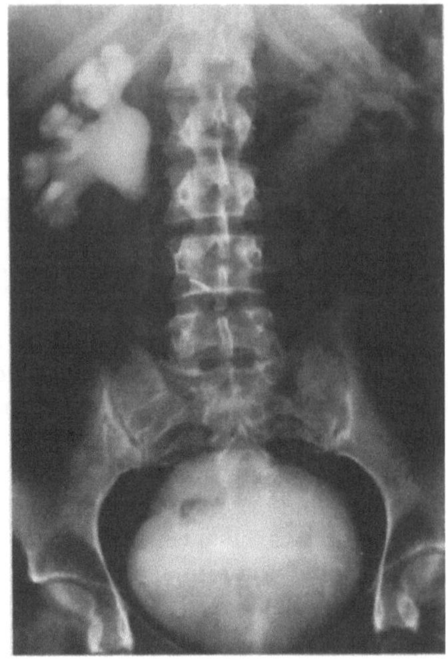

Fig. 2. Same patient as in Fig. 1, 15 min after frusemide.

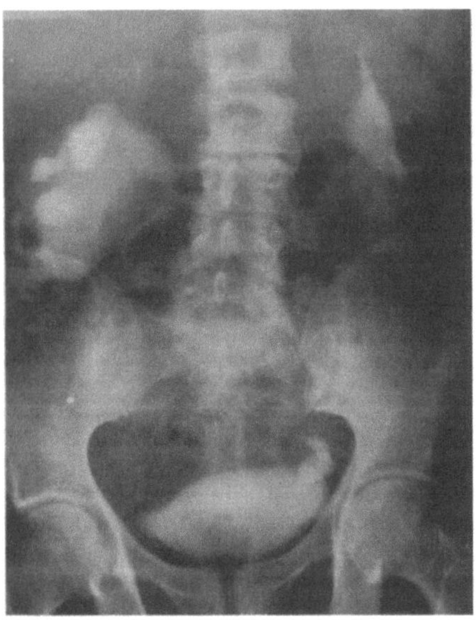

Fig. 3. Patient with bilateral PUJ obstruction, 20 min after contrast.

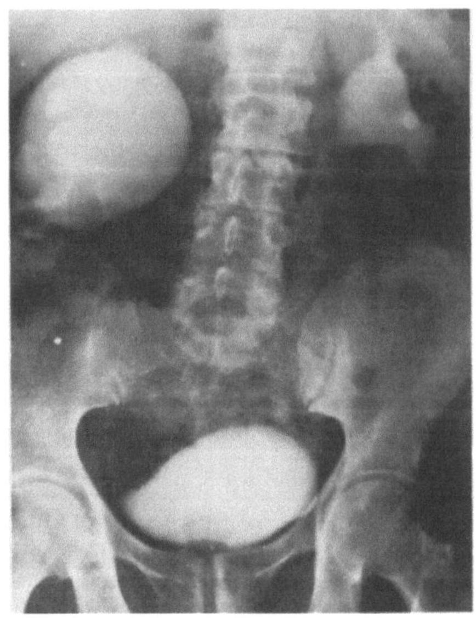

Fig. 4. Same patient as in Fig. 3, 15 min after frusemide.

Table 1. Comparison of diagnosis made on FIVU and pressure/flow studies.

		FIVU		
		Obstructed	Unobstructed	Equivocal
Pressure/flow studies	Obstructed	7	–	–
	Unobstructed	1	3	3
	Equivocal	–	2	–
	Failed	2	–	1
	Not done	1	–	–

Table 2. Comparison of diagnoses made on standard IVU and FIVU

	Standard IVU		
	Obstructed	Unobstructed	Equivocal
FIVU			
Obstructed	6	6	4
Unobstructed	5	3	4
Equivocal	2	0	0

Of the 41 patients who were investigated 26 underwent surgery. Pre-operatively the increase in the size of the renal pelvis varied between 0 and 106% with a mean of 51%. Measurement was impossible in one patient with poor renal function because of insufficient definition of the collecting system after contrast.

Twenty-four cases were studied post-operatively and the increase in the size of the pelvis after frusemide varied between 0 and 33% with a mean of 90%. Measurement was again impossible in one patient.

The results of frusemide urography were compared with the results of pressure/flow studies in twenty cases. The results of the two investigations correlated well (Table 1).

Thirty of the 41 cases studied had had standard urograms performed before being referred to our department. The diagnoses made by the radiologists after standard urograms was compared with the diagnoses made after frusemide urogramms.

In nine cases the diagnoses after standard and diuretic urography agreed, in 11 cases the diagnoses were reversed after frusemide urography and in eight cases in which standard urography was equivocal the diagnosis was made on frusemide urography; two cases remained equivocal after the diuretic urogram (Fig. 3, 4). In summary (Table 2) we see that in 30% of cases the two urograms gave similar results, in 37% of cases the diagnoses made after standard and frusemide urography were contradictory and in 27% in which standard urography was equivocal the diagnosis was made after frusemide urography.

There are disadvantages to urography in the diagnosis of PUJ obstruction: The radiation does is appreciable; in patients with poor renal function there may be insufficient defintion of the collecting system after contrast; where previous surgery has caused peri-pelvic fibrosis the compliance of the pelvis may be reduced and the criteria used for diagnosing obstruction become unreliable; intravenous urography is not a reliable measure of renal function.

Nevertheless, this study shows that although standard urography is unreliable in the diagnosis of PUT obstruction frusemide urography is as accurate as pressure/flow studies in differentiating between the obstructed and unobstructed system.

References

Covington T, Reeser W (1950) Hydronephrosis associated with over-hydration. Urol 63:438–440

Davis P, Woods KA, Evans CM, Gray WM, Kulatiliake AE (1978) The value of provocative and acute urography in patient with intermittent loin pain. Br J Urol 50:227–233

Johnson DE, Robison JR (1969) Dehydration-hydration excretory urography: use in clinical assessment of ureteropelvic junction obstruction. J Urol 101:408–410

Whitaker RH (1973) Diagnosis of obstruction in dilated ureters. Ann R Coll Surg Engl 53:153–166

Whitfield HN, Harrison NW, Sherwood T, Williams DI (1976) Upper urinary tract obstruction; pressure/flow studies in children. Br J Urol 48:427–430

Diagnostic Pressure Flow Studies of the Upper Urinary Tract

R. H. Whitaker

Introduction

For many years it has been assumed by urologists that a wide ureter, or large pelvis must be obstructed and the opposite to a refluxing ureter was an obstructed one. However, it was appreciated and discussed by Shopfner (1966), that not all wide systems are obstructed, but no proof for this belief was forthcoming until the work of Backlund and Reuterskiold (1969). These workers demonstrated non-obstructed wide ureters by showing low pressures on perfusion.

Similarly urodynamic evaluation of hydronephrosis was undertaken by Johnston (1969). It then became necessary for *obstruction* to be defined and in relation to the upper tract a definition was proposed (Whitaker 1973c): "a narrowing such that the proximal pressure is raised to transmit the usual flow through it". We found that it was impossible to define obstruction in any other terms than dynamic and this led to the concept that a diagnostic clinical approach must be on dynamic lines.

Early studies simply measured the pressure in the renal pelvis during a diuresis (Whitaker 1973b), but poorly functioning kidneys could not produce a sufficient pressure to overcome the obstruction and it was only by perfusing the system that a useful test emerged (Whitaker 1973a).

Clinical Pressure Flow Studies

The advantage of the study that we introduced in 1973 (Whitaker 1973a) was that a single cannula was introduced percutaneously into the collecting system of the kidney through which the fluid is perfused and also the pressure measured. The test has remained unmodified and was described again in detail in 1979 (Whitaker 1979b). The patient is mildly sedated and taken to the X-ray department. There a urethral catheter is passed and an intravenous injection of contrast medium given. In some very small children an anaestetic may be needed. The patient is turned prone and with the aid of fluoroscopic screening an 18 g cannula is passed vertically downwards, under local anaesthetic, into the kidney.

The bladder catheter is initially allowed to drain freely, but once the perfusion begins the bladder is allowed to fill from the perfused ureter. The bladder pressure is vital for calculating the result and must not be omitted. Contrast medium is perfused and its progress observed on the screen. The renal pelvic pressure is recorded via a transducer.

Although some workers find that these studies can be done with water manometers, I believe that a pen recorder is superior as it allows a permanent record and gives easy comparison from patient to patient. The equipment is simple and by modern-day standards inexpensive (Whitaker 1979 b).

A high flow rate (10 ml/min) is used initially to fill the system quickly, but if the pressure is high the flow can be adjusted to 5 or 2 ml/min. A high flow is essential to stress the system maximally and hence to detect obstruction if it is present. The screening during the test gives good visualisation of the anatomy and behaviour of the upper tract. It is essential to continue the perfusion until a steady-state is reached – the flow into the kidney being the same as the flow into the bladder.

If the bladder is abnormal the pressure within it may rise and then the renal pressure also rises. However, the differential pressure, or pressure drop between the kidney and bladder, and not the absolute renal pressure, dictates whether or not there is a true instrinsic obstruction at ureteric level.

Complications

Haematuria is sure to occur as the system has been penetrated, but this usually of a minor degree and of no clinical consequence. We have never needed to transfuse blood because of the procedure. Urinary tract infection is most unusual.

Interpretation of the Results

From the final pressure that is recorded in the renal pelvis must be subtracted the pressure needed to perfuse the cannula. Than the bladder pressure must be substracted to give the differential pressure form kidney to bladder. This pressure we term *"relative"*. We believe that the relative pressure should be no more than 12–15 cm water at 10 ml/min. In a neurogenic bladder the pressure in the kidney may be quite high, but the relative pressure may be normal suggesting that the upper tract dilatation is secondary to the hypertonicity of the bladder, but that there is no ureteric obstruction. We believe that pressure in excess of 22 cm water in the kidney are excessive and above this level operative relief is necessary.

Indications for Pressure Flow Studies

Any patient in whom there is the suspicion of an obstruction from a urogram, but in whom there is an element of doubt must be investigated further. Renography has advanced enormously over the last few years, but as yet is only 85% accurate in these equivocal cases. Pressure flow studies give an accurate assessment of the situation and allow a quantitative appraisal so that a logic clinical decision can be made. Despite the availability in our own unit of sophisthicated renography we still use the pressure flow study as a final arbitrator for the assessment of obstruction.

Results

Over 200 studies have now been performed in our unit, but others such as Dr. Richard Pfister in Boston have performed many more than this. Our first 170 studies were analysed recently (Whitaker 1979 a): 96% of these studies showed that there was quite definitely an obstruction (pressures over 22 cm water), or excluded an obstruction (less than 12 cm water). Only 4% of the 170 equivocal cases gave pressures in a range that might be described as "grey" – 15–22 cm water. This suggests that the test discriminates well between obstruction and non-obstruction.

More recent analysis of 75 patients with equivocal hydronephrosis showed that in 36 patients there was no obstruction. At flows of 10 ml/min the pressure varied between 2 and 14 cm water (mean 8 cm water). Thirty-nine patients showed obstruction and required a pyeloplasty. Their pressure at 10 ml/min exceeded 20 cm water. All but one patient had pressures in excess of 22 cm water. Thus again only one patient had pressures in excess of 22 cm water. Thus again only one patient had pressures of 15–22 cm water giving an unequivocal answer in 74 of 75 cases (98.5%).

In 20 of the 75 patients renography was also performed. In 12 of the cases there was full agreement, but for a variety of reasons, some obvious and others obscure, eight disagreed with the pressure study. An analysis of these studies is to be published elsewhere.

We concluded that although renography is becoming increasingly sophisticated it, as yet, cannot replace the accuracy of a pressure flow study.

Summary

Pressure flow studies have set the pace for an investigation of equivocal upper tract obstruction and as yet have not been superceded by other less invasive means in their degree of accuracy. The complications are few and not serious.

References

Backlund L, Reuterskiold AG (1969) The abnormal ureter in children. 1. Perfusion studies on the wide non-refluxing ureter. Scand J Urol Nephrol 3:219–228

Johnston JH (1969) Pathogenesis of hydronephrosis in children. Br J Urol 41:724–734

Shopfner CE (1966) Ureteropelvic junction obstruction. AJR 98:148–159

Whitaker RH (1973a) Methods of assessing obstruction in dilated ureters. Br J Urol 45:15–22

Whitaker RH (1973b) Diagnosis of obstruction in dilated ureters. Ann R Coll Surg Engl 53:153–166

Whitaker RH (1973c) The ureter in posterior urethral valves. Br J Urol 45:395–403

Whitaker RH (1979a) An evaluation of 170 diagnostic pressure flow studies of the upper urinary tract. J Urol 121:602–604

Whitaker RH (1979b) The Whitaker Test. Urol Clin North Am 6:529–539

Pressure Flow Diagnosis of Obstruction

R. Vela-Navarrete

The most elementary question that can be solved using urodynamic criteria, with reference to the upper urinary tract, is the following: *Is dilation due to the presence of obstruction?*

This is a common question when the upper dilated tract is readily visible after excretion urography and the indirect signs that usually accompany obstruction are not present. The term "equivocal dilatation" has been coined to define this circumstance. The equivocal dilatation may be localized at the calices, the pelvis, ot the ureter or may affect all of these structures.

When the upper tract cannot be demonstrated by excretion urography and dilatation is recognized by other techniques (retrograde or antegrade pyelography), the relation of dilatation to obstruction needs to be confirmed as well, at least in selected cases.

Various approaches to answer this basic question, i.e., what is the relation between dilatation and present obstruction, have been proposed. Whitaker (1973, 1975) suggested that this dilemma could be solved by using antegrade perfusion of a known flow (10 ml/min) with simultaneous monitoring of the resistance. Resistance was determined by measuring the differential pressure between the pelvis and the bladder. Although the Whitaker tests has several drawbacks (flow is unphysiologic, perfusion is done by machine, anatomy is disregarded, the limits of resistance are ill defined, etc.), it fulfills the criteria needed to recognize obstruction in the upper tract: flow and resistance are recorded simultaneously.

Since 1969 (Vela Navarrete 1970; Vela Navarrete and Robledo 1974), we have been using a procedure with the same objective whose scientific foundation can be summarized by examining these two simple questions:

1) Why is diuretic urography an inconclusive diagnostic procedure in cases of equivocal dilatation? We believe, in spite of the enthusiasm expressed by some authors, that diuretic urography cannot clarify the circumstances related to equivocal dilatation with certainty because flow is unknown during the entire procedure.

2) Will urography be considered a conclusive diagnostic test if flow is measured during the procedure? We are convinced that this is so, and we have developed a method which consists of antegrade perfusion of contrast dye, with variable but known flows and simultaneous radiographic control. The outstanding feature of this technique is that we are giving to urography a urodynamic support: the assurance that what we are observing on the X-ray screen happens with a perfectly established flow. In addition, we have optimal radiographic visualization, flow can be varied (usually between 1 and 12 ml/min), the test can be repeated during the same pro-

cedure as many times as necessary to reach a definitive conclusion (which is not the case with diouretic urography or isotopic renography), and resistance can be recognized by simply checking the drip.

The Technique

The test is begun by a transcutaneous puncture of the renal cavities. The patient lies in the prone position on an X-ray table with fluoroscopic control (Fig. 1). Local anesthetic is used in adults while in children anesthesia with ketamine (Ketalar) is used. A normal state of hydration is recommended. Before the examination adults should empty the bladder and children should have a catheter placed for free drainage.

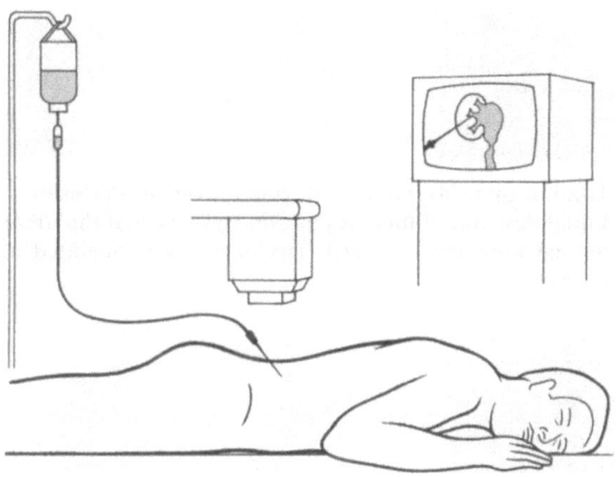

Fig. 1. Antegrade perfusion of contrast dye and radiographic control. This technique attempts to give a urodynamic support to urography by the assurance that the events observed on the radiographic screen take place at a perfectly known flow rate. The flow can be changed, increased, and repeated as many times as necessary during the same procedure until the diagnosis is reached.

The renal area is located by its anatomic relation, but if the initial attempt fails, excretion urography will facilitate the puncture. The following materials have generally been employed: a lumbar needle with a 14–16-gauge caliber and a Medicut cannula with 14–16-gauge caliber (Argyle).

Once the urine starts to drop from the needle, the baseline pelvic pressure is measured (simply by a connection with a graduated manometric tube which is maintained in a vertical position), and a few milliliters of urine are aspirated for analysis. Then the needle is connected through an intravenous set to a bottle containing normal saline with contrast dye or the appropriate commercial preparation. The bottle is situated at a height of 1 m above the skin level and perfusion is started. Low flows (1–2 ml/min) are excellent for observation of peristaltic activity. Higher flows (2–12 ml/min) are better for the detection of resistance. This may be so pronounced that some cases will not even tolerate a contant flow of 2–3 ml/min). In unobstructed cases we have reached over 10 ml/min without difficulty. Radiographic visualization on a fluoroscopic screen is mandatory during the whole procedure. Some films will be necessary for the record and for comparison. The final conclusion is based mainly on radiologic observation; therefore, it is essential to watch carefully and to have some experience in radiologic interpretation.

a

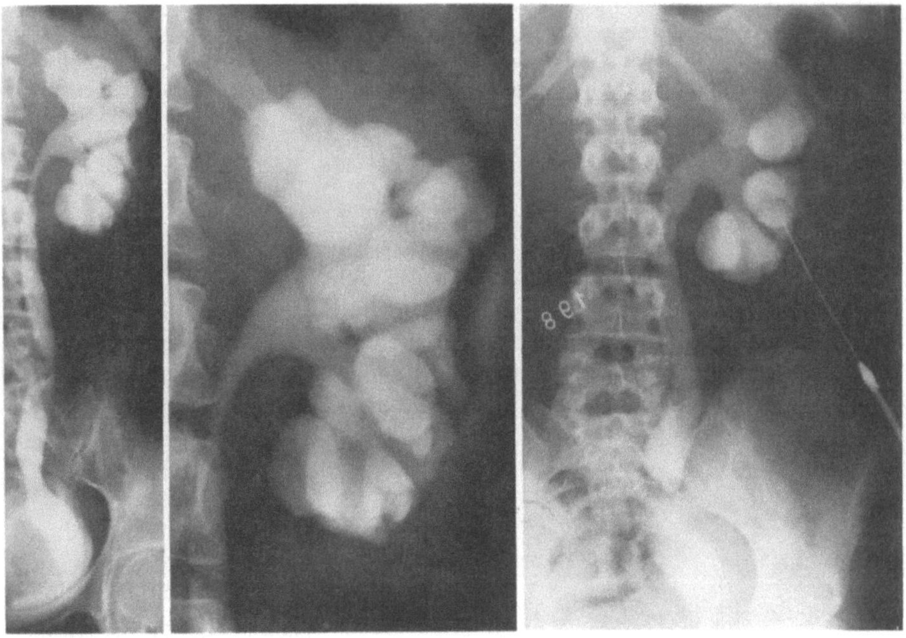

b, c

Fig. 2 a–c. Caliceal and ureteral dilatation in an asymptomatic young woman. Perfusion of 3 ml was sufficient to show increased dilatation and difficulties in urine transport at the ureterovesical junction. Resistance to increased flow was observed. The patient was operated on (ureteroneocystostomy) with excellent results.

a

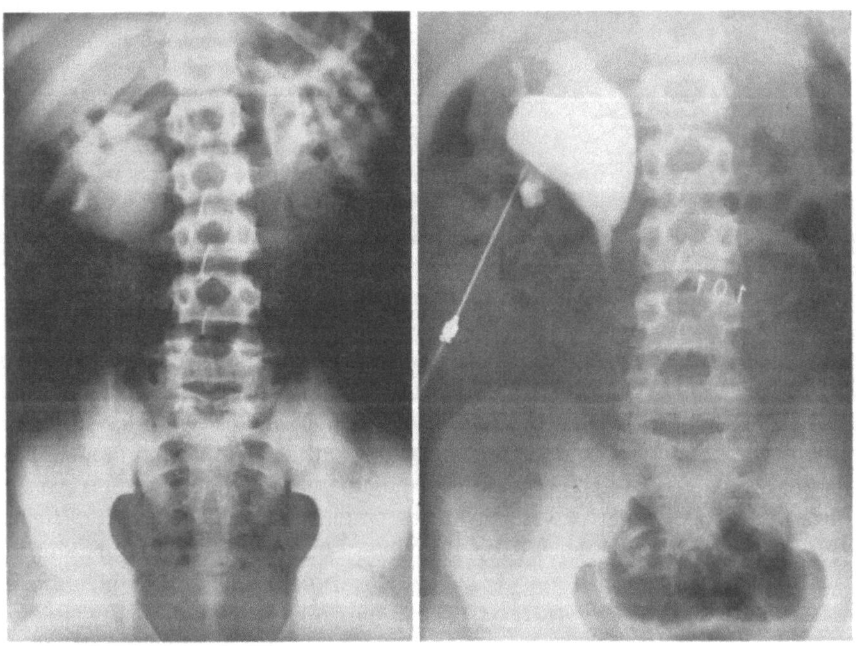

b

Fig. 3 a, b. Persistence of pelvic dilatation after a plastic procedure. Antegrade perfusion demonstrated a funnel-shaped pyeloureteral junction which tolerated flows of 6 ml/m in without important morphological changes, with synchronous pyeloureteral peristalsis and good ureteral transport of urine.

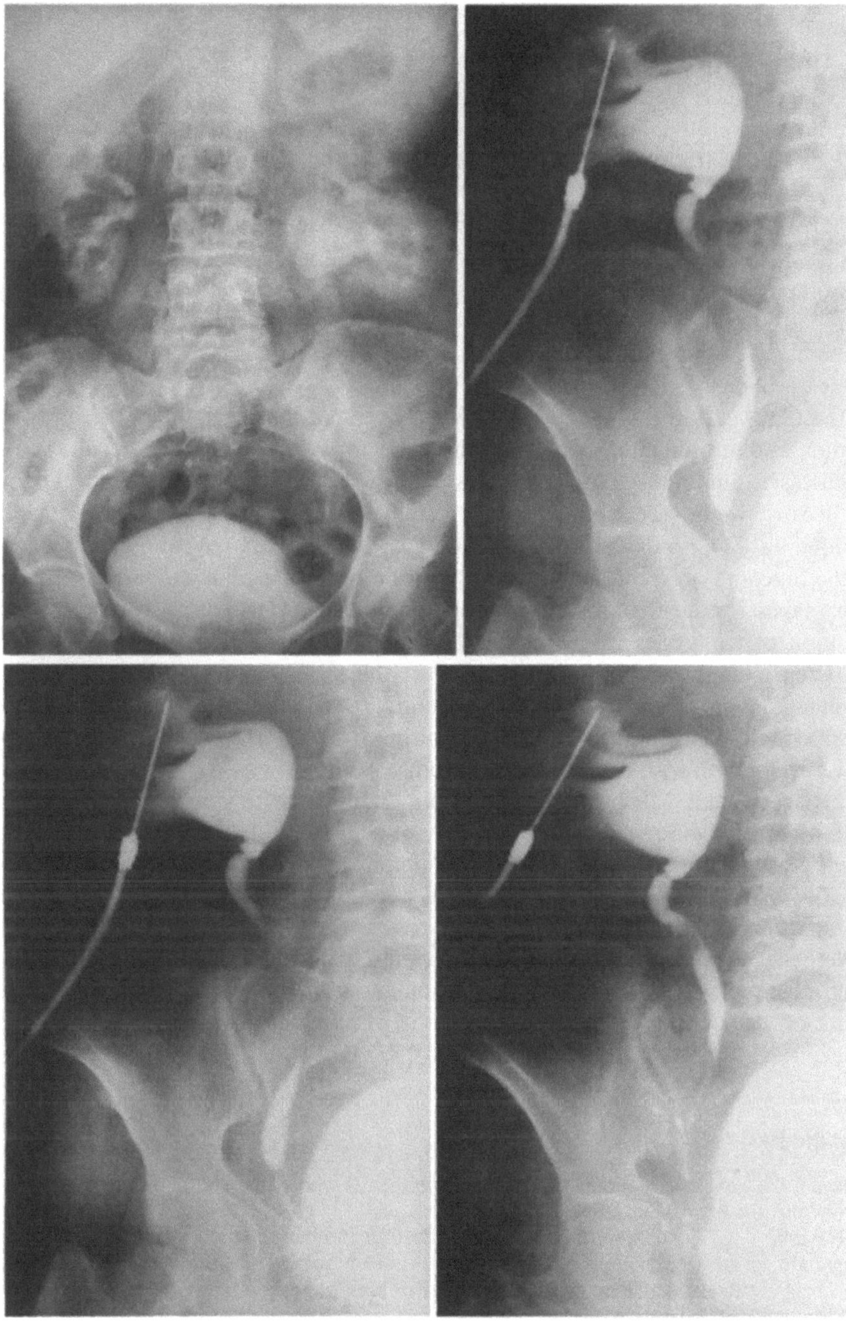

a b c d

Fig. 4 a–d. 60-year-old patient with polyuric renal failure and hyperparathyroidism. She had been operated on twice, on the left side (pyelolithotomy and iliac ureterolithotomy). High-dose excretion urography shows dilatation in the pelvis and upper ureter, without identifying the point of obstruction. Low flow perfusion allows the recognition of obstruction at the iliac ureter. In **a** and **b**, a normal peristaltic wave pushed the contrast bolus downward and beyond the point of obstruction. This peristaltic wave failed to force the whole bolus through the obstruction and a retrograde peristaltic wave was activated, thus refluxing part of the bolus back towards the pelvis (**c**). Attempts to increase the perfusion flow showed that this system did not tolerate a constant flow of 4 ml/min (**d**).

The Basic Urodynamic Study

The urodynamic evaluation of the upper tract should also help to answer other questions which are even more important than knowledge about obstruction. For example, in many cases it will be extremely important to know if there will be *reversibility* of upper excretory tract dilatation. This is essential in order to decide how much pelvis to be resected, how much ureter to be tailored, etc.

In other cases it will be necessary to know potential reversibility of obstructive nephropathy, once obstruction is corrected, to decide between radical or conservative surgery. We believe that the urodynamic evaluation can give a precise answer to these questions.

For many years minimal nephrostomy has been used to check the reversibility of dilatation and atrophic nephropathy with satisfactory results (Goodwin et al. 1955). In such cases, minimal nephrostomy was used as the least traumatic urinary diversion. Because we have used needle nephrostomy, not merely as a simple diversion technique but as a urodynamic tool (Vela Navarrete 1971 a, b), it is now our feeling that the outcome of needle nephrostomy can be predicted by a simpler procedure which makes needle nephrostomy obsolete and allows for a precise urodynamic evaluation of the upper urinary tract. This procedure is called *basic urodynamic study* (Vela Navarrete 1980) and consists of the simultaneous determination by transcutaneous puncture of these three parameters: (1) Baseline renal pelvis pressure, (2) solute concentration in aspirated urine from the renal pelvis, and (3) antegrade pyelogram, with or without perfusion.

This set of data will be sufficent in many conditions of obstruction and dilatation, when urodynamic circumstances cannot be clarified by other simpler means, to clearly establish the relation between dilatation and obstruction and predict reversibility of excretory tract dilatation and potential improvement of obstructive nephropathy.

We believe that this procedure represents the first attempt to understand upper tract urodynamics in conditions of obstruction and dilatation with a unified criteria, instead of developing a separate technique for each aspect of the problem (Figs. 2–4).

References

Goodwin WE, Casey WC, Woolf W (1955) Percutaneous trocar (needle) nephrostomy in hydronephrosis. J Am Med Assoc 157:891

Vela-Navarrete R (1970) Manometria, pielografia translumbar repetida y función renal por separado, en la valoración pronóstica del riñón hidronefrótico. Arch Esp Urol 23:163

Vela-Navarrete R (1971 a) Percutaneous intrapelvic pressure determinations on the study of hydronephrosis. Invest Urol 8:526

Vel-Navarrete R (1971 b) Repeat direct pyelography via needle nephrostomy. Acta Radiol [Diagn] (Stockh) 11:38

Vel-Navarrete R (1980) What is a urodynamic study of the upper urinary tract? Urology 15:93–98

Vela-Navarrete R, Robledo A Garcia (1974) El principio de la injección transcutánea en el estudio radio gráfico de la dinámica pieloureteral. Radiologia 16:51–56

Whitaker RH (1973) Methods of assessing obstruction in dilated ureters. Br J Urol 45:15

Whitaker RH (1975) Equivocal pelvi-uretic obstruction. J Urol 47:771

Non-Invasive Techniques in the Quantification of Ureteropelvic Junction Obstruction

U. Engelmann, G. Hutschenreiter, P. Alken, M. Marberger and F. Hahn

The search for an optimal procedure for diagnosing obstruction of the upper urinary tract is still going on. A variety of diagnostic methods are currently available. Whitaker's pressure flow studies (1977, 1978, 1979 a, b) give an adequate diagnosis of obstruction, but the question is whether the procedure is still a necessary one or whether it can be replaced by other methods, such as diuresis renography (O'Reilly et al. 1978; Lupton et al. 1979; Koff et al. 1979), frusemide intravenous urography (Whitfield et al 1979) or diuresis sonography.

Figure 1 shows a patient with a ureteropelvic junction (UPJ) obstruction, whose differential pressure was 20 cm H_2O at a flow rate of 5 ml/min, and almost 40 cm H_2O at 7.5 ml/min. After successful pyeloplasty, the respective values were 12 and 19 cm H_2O. According to Whitaker (1979 a), these values are on the borderline between obstruction and non-obstruction. In the same patient, diuresis renography no

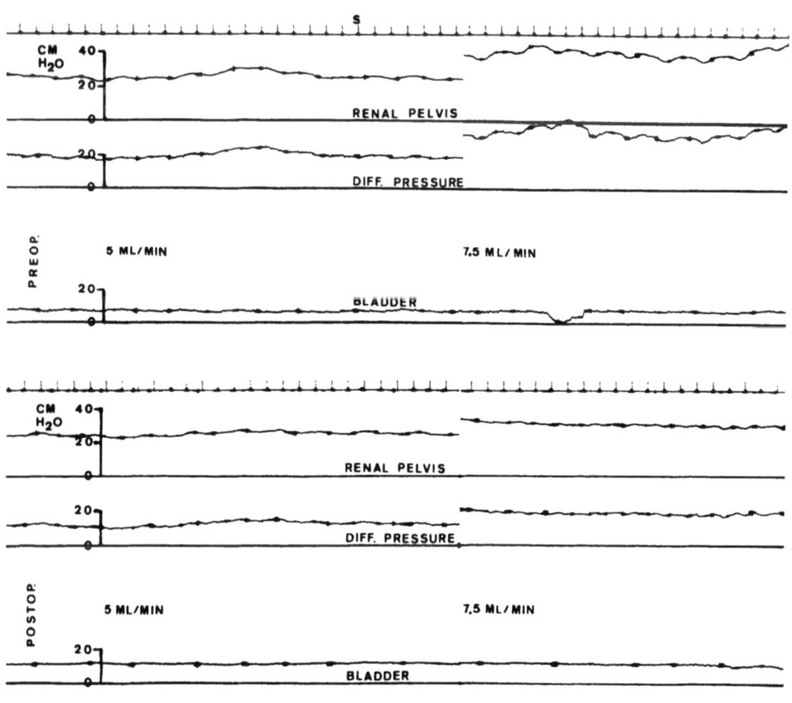

Fig. 1. Whitaker test before (*upper*) and after (*lower*) pyeloplasty.

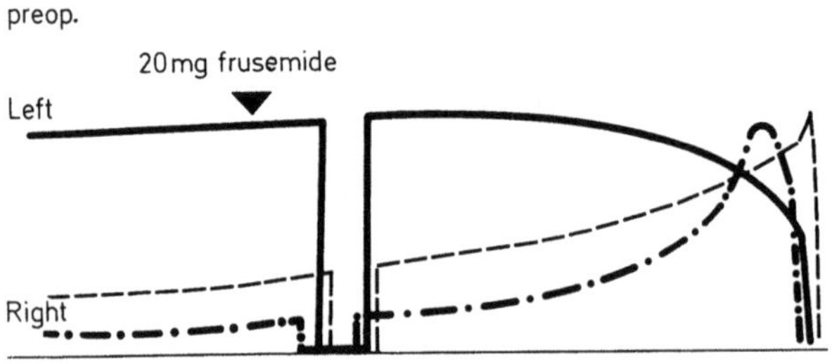

Fig. 2. Diuresis renography before pyeloplasty. Same patient as in Fig. 1.

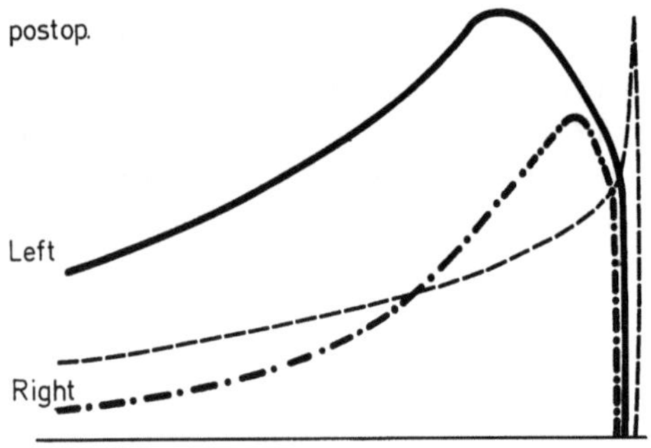

Fig. 3. Diuresis renography after pyeloplasty. Same patient as in Fig. 1.

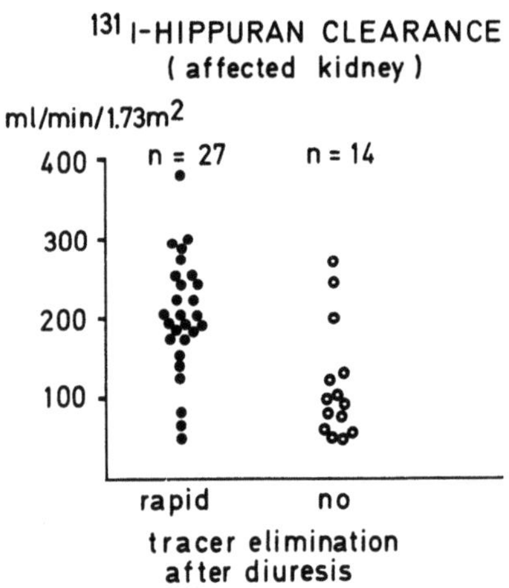

Fig. 4. Renal pelvic pressure versus ^{131}I-Hippuran clearance in patients with UPJ obstruction ($n = 14$).

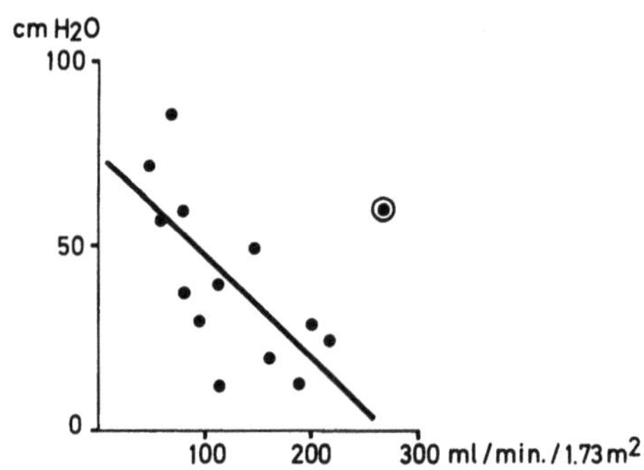

Fig. 5. Correlation between tracer elimination and kidney function.

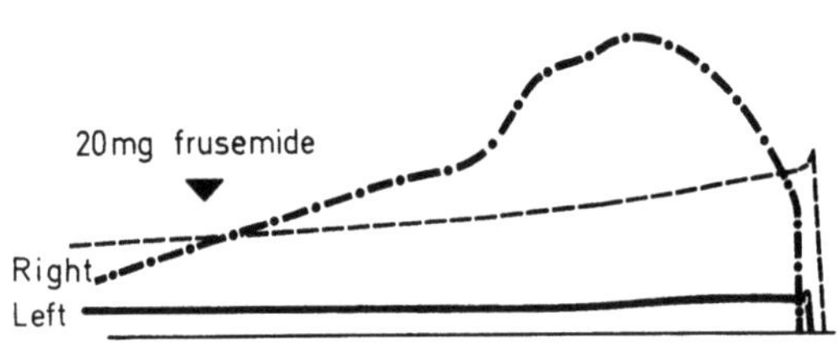

Fig. 6. Diuresis renography in severe, long-standing UPJ obstruction.

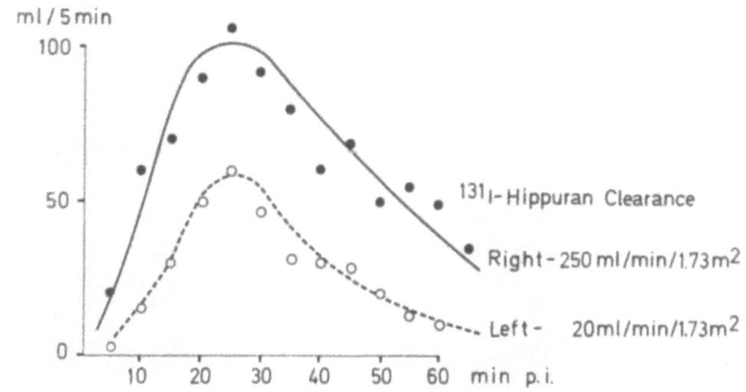

Fig. 7. Urine production after (20 mg i. v.) frusemide measured via a nephrostomy tube (left kidney) and an indewelling catheter (right kidney). Same patient as in Fig. 6.

longer demonstrated flow disturbances compared with the preoperative condition (Figs. 2,3).

When pelvic pressure is plotted against renal function (Fig. 4), adults show an inverse correlation between kidney function and pressure, that is, the higher the pressure, the worse the function. Put another way, the result of a long-standing, severe obstruction is a more rapid deterioration of renal function. Only in children can serious obstruction be found with relatively good renal function because of the short duration of the obstruction.

No tracer elimination after frusemide (Lasix) in diuresis renography is an indication of severe obstruction. The advantage of the method is that it measures renal function – but it also has its limits.

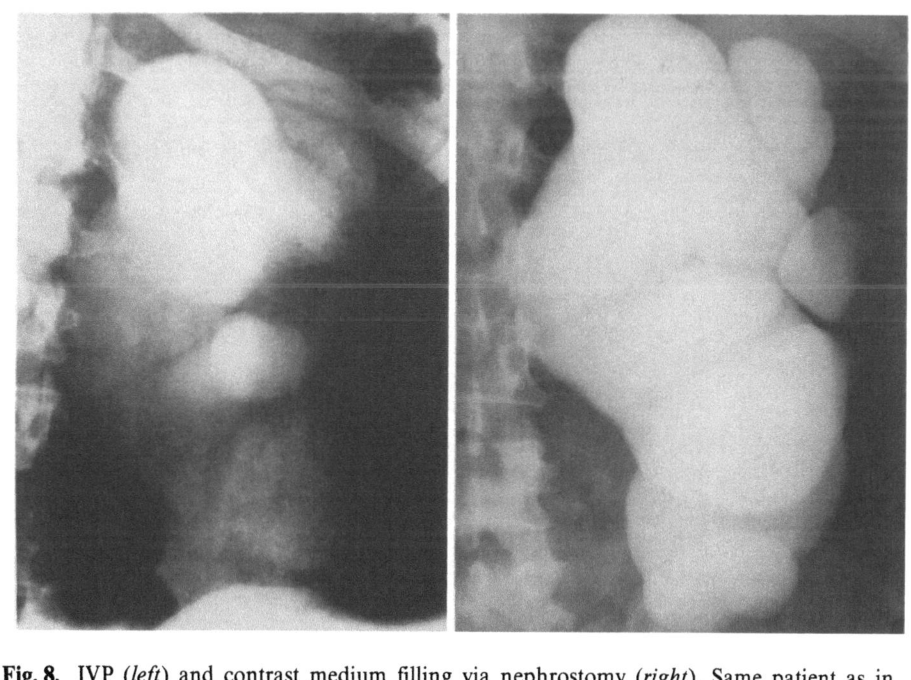

Fig. 8. IVP (*left*) and contrast medium filling via nephrostomy (*right*). Same patient as in Fig. 6.

a

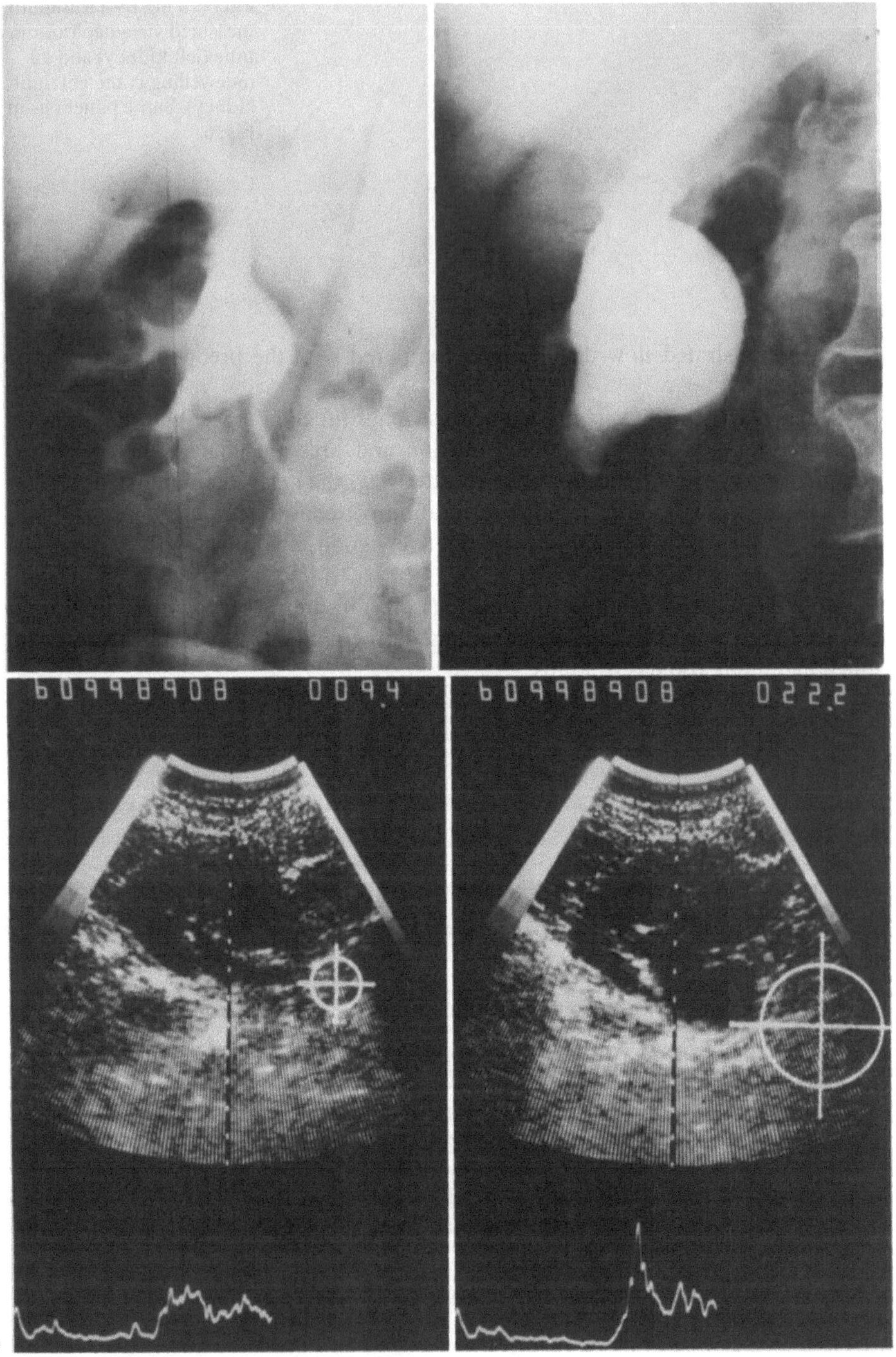

b

Fig. 9. **a** Diuresis IVP. **b** Diuresis sonography. Transverse prone scan of the left kidney before (*left*) and after (*right*) 20 mg frusemide. Same patient as in **a**.

It is obvious here that the lack of response to frusemide, that is, no tracer elimination after diuresis, almost only occurs in kidneys with poor absolute function (Fig. 5). But how should these results be interpreted?

Is this lack of response to frusemidc:

1) A sign of serious obstruction?
2) A sign of serious tubular damage in kidneys with low ^{131}iodine-Hippuran-clearance?
3) Or does the lack of response merely reflect the inaccuracy of this method in kidneys with poor absolute function?

Figures 6, 7 and 8 demonstrate this problem. Diuresis clearance shows no function on the left side and the corresponding lack of response to frusemide (Fig. 6). After frusemide administration, the hydronephrotic left kidney promptly responds with an increased urine production up to a maximum flow rate of almost 12 ml/min measured over a nephrostomy tube (Fig. 7). The severe obstruction is demonstrated as well by the intravenous pyelogram (IVP) (Fig. 8) as by the Whitaker test, which showed a pressure rise of 24 cm H_2O measured at 5 ml/min.

We can therefore conclude that a lack of tracer elimination in kidneys with poor function does not necessarily mean that there is a serious obstruction. The better renal function is, the better tracer elimination after frusemide can be demonstrated on the renogram.

Since both methos – the Whitaker test and diuresis renography – are limited in one way or another, the question arises whether a third study should be performed in addition to these two techniques, or wheter one can be omitted. One possibility is the diuresis IVP. However, this would mean an additional X-ray study, which can be avoided by diuresis sonography.

Sonographic surface and volume measurements of the dilated renal pelvis are sometimes difficult, firstly, because of the irregular form, and secondly, because of the often poor cranial outline behind the eleventh and twelfth ribs in pronounced hydronephrosis. In contrast to length, reproduction of maximal width and depth of the renal pelvis is superior with sonography (Fig. 9).

Frusemide diuresis does not lead to any measurable changes in non-dilated and intrarenal pelvises (Fig. 10) But, if the pelvis is extrarenal – as is usually the case with UPJ obstruction – dilatation depends on the degree of obstruction and function. The same is true for some kidneys in which clearance can no longer be measured: the increased production of isosthenuric urine leads to dilatation (Fig. 11). In kidneys which show no response to frusemide diuresis, there is no increase in diameter, just as in normal kidneys without obstruction (Fig. 12).

In 29 measurements carried out on obstructed kidneys, the average increase of the maximal depth and width diameters of the renal pelvis after frusemide diuresis was 53% (Fig. 13). As a rule, width increases more than depth. An increases in diameter of 30% or more is a clear criterion of obstruction, corresponding to the Whitaker Test and diuresis renography.

Our conclusions are as follows:

1) The Whitaker Test, which is invasive and provides no information on renal function, no longer seems necessary for clarification of UPJ obstruction.

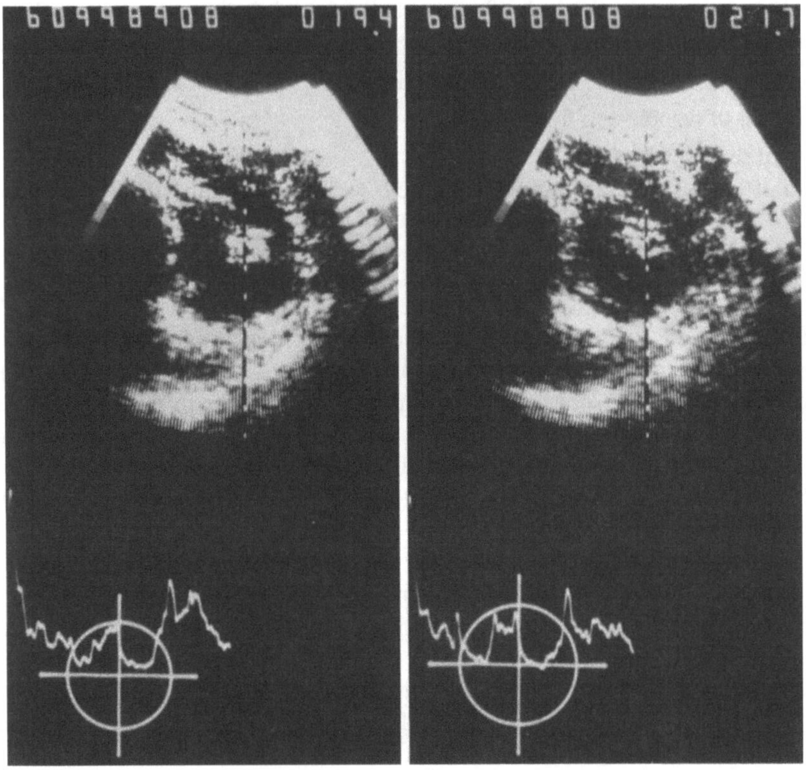

Fig. 10. Diuresis sonography. Transverse prone scan of non-obstructed left kidney.

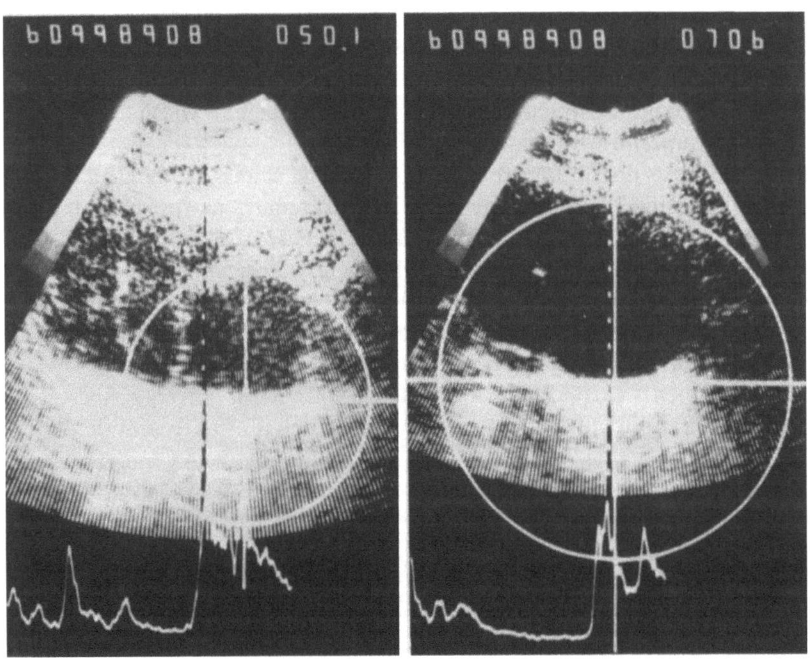

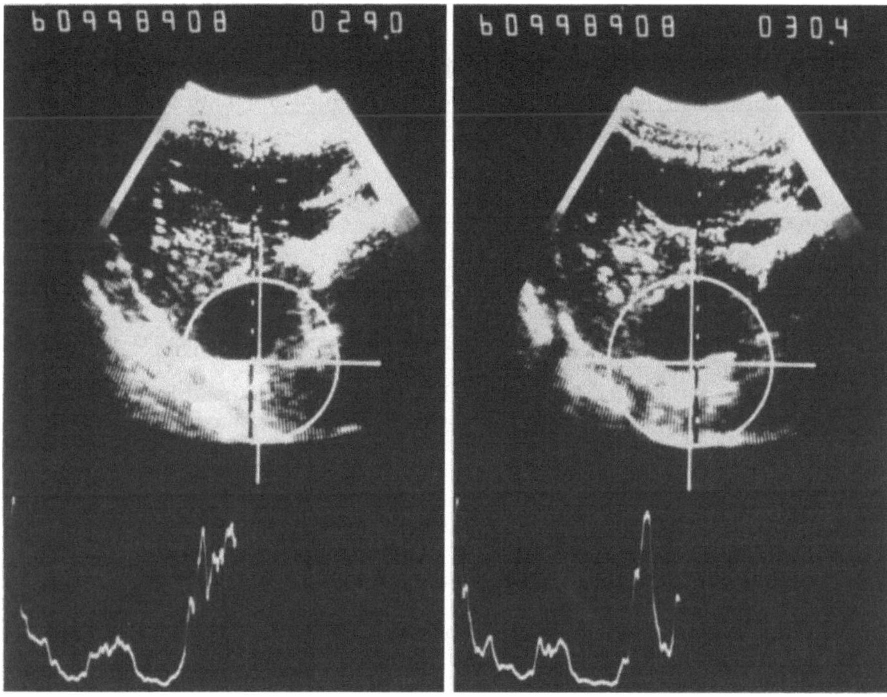

Fig. 12. Diuresis sonography. Transverse supine scan of right kidney. No response to frusemide diuresis.

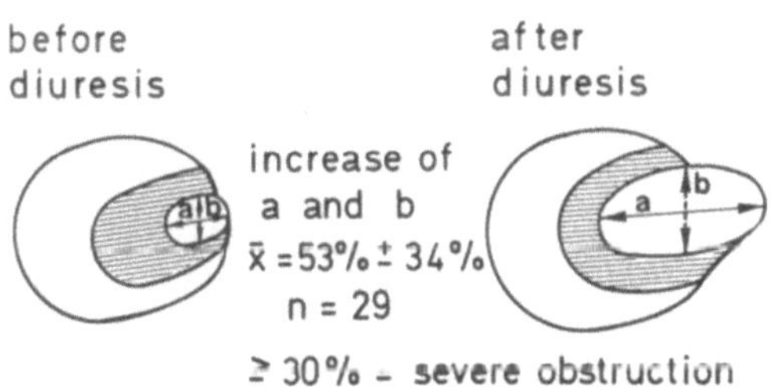

Fig. 13. Diuresis sonography. Increase of width and depth in transverse scan after frusemide diuresis.

2) Diuresis renography is the method of choice, as it gives adequate information about the degree of obstruction. However, the renal function determinations should be interpreted with great care, as an overestimate of function is possible (Doppelfeld and Weißbach 1979), and there is one exception:

3) Kidneys with poor function may respond to frusemid with water diuresis which is not registered by diuresis renography. In these cases the method is inaccurate.

Fig. 11. Diuresis sonography. Transverse prone scan of severely obstructed left kidney. Same patient as in Figs. 6–8.

4) An adequate supplement to diuresis renography could therefore be diuresis sonography, as it is non-invasive and can identify obstruction in kidneys with poor function, but further investigation in this field is needed.

For diagnosis of UPJ obstruction, a combination of conventional IVP, diuresis renography and sonography is recommended.

References

Doppelfeld E, Weißbach L (1979) Untersuchungen zum Einfluß von Harnabflußstörungen auf die Ergebnisse der katheterlosen seitengetrennten Bestimmung der renalen Hippuran-Clearance. Aktuel Urol 10:85

Koff SA, Thrall JH, Keyes JW Jr (1979) Diuretic radionuclide urography: A non-invasive method for evaluating nephroureteral dilatation. J Urol 122:451

Lupton EW, Testa HJ, Lawson RS, Edwards EC, Carroll RNP, Barnard RJ (1979) Diuresis renography and the results of pyeloplasty for idiopathic hydronephrosis. Br J Urol 51:449

O'Reilly PH, Testa HJ, Lawson RS, Farrar DJ, Edwards EC (1978) Diuresis renography in equivocal urinary tract obstruction. Br J Urol 50:76

Whitaker RH (1977) Pressure-controlled nephrostography. Eur Urol 3:145

Whitaker RH (1978) Clinical assessment of pelvic and ureteral function. Urology 12:146

Whitaker RH (1979a) The Whitaker Test. Urol Clin North Am 6:529

Whitaker RH (1979b) An evaluation of 170 diagnostic pressure flow studies of the upper urinary tract. J Urol 121:602

Whitfield HN, Britton KE, Hendry WF, Wickham JEA (1979) Frusemide intravenous urography in the diagnosis of pelviureteric junction obstruction. Br J Urol 51:445

Analysis of Peristaltic Urine Transport in the Ureter by ^{123}I-Hippuric Acid

K. U. Laval, K. Vyska, Ch. Freundlieb, and L. E. Feinendegen

Clinical investigations of ureteral peristaltic transport function are usually done by endo-ureteral techniques, e.g. pressure (Lapides 1948; Lutzeyer 1963; Boyarsky and Labay 1972) and flow (Melchior and Simham 1971) measurements, or by radiographic methods, e.g. videodensitometry (Tscholl et al. 1974; Weinberg and Labay 1977) and cineradiography (Durben et al. 1980). Ureteral catheterisation carries the risk of infection whereas radiographic procedures have the well-known disadvantages of reaction to radiopacity (Shehadi 1975) diuretic effects and radiation charge.

Methods

For our investigation we used ^{123}I-hippuric acid (Cyclotron from E.I.R., Würenlingen, Switzerland). The ^{123}Iodine used as the tracer was derived from the reaction: ^{127}I(d, 6n) ^{123}Xe(ß, EC) ^{123}I (Stöcklin 1977). The investigation was done in the supine position by means of a gamma camera (Nucl. Chicago LFOV) equipped with a high-resolution parallel hole low-energy collimator. The data were first computerised with the list-mode-technique (Digital Equipment pdp-50). The data processing was usually done by printing series of matrices with a frequency of one matrix per second. On integral images of about 30 matrices we marked regions of interest over the mid-ureter and the peri-ureteral background tissue. From these regions activity curves were registered from the 4th to 500th second after application.

The examinations were done on five healthy volunteers with no special preparation or diet. All individuals received 2 mCi ^{123}I-hippuric acid intraveneously. The maximal radiation charge was calculated for the bladder as critical organ with 100 mrad.

Results

Figure 1 shows an activity curve registered from a mid-ureter segment. The analysis is done by activity calculation for each second. The registration starts with the activity almost constantly on background level. Beginning from the 190th second after application rhythmic changes of activity are recorded with a frequency of 1.5 to 2 waves per minute. The minima points of the curve are still on background level, while the oscillating curve is superimposed upon this level. The curve maxima reach

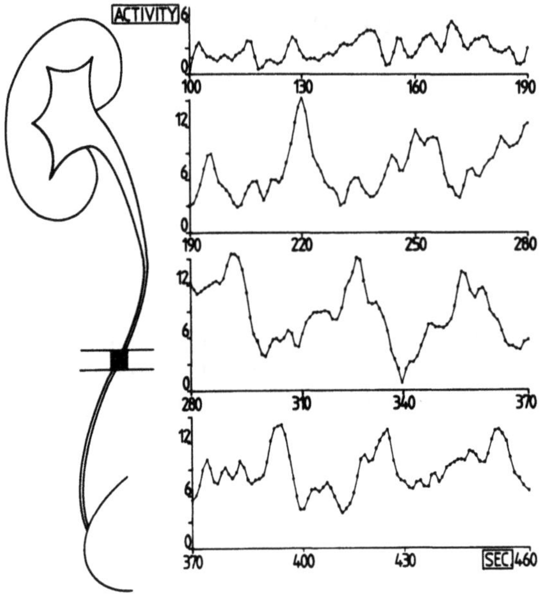

Fig. 1. Activity curve registered from a mid-ureter segment, schematically drawn.

almost equal height. After the minimum the activity curve regularly shows a slow increase up to the maximum, which is then followed by an abrupt decrease to the next minimum. The profile of the activity curve between two minima correlates to a urine bolus.

Figure 2 shows the shape of the activity profile of a single urine bolus. The profile shows a slow and steady increase to the maximum, which is followed by an

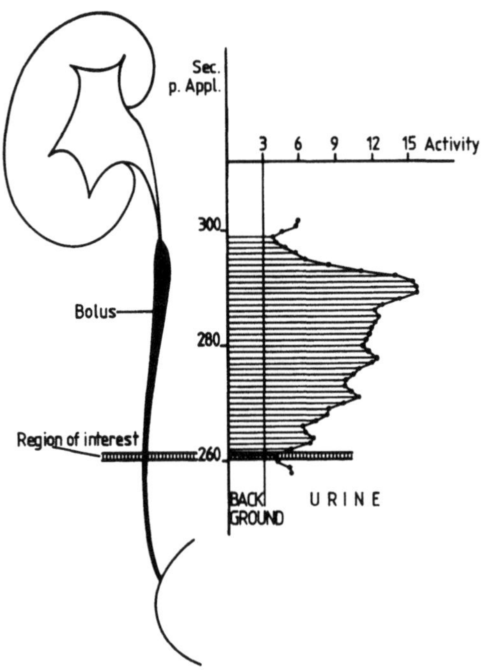

Fig. 2. Shape of the activity profile of a single urine bolus. According to the activity level, the bolus is drawn schematically within the ureter. The shape is part of the curve presented in Fig. 1.

abrupt decrease to the next minimum. The minimum corresponds to the contractile ring of the ureter propagating the urine bolus through the region of interest towards the bladder.

Discussion

All non-invasive techniques for investigation of ureteral transport function use the endo-ureteral volume distribution during time as the only source of information. Therefore a homogeneous distribution as well as a constant concentration of the tracer material in the urine is mandatory. Under this condition the registered activity is in proportion to urine volume, and the changes of activity with time are proportional to volume changes with an adequate time constant.

The computer analysis of the activity signals from the mid-ureter show the following typical features:

1) The low plateau at the start of recording is equal to the background activity and the late rise of the activity level is due to the physiological transit time of hippuric acid through the kidney and proximal ureter. Thus, the shape of the recording demonstrates the proper identification of the ureter within the region of interest.

2) The minima of the ureteral activity curve are almost exactly at background level, which proves that for these moments of time the ureter is empty and there is no tracer volume in this segment of ureter. This happens when the active contractile ring passes the region of interest. From the minima the frequency of peristalsis is derived, which in our cases was between 1.5 and 2/min. The activity rise between these minima provides information about the shape of a bolus moving through the region of interest towards the bladder (Fig. 2). The activity profile of a bolus shows a rather slow increase of bolus diameter compared with the rapid decrease following the maximum. The maxima or different boli show approximately the same activity level.

References

Boyarsky S, Labay PC (1972) Ureteral dynamics. Williams & Wilkins, Baltimore

Durben G et al. (1980) The time distance diagram: a new method to analyse ureteral peristalsis by cineradiography. Invest Urol (to be published)

Lapides J (1948) Physiology of the intact human ureter. J Urol 59:601–637

Lutzeyer W (1963) Harnleiterdruckmessungen. Urol Int 16:1–15

Melchior H, Simhan KK (1971) Zur Problematik der Uro-Rheomanometrie. Biomed Tech (Berlin) 16:99–102

Shehadi WH (1975) Adverse reactions to intravascularly administered contrast media. A comprehensive study based on a prospective study. AJR 124:145–152

Stöcklin G (1977) Bromine-77 and Iodine-123 radiopharmaceuticals. Int J Appl Radiat Isot 28:131

Tscholl R et al. (1974) Measurement of the velocity and rate of ureteral contraction with a video integrator in a model, in animals and in humans, peroperatively and with intact body surface. Invest Urol 12:224–232

Weinberg SL, Labay P (1977) Ureteral function. The urometrogram at increased urine output. Invest Urol 14:307–311

Urodynamic Investigation of Urinary Incontinence

E. S. Glen

Accurate diagnosis is essential for the proper management of any disorder, and incontinence is no exception. A detailed clinical history and examination are required. Do not be misled by those who claim that urodynamics may replace careful routine investigation. The overall picture must be appreciated before embarking upon specialised investigation. For example, incontinence may be the presenting symptom in the following conditions:

1) Urinary tract infection, especially in children;
2) diabetes;
3) neurological disorders such as multiple sclerosis, early spinal cord compression etc. Lumbar disc protrusion may present in this way, progressing to chronic retention with overflow incontinence;
4) fistula and ectopic ureteric communication with urethra;
5) psychiatric disorders including alcoholism;
6) iatrogenic causes such as excessive sedation in the elderly or injudicious use of diuretic.

If incontinence is not due to any of these conditons, or if it persists after appropriate treatment, then urological and urodynamic investigations are necessary. Recent experience has shown that excretion urography is not necessary unless there is a clear indication such as haematuria or proven chronic urinary tract infection (Glen 1980, unpublished). However, if cystometry demonstrates a high pressure system in the presence of poor voiding, excretion urography is advisable since renal damage may have occurred due to vesicoureteric reflux. Cystourethroscopy is useful, and in our series has demonstrated relevant abnormalities in about 50% of 400 women with incontinence referred to the Uro/Gynaecological Clinic.

Urodynamic Investigations. The word urodynamic is used loosely, and is applied to some investigations that are properly defined as static measurements. Accepting common usage however, the investigations currently available are listed in Table 1. These investigations and their relative values will be discussed.

Cystometry. This is the single most useful investigation, simple to perform and easy to interpret. Early techniques involved incremental filling, with pressure being recorded after each installation of fluid. This was mainly due to the limitations imposed by available equipment. Continuous flow cystometry is preferable, pressure being recorded throughout filling. The International Continence Society (I.C.S.) created a committee to standardise nomenclature in urodynamics. The first three reports have been published in all major urological journals and are collated in the *Jour-*

Table 1. Investigations currently available in urodynamic clinics. Cystometry and bladder emptying flowrate measurement are the most popular basic screening tests. Calculation of intrinsic detrusor pressure (intravesical pressure minus intra abdominal pressure) provides greater accuracy in cystometry and UCPP measurement when provocative measures are employed, such as change of posture, coughing or other patient activity. This refinement is essential in procedures 3 and 4 to identify the relative roles of detrusor contraction and increased intra-abdominal pressure.

1) Cystometry
2) Bladder-emptying flow rate measurement
3) Flow measurement combined with bladder pressure measurements (CPF)
4) CPF plus simultaneous voiding cystourethrography (VCU)
5) Urethral closure pressure profile measurement (UCPP)
6) Electromyography combined with one or several of these procedures
7) Urine loss measurement by the "recording nappy"

nal of Urology (Bates et al. 1979). The reports include recommendations regarding standard reference points in urodynamic measurements and are essential reading for anyone working in this field.

The use of gas as a filling medium is favoured in North America, perhaps because of its convenience in office practice. However, if used it should be reserved for rapid screening of patients with suspected neurological disorders since it is liable to produce artefacts, more so than water, and is not so reliable in general practice. The gas dries the bladder mucosa and may cause pain in patients with normal sensation.

The rate of filling is important in some patients, and if possible cystometry should be performed at two rates to provide maximum information. Our own practice is to use a filling rate of about 20 ml/min. (medium fill in I.C.S. terminology) followed by rapid fill cystometry of 100 ml/min or more as a provocative cystometrogram (Glen and Rowan 1973). Rapid filling may provoke uninhibited contraction in some individuals, for example in multiple sclerosis. Recording a medium-fill followed by a fast-fill cystometrogram is convenient in that other urodynamic investigations are facilitated at the same attendance. For example, urethral closure pressure profile measurement (UCPP) is performed with the bladder empty and again when it is full. Bladder-emptying flow rate is measured on arrival at the clinic, and again when a known volume has been instilled. Cystometry is recorded during rapid installation prior to the final recording of flow.

Cystometry can be performed in various ways:

1) Two fine urethral catheters may be employed, one for filling and the other for recording. The insertion of these catheters can be painful especially in males, and this technique is not recommended.

2) A double lumen catheter permis simultaneous filling and recording. A suitable catheter is available from Portex Limited, Hythe, England.

3) Suprapubic catheters. When cystometry is combined with flow studies, a modern suprapubic cannula is ideal for the measurement of bladder pressure. It will not inhibit voiding, nor interfere with the direction of urine flow into the flow meter unlike the urethral catheter used by so many clinicians today. Several suitable suprapubic catheters are already available, our own preference at present being for that produced by Dow Corning Ltd.

4) Cystometry combined with intra-abdominal pressure recording is used to estimate the subtracted or intrinsic detrusor pressure (intravesical pressure minus intra-abdominal pressure). It is recognised that intra-abdominal pressure is variable and depends on the site or recording and the activity of the subject. For convenience, intra-abdominal pressure is usually estimated by means of a simple cannula in the rectum. The terminal openings at the rectal end are protected by a rubber cover. Care must be taken to extract all air from the system to obtain the maximum frequency response, a water-filled system providing the most useful technique.

Subtraction of intra-abdominal pressure is advisable when cystometry is attempted during coughing, alteration in posture etc. Otherwise changes in intra-abdominal pressure may simulate or conceal uninhibited bladder activity.

5) Transducer-Tipped Catheter (TTC). These catheters offer a better frequency response improving accuracy but are fragile and expensive. In males there is an additional disadvantage in that the TTC is stiff and may be difficult to insert into the bladder. Professor Rossier, Boston, overcomes this difficulty by introducing the TTC within a split, soft urethral catheter which can then be withdrawn leaving the TTC in place. The current cost of about £ 1550 is a major disadvantage, as is the time-consuming sterilisation technique. If a robust and less expensive TTC can be produced it will probably replace the other measurement systems.

6) Other systems have been tried but found deficient. For example, the radio transmitter "pill" placed in the bladder proved unreliable and was difficult to insert. The incrased interest shown by manufacturers may produce new and better instruments.

Incremental filling should now be reserved for the measurement of bladder compliance. This is not a routine procedure but can be used to estimate the quality of the bladder wall.

Bladder-Emptying Flow Rate Measurement. It is true that it is sometimes possible to observe the stream of urine voided by patients and derive useful informations as to strength of flow, presence or absence of hesitancy, intermittent or prolonged flow, and terminal dribbling. However, voiding in public presents difficulties for many apparently normal males, and no one has satisfactorily described how flow can be observed in females. For these reasons, flow meters are proving to be invaluable. The most reliable currently available is made by Disa Limited. It consists of a transducer at the base of a collecting funnel. The urine flow directed into the funnel falls on a rotating disc. The flow tends to slow the rotation, producing an electrical signal which is recorded on heat-sensitive paper. The flow meter records the maximum flow rate, the flow time, volume voided and also reproduces the pattern of flow. Interpretation should be based on all of these measurements, preferably after several flows. Provided reasonable care is taken to ensure an adequate volume in the bladder before voiding, privacy and familiarity in using the apparatus, reliable and valuable information can be obtained (Rowan et al. 1977). The flow meter can be used for diagnosis and assessment of bladder-emptying problems that may be associated with incontinence.

Flow measurement combined with bladder pressure measurements (CPF): Measurement of intravesical pressure and intrinsic detrusor pressure (intravesical minus intra-abdominal pressure) together with simultaneous measurement of flow rate and volume voided provides valuable information about bladder function in problem cases. For example, poor voiding may result from weak detrusor contraction, micturition being dependent on the use of intra-abdominal pressure. The investigation may demonstrate normal flow measurements associated with an abnormally high detrusor pressure. These patients are at risk in terms of upper urinary tract obstruction or reflux, leading to renal damage.

CPF plus simultaneous voiding cystourethrography (Bates et al. 1970): It is fashionable to combine CPF with micturating cystography, commonly called voiding cystourethrography (VCU). By means of two television cameras and an electronic mixer, the pressure and flow measurements are recorded simultaneously on videotape. While this is convenient for teaching purposes, the combination is probably unnecessary and imposes additional problems on the patient with difficulty in voiding. The apparatus is expensive and the patient is subjected to relatively high levels of radiation, especially if lateral views are taken. VCU is probably best reserved for patients with a high bladder pressure where reflux is suspected. Even then it is not essential to combine VCU with pressure measurements, although the combination does have an academic attraction.

Urethral closure pressure profile measurement (Rowan and Glen 1979): This measurement records the length of the urethra in centimeters and the yield pressure within the urethra exerted along that length, expressed in centimeters of water.

The investigation is of particular value in women, interpretation being more difficult in men because of the more complex shape of the posterior urethra. The procedure has been somewhat neglected due to earlier inadequate techniques performed by workers who did not take the precaution of continuing cystometry during profile measurement. It is pointless to record UCPP when the bladder is contracting, since detrusor activity is likely to produce reflux urethral relaxation as the first step towards voiding. The UCPP will obviously be affected. It is also helpful to measure UCPP with the bladder empty and again when it is at its functioning capacity as determined by filling cystometry. The normal UCPP shows either improvement as the bladder fills, or is already at a high level when the bladder is empty. The practice of using a standard volume, for example 150 ml in the bladder, can be misleading since this volume may represent the functioning capacity in one individual, and only a fraction of the capacity in others.

Deterioration in profile as the bladder fills is an indication for physiotherapy and/or surgery in incontinent women in whom cystometry is normal. However, a fibrosed urethra acts as a rigid tube and UCPP may then be inaccurate. The presence of such a frozen urethra is easily detected by palpation and cystourethroscopy. Details of technique are well-described in the literature. The principal methods employed are described in Table 2.

EMG. Measurement of sphincteric EMG is difficult since localisation of the sphincter is rather subjective and interpretation highly subjective. Measurement of EMG of the detrusor is invasive and not particularly useful. Where neurological disease is suspected, EMG and the provocative stimulus of cold infusion during cystometry can be useful. EMG is best performed by means of suitably positioned needle electrodes. In patients with normal sensation, the needles may cause discomfort initially.

Table 2. Principal catheter systems used for urethral closure pressure profile (UCPP) measurements. There are multiple variations but the principal techniques are described.

1) *Simple catheter with two or more side openings at the distal end*
A continuous flow of 2 ml/min passes through one arm of a "Y" connector, along the catheter. Initially this fluid column measures bladder pressure. The recording channel is connected to the second arm of the "Y" connector. When the catheter is withdrawn slowly, the side openings enter the urethra and the UCPP is recorded

2) *Catheter with side openings for UCPP, with the addition of a separate lumen opening into the bladder*
This permits continuous cystometry during UCPP measurement. In this way artefact produced by detrusor contraction can be detected

3) *Catheter with side openings covered by a membrane*
This system is inferior, the membrane tending to cover a relatively wider area of urethra making measurements less precise. Bonding of the membrane to the catheter can create an irregular surface. The frequency response of the membrane itself may vary, especially if the catheter is subjected to re-sterilisation

4) *Catheter with recording points spaced at intervals along its length*
The measuring points may also be open or covered by a membrane. It is claimed that these points at set intervals enable reliable measurements to be carried out simultaneously, for example at bladder neck and external urethral sphincter. This is difficult to accept since the bladder neck alters during filling or the initiation of micturition and the distance between bladder neck and the sphincter is not static

5) *Catheters with built-in micro-transducers*
These are ideal in theory but at present are expensive and delicate. In time, these problems may be overcome and the system could than be more widely employed

It is sometimes necessary to use local anaesthetic. Surface electrodes do not provide accurate although they are used by some workers. Interference due to movement of electrodes, adjacent muscle activity and electrical interference in the vicinity can all present problems.

Urine Loss Measurement. Rough and ready estimation of incontinence may be made by counting the number of incontinence pads used and weighing discarded pads to assess the volume of urine absorbed. The Uriloss detector pad is more convenient but requires the patient to be linked by wire to a recorder. The commercially produced device is less accurate than the original described by James et al. (1971) but does provide greater accuracy than any other available system.

In conclusion, it is essential to realise that the diagnosis of the cause of incontinence is based on multiple investigations and full clinical assessment. No single test will give the answer. Urodynamic investigations supplement and do not replace routine clinical assessment and investigation.

References

Bates CP, Whiteside G, Turner Warwick R (1970) Synchronous cine/pressure/flow cysto-urethrography with special reference to stress and urge incontinence. Br J Urol 42: 714–723

Bates P, Bradley WE, Glen ES, Griffiths D, Melchior H, Rowan D, Sterling A, Zinner N, Hald T (1979) Standardisation of terminology of lower urinary tract function. Collation of first three reports. J Urol 121:551–554

Glen ES (1980, unpublished) Evaluation of role of urodynamics. Interim Report to Biomedical Research Committee, Scottish Home and Health Department

Glen ES, Rowan D (1973) Continuous flow cystometry and urethral pressure profile measurement with monitored intravesical pressure: A diagnostic investigation. Urol Res 1:97–100

James ED, Flack FC, Caldwell KP, Martin MR (1971) Continuous measurement of urine loss and frequency in incontinent patients. Br J Urol 43:233–237

Rowan D, Glen ES (1979) Clinical investigation and evaluation of urinary stress incontinence. In: Cantor EB (Ed) Stress incontinence. Thomas, Springfield, Ill., pp 61–104

Rowan D, McKenzie AL, McNee SG, Glen ES (1977) A technical and clinical evaluation of the Disa flowmeter. Br J Urol 49:285–291

Urodynamic Investigations in Neuromuscular Disorders of the Lower Urinary Tract

T. Hald

A precise diagnosis of neuromuscular bladder disorder cannot be made without appropriate testing. On the other hand the test situation may yield findings which are not relevant to the habitual voiding situation of the patient. It is therefore important to evaluate urodynamic findings and the clinical situation and never to rely on only one of these complementary sources of information.

The level of a neurological lesion serves as a guide to the type of dysfunction, but it cannot predict the exact outcome of the behavior of the lower urinary tract. A number of tests have been devised in the last few years. My purpose is to evaluate the clinical yield of some of these tests and delineate the areas of indication.

Screening

A natural choice for screening or initial investigation is cystometry and electromyography (EMG) from the urethral sphincter and flowmetry. In neurological bladder dysfunction, CO_2-cystometry has the advantage over ordinary water cystometry in its speed and therefore repeatability. A series of cystometrograms with the patient sitting, lying, standing, etc., will allow the test situation to mimic real life. The only information which is truly helpful is the finding of ± sensation and ± reflex contraction and whether the latter is under voluntary control. The addition of simultaneous sphincter EMG allows for the detection of voluntary control, detrusor-sphincter dyssynergia and uninhibited sphincter relaxation. Also, the EMG serves as a security that the patient follows instructions (relax, hold, let go). Flowmetry is primarily a screening for detrusor-urethral balance. A normal flow curve is, however, sometimes found in patients with neurogenic bladders, especially the suprasacral types, or in females with infrasacral lesions and a very low urethral resistance.

The combination of cystometry, EMG, and flowmetry will suffice for 75% of all patients and should be available in all urological institutions.

Additional Testing

Further testing depends on the problem suspected. The preliminary diagnosis will be one of the following:

1) Infravesical obstruction,
2) nonneurological incontinence,

Table 1. Selection of tests in neuromuscular bladder disorders.

Screening	Problem	Additional test
		Momentum flux
	Infravesical obstruction	Pressure/flow/EMG
		MCUG
Flowmetry		Urethrocystometry
	Incontinence	UCCP
		Cystometry–EMG
Cystometry		Pharmacological test
	Neuropathic bladder	Evoked responses
		Cystometry in anesthesia
		EEG
	Psychological	Psychiatric evaluation
		Personality test

3) neurogenic bladder sensu stricto,
4) psychological disorder.

Additional tests are useful for detecting these problems and overlap one another in their indications. These are shown in Table 1.

The *infravesical obstructions* are best studied by a simultaneous pressure/flow study. The addition of EMG and X-ray monitoring is useful but not mandatory in all cases.

In *primary incontinences* the main issue is to separate motor urge incontinence and genuine stress incontinence. Urethrocystometry is the superior test. The closure pressure profile is overrated, the tremendous spread in values of maximum urethral closure pressure having been neglected. In many incontinence situations the crucial urodynamic happenings in the lower urinary tract may be extremely short lived and are easily missed. The lateral MCUG is especially helpful in showing the type of bladder suspension defect present, and is therefore especially indicated in genuine stress incontinence.

When a true *neuropathic bladder* is suspected, cystometry and EMG should be supplemented by pharmacological tests (carbachol, noradrenalin) to diagnose denervation supersensibility and give a guide to treatment (α- and β-blocking agents, ephedrine).

Evoking the bulbocavernosus reflexes can be used to document peripheral neuropathy and anatomical interruption of the pelvic reflexes.

Table 2. Clinical yield from selected urodynamic tests.

Problem	Method						
	Cystometry	Sphincter EMG	Pressure/flow study	Evoked potentials	Urethro-cystometry	UCPP	Pharmacological testing
Detrusor reflex testing	+ + +	+	0	0	+ +	0	+ +
Striated sphincter function	0	+ + +	+ +	+	+ + +	+ +	0
Detrusor-sphincter coordination	+ + +	+ + +	+ + +	0	+ + +	0	0
Continence	+ + +	+	(+)	+	+ + +	+	+ +
Voiding efficiency	0	+	+ + +	0	0	0	+ +

+ + +, Method of choice. + +, Useful. +, Sometimes valuable. (+), Doubtful value. 0, Not applicable.

Electroencephalography (EEG) may be employed in cases of enuresis, where epileptiform patterns may be seen, leading to proper treatment. *Psychological bladder problems* are very difficult to evaluate. Early psychiatric assistance is mandatory to avoid fixation of the person in the patient role by superfluous multiple urodynamic tests. Psychological tests (e. g., the MMPI personality test) are attractive to all of us who are not too well versed in the intricacies of psychiatry. Cystometry in light anesthesia seems to be of value in evaluating female urinary retention. The finding of a preserved reflex, when cortical inhibition is lost, is indicative of a psychological disorder when a urethral obstruction or irritation can be ruled out. Table 2 shows the usefulness of some of the more common tests.

Conclusion

The following questions should be answered in all cases:

1) Is there a detrusor reflex and is it under voluntary control?
2) Is there detrusor-sphincter coordination?
3) How is the voiding efficiency?
4) Which continence mechanism is at fault?

The urodynamic testing of a patient need not be lengthy, expensive, traumatic, or unpleasant. By employing a few properly selected tests the whole spectrum of functional and anatomical voiding and continence disorders can be evaluated.

Sphincter Electromyography in Female Incontinence

R. L. Vereecken, G. De Meirsman, and B. Puers

Most surgical treatments of stress incontinence act by a passive supports of the bladder neck; they have failure rates of between 5% and 20%. On the other hand, recent studies have drawn attention to excellent results which can be obtained by active perineal muscle training. Techniques should therefore be available to select patients for each group of treatment and to predict the final successes of both. Such a test could be electromyography (EMG) of the striated pelvic floor musculature. However, EMG by means of surface electrodes mounted on an anal plug as usually performed in the urodynamic evaluation of troubles of the bladder-urethral coordination system is too rough. In order to obtain exact information about the urethral and anal sphincter efficiency, we recorded the electrical activity by means of coaxial electrodes. The value of this technique has already been proved in many neurological lesions (Chantraine 1966; Allert 1974).

Material and Methods

One hundred and thirty-four incontinent women, aged between 21 and 76, were investigated. Patients with known neurogenic (e.g. multiple sclerosis, discus pathology) or metabolic (e.g. diabetes) diseases were excluded from this series. Gynaecological and obstetrical histories were carefully recorded as objectively as possible: previous vaginal interventions, suprapubic surgery, number of births, weight of neonati and dystocia (forceps, lacerations, episiotomy). Since in the small group of patients a correlation with each of these factors seperately could introduce erroneous conclusions, we gave a point to each of these factors and divided in this way the patients into three categories of appreciation of possible local injury to the urethra. Classical cystometry is performed by bladder filling at 20 ml/min; the intraluminal pressures are measured with the Gaeltec microtip sensor; for the urethral pressure profile the catheter is withdrawn at a velocity of 5 cm/min. During bladder filling, 43 cases showed spontaneous non-inhibited bladder contractions of more than 15 cm of water and were classified as urgeincontinence. Ninety-one women showed stable bladder curves as occur in the stresstyp of incontinence.

Of the 91 stressincontinent women, 59 were treated for more than 6 months, 52 were cured and seven women claimed an incomplete regression of the incontinence. Coaxial electrodes (Medelce) were introduced into the ventral peri-urethral striated musculature and into the anal sphincter; different sites of the sphincters were explored if the activity was low or abnormal. Reflex activation of the sphincters was studied at cough, and after electrical stimulation of the bladder neck or anus by electrodes mounted on a urethral catheter or an anal plug respectively. The pudendal reflex time is studied by measuring the latent period and duration of the reflex response in the sphincters after supramaximal electrical stimulation of the bladder neck or anus. This technique has been presented at the ICS Congress in Rome (Vereecken et al. 1979) and will be published in detail elsewhere; it differs from the technique of Bradley (1972) by the fact that optical superimposition of a few responses is made instead of a computerised analysis of very large numbers of responses. Voluntary activation of the sphincters was explored by a prolonged maximal contraction or by a series of short maximal contractions (3) separated by short relaxations (3).

A frequency power spectrum of the EMG action potentials was made according to the previously described technique. In this technique the total power emitted at each frequency for a fixed small period of EMG activity is calculated by means of a microprocessor.

Results

Twenty-five out of 91 stress incontinent and only 6 out of 43 urge incontinent patients showed signs of partial peripheral denervations and one of following abnormal patterns: bizarre high frequency potentials (Fig. 1) accelerated firing frequency, polyphasic potentials, fibrillations and fasciculations. Exceptionally low tone activity was noted in four cases and in three patients no activity at all could be detected in the urethral sphincter despite multiple insertions and our large experience of sphincter EMG. If a pathological EMG was detected, a control insertion of the needle at the contralateral site was performed; in this way we frequently observed asymmetry of the degree of injury. In 57% only the urethral sphincter was involved, in 12% only the anal sphincter and in 21% both sphincters with a more pronounced abnormality in the urethral sphincter.

There was a clear correlation between EMG pathology and the estimated intensity of the previous trauma as can be observed in the following list:

Class I	61 patients	2 pathological EMGs;
Class II	47 patients	9 pathological EMGs;
Class III	30 patients	27 pathological EMGs;
Total:	134 patients	38 pathological EMGs.

Six out of seven failures of 59 surgically treated stress incontinent women had markedly abnormal EMG curves. In the stress incontinent group 39 patients exhibited a poor voluntary and selective maximal activation of the sphincters. The sphincter contraction was a part of a general contraction of abdominal, gluteal and leg muscles, or the activation was of poor intensity (a few motor units instead of a rich interferential curve) and of short duration (no more than 10).

Reflex sphincter activation during coughing and Valsalva manoeuvre were also reduced in 59% of stress incontinent women.

We did frequency power analyses of several fragments of the EMG of 14 patients with stress and five patients with urge incontinence. The latter group showed a normal pattern with a peak of activity at rest at 200 Hz and during activation peaks at 400 and 800 Hz. On the contrary 9 of the 14 patients with stress inconti-

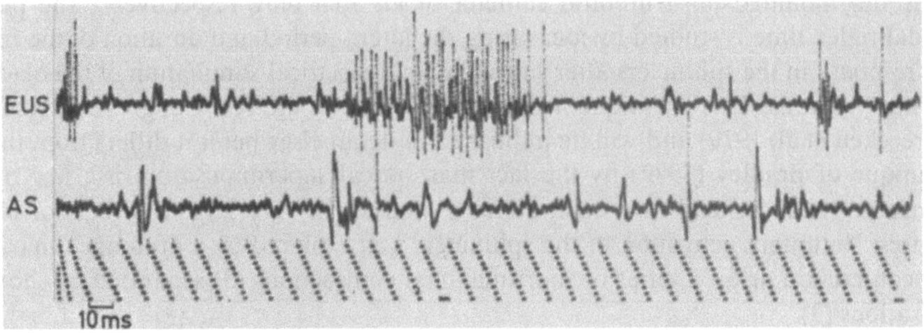

Fig. 1. Bizarre high frequency potentials in the peri-urethral striated musculature of a 45-year-old woman with stress incontinence. *EUS*, Urethral sphincter. *AS*, Anal sphincter.

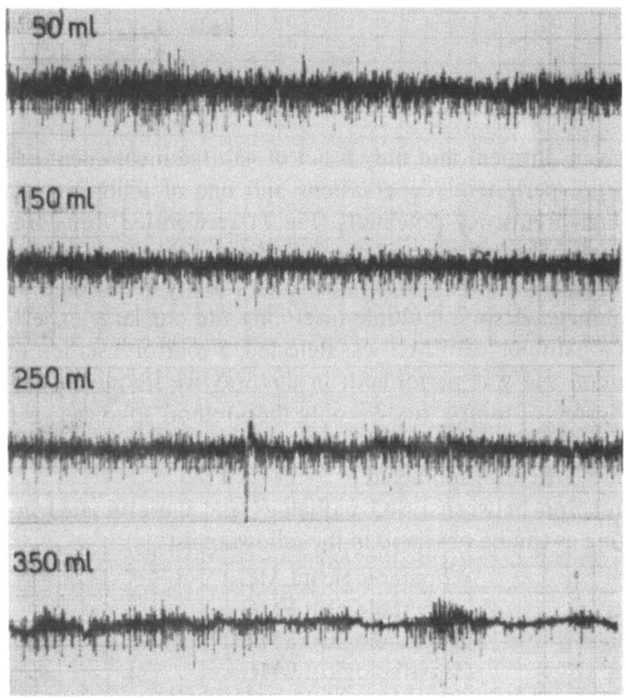

Fig. 2. Decrease of EMG activity in the peri-urethral striated musculature during bladder filling in a stress incontinent woman.

nence showed a shift to the lower frequencies while the power at frequencies above 400 Hz was very low even during maximal contraction.

In 12 stress incontinent and 13 urge incontinent women the EMG activity gradually decreased with increasing bladder volumes (Fig. 2); this was not due to a dislocation of the EMG electrodes since normal interferential activity remained at cough and voluntary contraction.

In unstable bladders two opposite patterns of EMG could be observed during the abnormal bladder contractions: in 14 patients a simultaneous significant in-

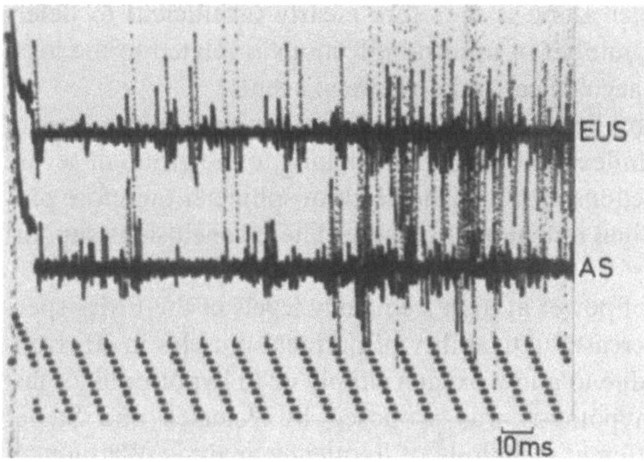

Fig. 3. Electrical stimulation of the anal mucosa evokes a delayed (100 ms) reflex response in both urethral (*EUS*) and anal (*AS*) sphincters. (30-year-old patient with stress incontinence).

crease of EMG activity at the beginning or during the whole period of increased bladder pressure arose; in the other patients the bladder hypertension immediately inhibited all sphincter activity as during normal voiding.

In most patients the reflex contraction of both anal and urethral sphincter after electrical stimulation of the bladder neck and/or anus fell within the normal latent periods of 55–80 ms. However, in 26 of 85 stress incontinent women the latency was increased up to values of 140 ms (Fig. 3). In seven patients the latency in the anal sphincter was more delayed than in the urethral sphincter. An increase of latent periods was also observed in 15 of 34 unstable bladders. Reaction to anal ring stimulation was usually more pronounced in the anal than in the urethral sphincter.

Discussion

Until now the main indication for recording EMG of perineal muscles has been the detection of detrusor-sphincter dyssynergia in neurogenic diseases (Vereecken and Verduyn 1970; Vereecken et al. 1977), or in external sphincter spasms by infection (Tanagho et al. 1971). For this aim many urologists record the total perineal activity by anal plug electrodes. Another application, trusted to the electromyographists, is the follow-up of recuperation or stabilisation of muscle activity after surgical interventions for myelomeningocele, cauda equina tumours, etc. (Chantraine 1966; Allert 1974); individual examination of each muscle by coaxial electrodes is then required. Very few studies report EMG patterns in stress and urge incontinence. Recently Papy et al. (1977) reported a good relation between sphincter EMG abnormalities in stress incontinent women and results of surgical treatment.

The most unexpected result of this study is the large number of EMG abnormalities in the urethral sphincter; these were not suspected by other anamnestic or clinical symptoms. Even if we accept that the external sphincter as a small musculature plays only a minor role in continence – the bladder neck being the most important structure in this respect – it cannot be denied that EMG abnormalities probably reflect the deficiency of the urethra, of which the striated component is easier to measure than the smooth muscle component. We found a much higher frequency of abnormalities in the urethral sphincter than in the anal sphincter (78% against

33%). EMG of the anal sphincter alone is therefore clearly insufficient to detect sphincteral injuries. The higher number of urethral affections is related to the local trauma of the vagina during gynaecological and obstetrical events.

There exists a close correlation between EMG abnormalities and failure rates of surgery for stress incontinence. Indeed, all bad results belong to the group of severe and bilateral urehtral EMG affections. EMG of the urethral sphincter therefore provides a basis for predicting the final outcome of surgery. These conclusions support the results of Papy et al. (1977).

We considered the absence of power at high frequency levels of the EMG spectrum as an expression of the increased fatigability of perineal muscles in stress incontinent women. This may be due to a low oxygen supply or to hypotrophy of fast muscle fibres. An analogous hypothesis was proposed by Petersen and Stener (1970), who used, however, a different technique of frequency analysis. We found a surprisingly high number of delayed latency periods after electrical stimulation of the bladder neck in anal mucosa. Extraspinal nerve lesion may be an important factor in elder patients and in those with bilateral pathological EMG findings in the sphincters. There is, however, still a large group without explanation of the phenomenon. A weak central reflex loop due to insufficient training is a plausible explanation. If so, beneficial effects can be expected from electrostimulation with pacemakers, which could facilitate reflex pathways. Anyway it may indicate that these patients are unable to achieve a strong reflex perineal contraction fast enough to counteract an increased intravesical pressure during coughing. Clinical experience has shown that some women are incontinent at cough only, while others are wet during walking without losing more water during coughing. In as much as active perineal contraction reinforces urethral competence during sudden stress, its delay will permit urine loss. Futhermore, the reflex activity is very often reduced.

EMG monitoring of the sphincters can also be a useful help for training perineal musculature. We observed that during repeated urodynamical sessions the patients became more conscious of the way they could selectively activate their sphincters.

References

Allert, Max L von (1974) Diagnostik neurogener Blasenstörungen durch Elektromyographie. Thieme, Stuttgart

Bradley WE (1972) Urethral electromyography. J Urol 108:563–564

Chantraine A (1966) Etude électromyographique chez le spina bifida avec myéloméningocèle, avant et après opération. Electromyogr Clin Neurophysiol 6:257–262

Papy JJ, Benaim LJ, Conte Devolx J, Serment G (1977) Electromyography of anal and urethral sphincters in female urinary stress incontinence. Internat. Feder. EEG Neurophys. Clin.; 9th Cong., MO 96, p 610

Petersen K, Stener I (1970) An electromyographical study of the striated urethral sphincter, and the levator ani muscle during ejaculation. Electromyogr Clin Neurophysiol 10:23–44

Tanagho EA, Miller ER, Lyon RP, Fisher R (1971) Spastic striated external sphincter and urinary tract infection in girls. Br J Urol 43:69–81

Vereecken RL, Verduyn H (1970) The electrical activity of the paraurethral and perineal muscles in normal and pathological conditions. Br J Urol 42:457–463

Vereecken RL, Ketelaer P, Joossens J, Leruitte A (1977) Frequency analysis of the electromyographic activity in striated pelvic floor muscles. Eur Urol 3:333–336

Vereecken RL, De Meirsman P, Puers B, Slaets J (1979) Electrophysiological exploration of the central reflex centers. In: Guido Guidotti (ed) Proc. IXth Ann. Meeting ICS, Rome, pp 233–234

Transurethral Electromyography of the Striated Sphincter of the Urethra

J. De Leval and R. Piscart

The urethral profile is an important contribution to the urodynamic study of the lower urinary tract. This is a comprehensive exploration, in which the curve obtained is a function of four factors: the smooth muscle, the striated muscle, the abundant fibroelastic tissue, and the vascular bed.

For the purpose of selectively studying the striated muscle component of the posterior urethra, we have developed a new electromyographic technique. We do not use the needle electromyography (EMG), which permits a qualitative study leading to a diagnosis and a localization of the lesion with respect to Budge's parasympathetic center, but rather we use a contact type EMG, which registers the activity of striated muscle fibers by means of two electrodes, thus giving us a quantitative idea of the segment studied.

Very rapidly we decided to discard the double ring electrodes fixed to a catheter which we withdraw at a constant velocity, because this system produced too many artifacts. We abandoned it in favor of catheters outfitted with a number of paired electrodes which would allow us to register simultaneously the electrical activity at different levels and thereby give us a static electrical profile of the urethra.

Apparatus and Materials

The electromyographic study is always combined with a radiological exploration. In order to visualize the striated urethral sphincter, we use a latex bougie, which has walls 1 mm thick, a caliber of 16 charriere, and an external surface graduated lengthwise by means of radiopaque markers, each graduation measuring 2.5 mm. The bougie is filled with a radiopaque product and the system is brought to a pressure of 70 cm H_2O. The electromyographic apparatus includes different kinds of catheters outfitted with contact electrodes and an electronic registering system for recording the results.

The catheters are constructed from a tube of Plexiglas 6.5 mm in diameter and 27 cm long. The recording electrodes are fashioned from a small silver metallic bar 8 mm wide and 4 mm long; they are arranged in pairs, each member separated from the other by 3.5 mm. The pairs are arranged on the catheters, on the anterior and posterior aspects at 1 cm intervals. Several prototypes were devised with a variable number of paired electrodes (eight anterior, eight anterior; eight posterior, four anterior; four posterior, one anterior; one posterior). Each pair of electrodes is linked to a relay situated at the extremity of the catheter (Fig. 1).

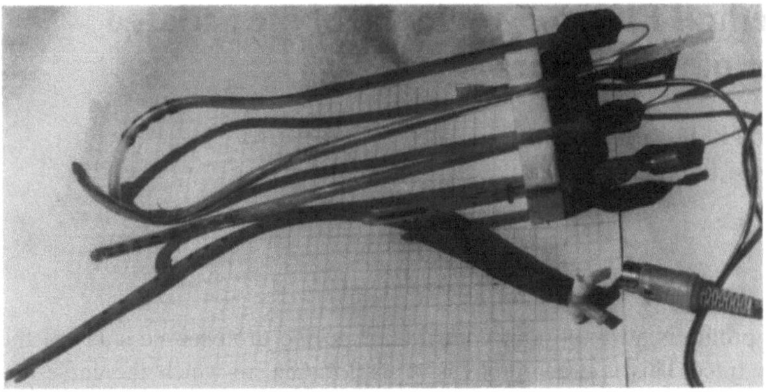

Fig. 1. Catheters with variable numbers of paired electrodes.

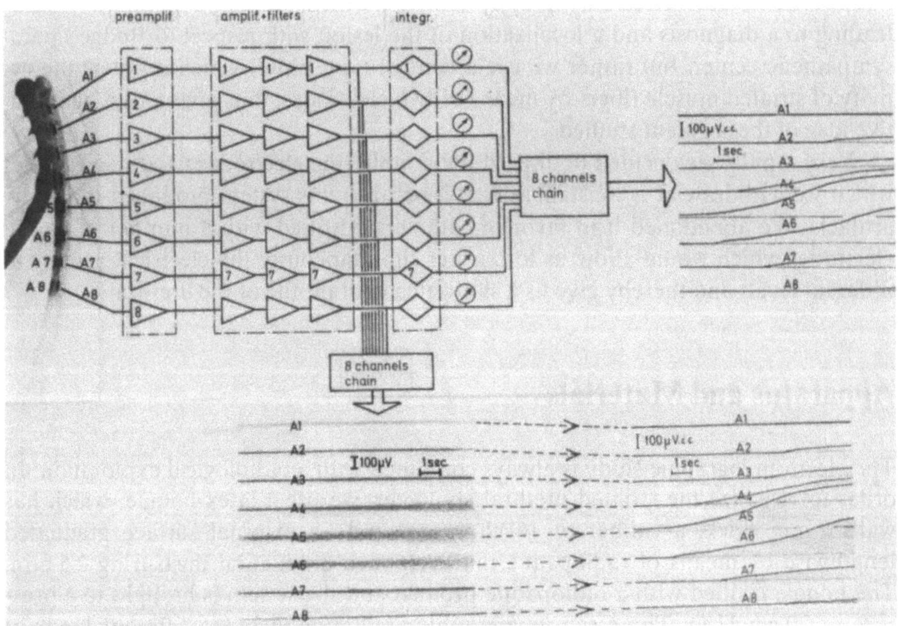

Fig. 2. Synoptic system of the eight channels chain.

The Electronic System. Our setup allows the simultaneous study of eight different territories; the electromyographic signals of the eight regions are preamplified, then filtered. By means of an electronic commutator which registers at very high speed the activity of each of the eight channels, we are able to obtain eight tracings registered as such or after integration (the Medelec recorder on photosensitive paper) (Fig. 2).

The Exploration Procedure

After having filled the patient's bladder with 100 g radiopaque substance and after having inserted in the patient's urethra the bougie described above, we ask the patient to contract his sphincter. This allows us to visualize the contraction and to ascertain, by mens of a strict lateral X-ray film, the distance separating the urogenital diaphragm from the bladder neck (Fig. 3). As well, anterior-posterior (A-P) and three-quarter obliques are interesting for the morphological study of the contraction.

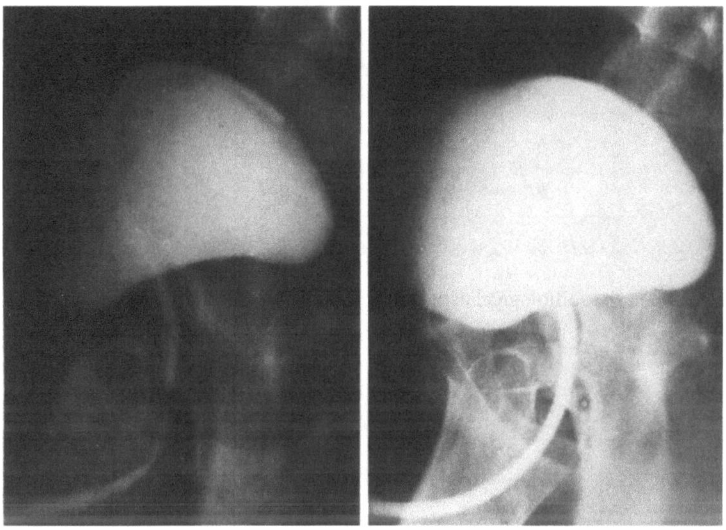

Fig. 3. View of the contraction of the striated sphincter.

After withdrawal of the bougie, we instill a sterile electrolytic gel into the urethra and then insert the multielectrode catheter. The latter is positioned so that the first pair of electrodes is located at the level of the bladder neck. The electromyograph is connected.

An A-P X-ray film is taken and then the electrical activity is recorded first at rest, then during a progressive contraction until the latter is maximal.

Results

The maximal activity of the striated sphincter is located at the level of the urogenital diaphragm, which is situated 5 cm from the bladder neck. The activity at rest is present from the 4th to the 6th cm and is at a maximum at the 5th cm. This activity averages 30 MV. During maximal contraction, this activity reaches values of 120 MV at the level of the UM zone (zone of maximal urethral activity) 5 cm from the neck of the bladder. The active zone is at this moment much longer: it stretches

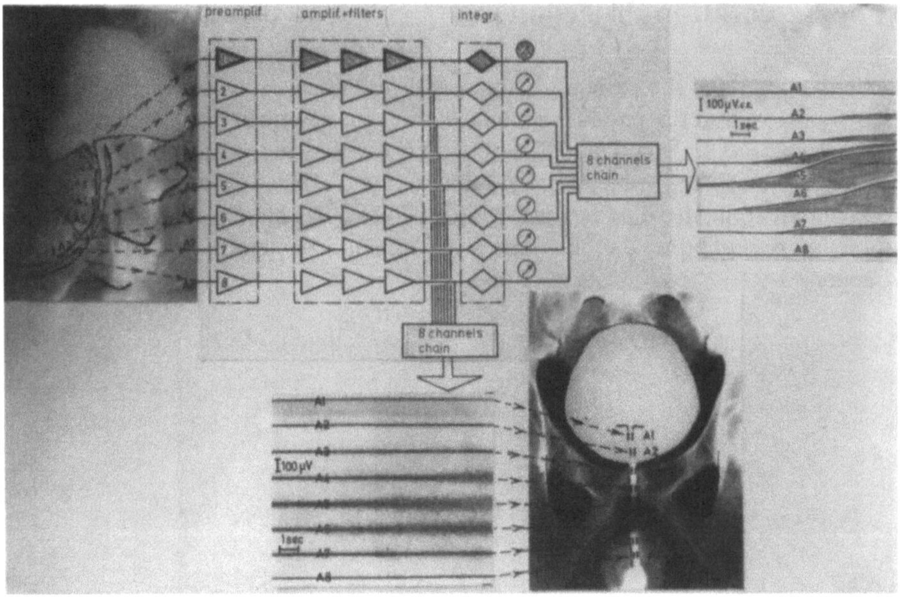

Fig. 4. Correlation between the radiological aspect of the urethral contraction and its electrical activity.

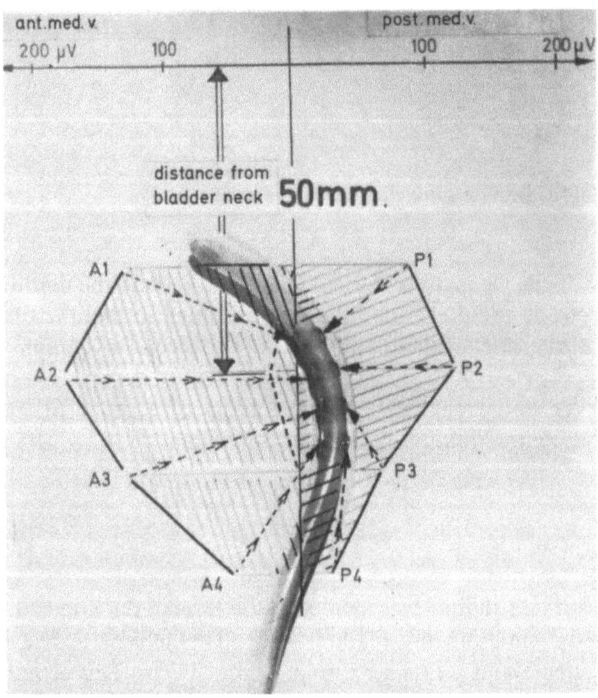

Fig. 5. Electrical profile of the anterior and posterior face of the urethra. The UM zone is at the 5th cm.

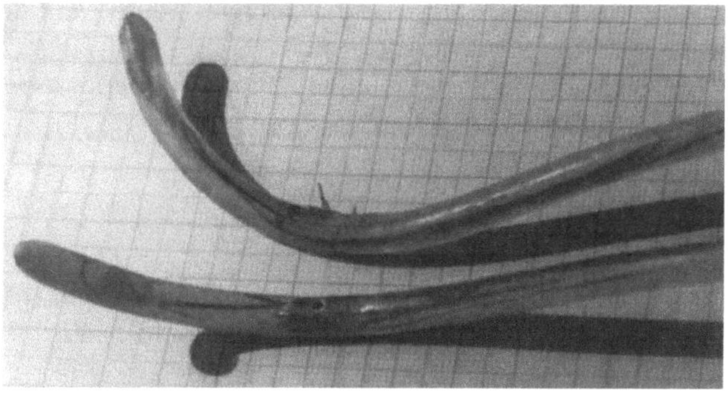

Fig. 6. The catheter for sphincteric infiltration.

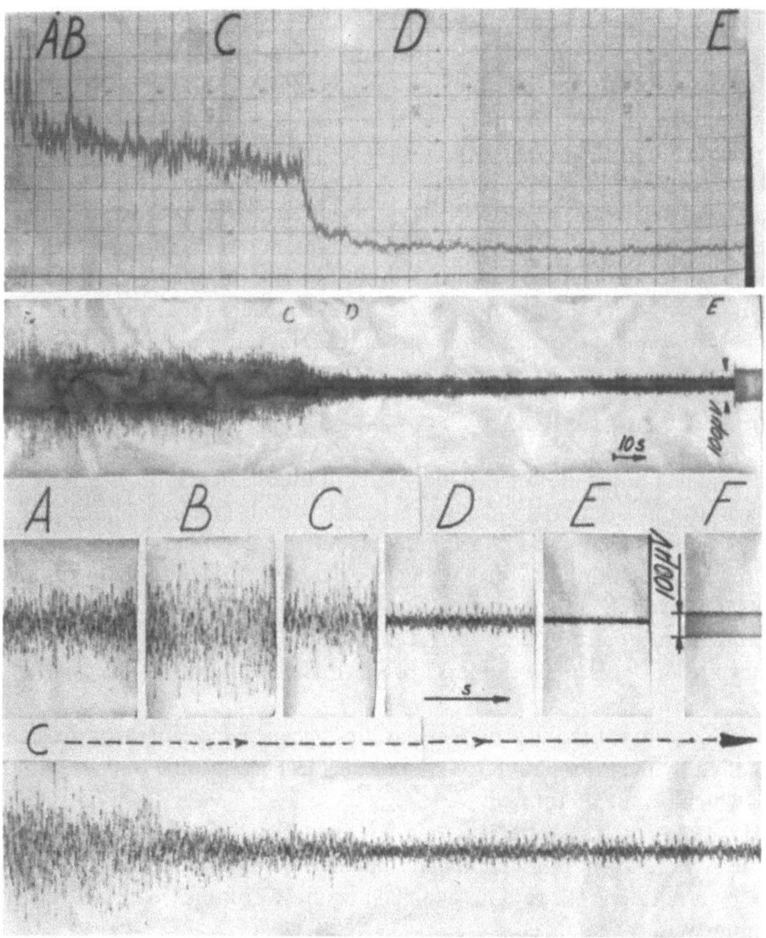

Fig. 7. Detail and results of an intrasphincteric infiltration.

proximally to near the bladder neck, where we record a discrete activity, and distally to 1.5 cm from the urogenital diaphragm (Fig. 4).

The electrical activity registered is always more important at the anterior aspect then at the posterior aspect, at rest, as well as during active contraction (Fig. 5).

Applications

In the case of striated sphincter disease, it is generally agreed that a period of spasticity precedes the installment of definitive fibrosis. The affection can be reversible if parasphincteric infiltrations are realized at the outset.

Since there exists a zone of maximal activity at the anterior aspect, it seemed to us preferable to infiltrate the striated sphincter at this point. To accomplish this, we use a catheter outfitted with only one pair of electrodes situated anteriorly 7 cm from its extremity. Inside this instrument there is a conduit, which terminates near the two electrodes (Fig. 6). We insert into this conduit a catheter with a mandrin, at the end of which we have mounted a needle. This whole system is inserted into the urethra of the patient with the needle retracted and as soon as the most active zone is located with the help of the electromyograph, we plunge the catheter with its mandrin; the needle can thus penetrate the UM zone to a depth of about 5 mm. During the penetration of the needle, we most often record a surge of activity. The mandrin is withdrawn and then 2 cc lidocaine (Xylocaine) 1% is instilled. We obtain a virtually immediate electrical silence (Fig. 7).

Activity resumes most often after 30–45 min without, however, attaining its original level. At this time the needle is withdrawn into the interior of the catheter and the latter is withdrawn from the urethra. These procedures are repeated depending on the clinical evolution and the measurements of residual urine.

Discussion and Conclusions

This new urostatic technique allows a spatial study of the striated sphincter. The result obtained confirm in a remarkable way previous anatomic and histologic studies. The striated sphincter is composed of a thick sleeve of striated fibers located at the level of the urogenital diaphragm with the density of fibers sometimes bein less important at the posterior aspect (Grannum and Sant 1972). With regard to the periurethral musculature, certain fibers go all the way up to the bladder neck (Manley 1966). They are not present at the level of the first centimeters of the posterior urethra.

This study shows that there is a perfect parallel between the length of the contraction objectified by the radiopaque sound and the electrical profile of the urethra, the activity of which can be quantified.

In physiopathology this apparatus makes possible the diagnosis of cystosphincteric dyssynergias, notably sphincter spasticity, which can be immediately treated by the incorporated infiltration system. The efficacy of this treatment can, in addition, be immediately visualized.

As far as long-term results are concerned, they seem to us very positive since only exceptionally now do we resort to sphincterotomy.

Finally, this is an invaluable instrument for the pharmacological study of the striated sphincter and the first results obtained leave no doubt as to the interest of the technique.

References

Andersen JT, Bradley WE (1976) The urethral closure pressure profile. A new technique using gas and simultaneous EMG-recording from the urethra. Br J Urol 48:341

Andersen JT, Bradley WE (1977) Urethral pressure profilometry: assessment of urethral function by combined intraurethral pressure and electromyographic recording. J Urol 188,77:423–427

Andersen JT, Bourne RB, Bradley WE (1976) Combined electromyography and gas urethral pressure profilometry before and after transurethral resection of the prostate. J Urol 116:622

Archimbaud JP (1974) Les dysfonctionnements vésico-sphinctériens neurologique, Masson, Paris, pp 112–121

Bradley WE, Timm GW (1976) Combined electromyographic and gas urethral pressure profilometry. J Urol 115:433

Brown M, Wickham JEA (1969) The uretral pressure profile. Br J Urol 41:211

Caine M, Edwards D (1958) The peripheral control of micturition: a cineradiographic study. Br J Urol 30:34

Chantraine A (1966) Electromyographic des sphincters striés uréthral et anal humains. Etude descriptive et analytique. Rev Neurol (Paris)115:396–403

Chantraine A, Lloyd K, Swinyard DA (1966) The sphincter ani externus in spina bifida and myelomeningocele. J Urol 95:250–256

De Leval J (1979) New technic for infiltration of the urethral external sphincter. 12 May, New York, American Urodynamic Association

De Leval J, Piscart R (1973) Etude radiodynamique du sphincter strié de l'urèthre. Technique nouvelle. Acta Urol Belg 41:509–518

De Leval J, Piscart R (1980) Infiltration élective du sphincter strié de l'urèthre au lit du malade. Acta Urol Belg 48:303–310

Francois N, Maury M, Cukier J (1976) Les infiltrations para-sphinctériennes. J Urol Nephrol (Paris) 10/11:813–820

Franksson C, Peterson I (1955) Electromyographic investigation of disturbances in the striated muscle of the urethral sphincter. Br J Urol 27:154

Gil-Vernet S (1968) Morphology and function of vesicoprostato-urethral musculature. Treviso: Canova 11:245–269

Grannum R, Sant BA (1972) The anatomy of the external striated urethral sphincter. Paraplegia 10:153–156

Grondard E, Francois N, Maury M, Cukier J (1978) Les infiltrations parasphinctériennes anesthésiques du strié de l'urèthre chez le paraplégique. J Urol Nephrol (Paris) 3.207–214

Hutch JA (1972) Anatomy and physiology of the bladder, trigone, and urethra. Butterworths, London, pp 1–132

Lapides J, Ajemian EP, Stewart BH, Breakey BA, Lichtwardt JR (1960) Further observations on the kinetics of the urethrovesical sphincter. J Urol 84:1

Manley CB (1966) The striated muscle of the prostate. J Urol 95:234

Nordling J, Meyhoff H, Walter S, Andersenn JT (1978) Urethral electromyography using a new ring electrodes. J Urol 120:571–573

Vereecken RL, Verduyn H (1970) The electrical activity of the paraurethral and perineal muscles in normal and pathological conditions. Br J Urol 42:457–463

Whitmore WF, Fam BA, Yalla SV (1978) Experience with anteromedian (12 o'clock) external urethral sphincterotomy in 100 male subjects with neuropathic bladders. Br J Urol 50:99–101

Yalla SV et al. (1977) Anteromedian external urethral, sphincterotomy: technique, rationale and complications. J Urol 117:489–493

A New, Simple Urodynamic Apparatus

P. Abrams, P. J. R. Shah, and R. C. L. Feneley

Urodynamic studies now have an accepted place in the investigation of many urological, gynaecological, geriatric and neurological patients with lower urinary tract symptome. Like all new investigation techniques urodynamic studies are taking a time to achieve widespread acceptance. This may be partly due to the relative complexity and expense of the recording equipment required. However, it has been the reliability and accuracy of the equipment, which has become available in the last 10 years, that has made routine urodynamic studies worthwhile. Continuous pressure measurement by robust transducers and the use of chart recorders represents a considerable advance on hand-drawn cystometrograms constructed using incremental bladder filling and pressure recorded by a water manometer.

The system described represents an attempt to reduce the complexity of urodynamic recording, to reduce the purchase price of such systems, to produce such a system without loss of information and to present the recorded data in a form more suitable for inclusion in case notes than the long traces produced by the traditional moving chart recorder. By producing a simple system it is hoped to encourage more clinicians to adopt urodynamic studies as a routine part of their clinical evaluation of patients with voiding disorders.

The system described here is based on the recording of a pressure-volume loop of the micturition cycle as described to the International Continence Society in 1976 (Abrams and Torrens) and used to calculate bladder work. It will be shown that using a simple system it is possible to obtain the same information usually recorded on a five-channel moving chart recorder; that is, rectal pressure, bladder pressure, subtracted detrusor pressure, bladder volume and urine flow rate. The simple apparatus can also be used to record free flow rates and urethral pressure profiles.

Methodology

Pressure Measurement. Bladder and rectal pressure are measured using similar Gaeltech (5F, Type 12Ct) catheter-tip transducers. The tip of the rectal catheter is protected by a finger cot. The subtracted detrusor pressure (bladder pressure minus rectal pressure) is derived by electronic subtraction. Catheter-tip transducers have several advantages over the normal system where the catheters in bladder and rectum are connected by fluid-filled tubes to external transducers. As the catheter-tip transducer lies within the patient, artifacts due to movement are considerably reduced. Calibration is easier. Sterilisation is possible as the transducer can be kept in Cidex. Furthermore catheter-tip transducers are more accurate and result in a pressure-measuring system with a better response time.

Bladder Volume and Urine Flow Rate Measurement. After experimenting with several systems a two-transducer method is now used to record bladder volume and hence urine flow rate. The saline bag for bladder filling is hung from a force transducer (Lectromed UF2) and, therefore, inflow volume is known. The voided volume and urine flow rate is recorded using a capacitance flow meter (Lectromed 4911). By electronic subtraction of output volume (flow meter) from input volume (force transducer) the bladder volume is known continuously. Urine flow rate is derived by differentiation of volume with time.

Urine flow rate can also be calculated from the pressure volume loop by the addition of a 1s time marker on the outflow trace. The maximum distance between two consecutive marks is the maximum urine flow rate.

Recording Equipment. An XYt plotter (Bryans Southern Instruments 26000 series) has been used. This instrument is a flat bed recorder in which A4-size paper is used. In contrast to the more usual moving-paper, static-pen, multichannel-chart recorder the XYt plotter has static paper and a single moving pen. The XYt plotter can be used in two modes: XY and XYt. In the XY mode the pen moves to any point on the paper dependent on the values of the parameters on the X and Y axis. However in the XYt mode only one variable can be used and is presented on the vertical (X) axis. In the XYt mode the pen moves horizontally across the paper at a fixed rate. The advantages of using an XYt plotter are that the capital cost is far less than for a multichannel recorder and that the recording paper (A4 size) is more manageable than that produced by the conventional chart recorder and suitable for direct filing in case notes.

Free-Flow Rate Estimation. With a full bladder the female sits and the male stands to void. The urine flow rate is recorded using the XYt mode of the plotter with flow rate on the X axis.

Urethral Pressure Profile Measurement. The pressure catheters are introduced into rectum and bladder with the patient supine. These recordings are also made using the XYt mode of the plotter with urethral pressure on the X axis. A catheter withdrawal machine (Lectromed) is used for accurate profile measurement.

Pressure Volume Loop Recording. A filling catheter is passed into the bladder and the residual urine estimated. The patient then transfers to a commode for the filling and voiding cycle. Saline is pumped into the bladder (Watson Marlowe peristaltic pump) at 60 ml/min until the patient says he has a full bladder. After removal of filling catheter the patient is asked to attempt to void to completion. Subtracted detrusor pressure is recorded on the X axis and bladder volume on the Y axis, the XY mode of the recorder being used.

'Off-line' Recording. By the use of memory stores the urine flow rate and a second pressure volume loop using total bladder pressure can be recorded on the XY plotter.

The data presented in Table 1 not differ from that recorded in a traditional multichannel urodynamic investigation (Bates et al. 1970). However it is suggested that there are advantages in ease of operation, in reduction of capital and service cost and in presentation and storage of data.

Table 1. Summary of recorded data.

1) On-line recording
   a) In the XYt mode (Fig. 1)
      Free urine flow rate
      Urethral pressure profile (residual urine)
   b) In the XY mode (Fig. 2)
      Pressure (subtracted) volume loop
      Urine flow rate
2) Off-line recording
   a) In the XYt mode
      Urine flow rate
   b) In the XY mode
      Pressure (bladder) volume loop

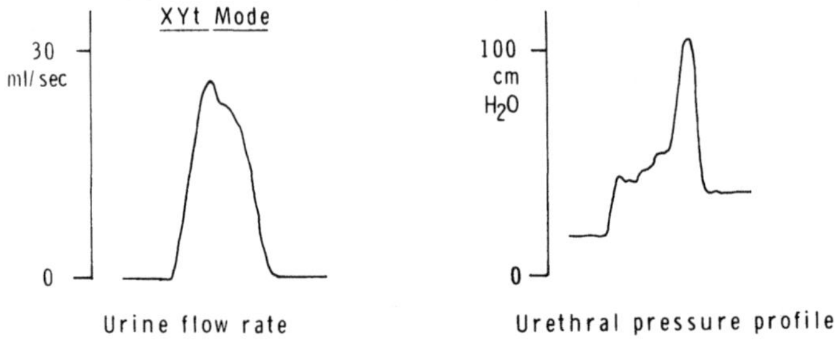

Fig. 1

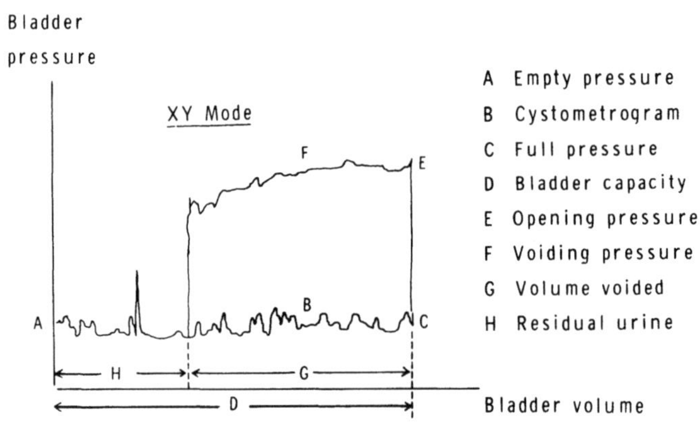

Fig. 2

Acknowledgements. We should like to record our appreciation for the help given by Ormed Engineering in the continuing development of this apparatus. Our thanks go to Miss Daphne Beckett who typed the manuscript.

References

Abrams PH, Torrens MJ (1976) Bladder work calculation in the assessment of intravesical obstruction. Communication to the International Continence Society, Antwerpen

Bates CP, Whiteside CG, Turner Warwick R (1970) Synchronous cine/pressure/flow cystourethrography, with special reference to stress and urge incontinence. Br J Urol 42:714–722

List of Contributors

Abbou, C. C., Service d'Urologie, Hôpital Henri Mondor, 51, Ave du Maréchal De-Lattre-De-Tassigny, F-94010 Creteil (pp. 185, 225)

Abrams, P., Department of Urology, Norfolk and Norwich Hospital, Brunswick Road, GB-Norwich, Norfolk NR1 3SR (p. 326)

Albrecht, K. F., Urologische Klinik der Städtischen Krankenanstalten, Heusnerstr. 40, D-5600 Wuppertal-Barmen (p. 80)

Alken, P., Urologische Klinik, Universität Mainz, Langenbeckstr. 1, D-6500 Mainz (pp. 243, 293)

Auvert, J., Service d'Urologie, Hôpital Henri Mondor, 51, Ave du Maréchal De-Lattre-De-Tassigny, F-94010 Creteil (pp. 179, 225)

Belgrano, E., Clinica Urologica Università, Viale Benedetto XV, I-16132 Genova (p. 197)

Bodart, P., Service de Radiologie, Cliniques Universitaires St. Luc, Université Catholique de Louvain, Avenue Hippocrate, 10, B-1200 Bruxelles (p. 1)

Bollack, C., Service d'Urologie, Centre Hospitalier et Universitaire, Hospices Civils, F-67005 Strasbourg (p. 239)

Bornes, J. C., Service de Radiologie, Hôpital Henri Mondor, 51, Ave du Maréchal De-Lattre-De-Tassigny, F-94010 Creteil (p. 179)

Botto, H., Service d'Urologie, Hôpital Henri Mondor, 51, Ave du Maréchal De-Lattre-De-Tassigny, F-94010 Creteil (pp. 179, 185)

Braedel, H. U., Universitätsklinik des Saarlandes, Röntgenabteilung der Urologie, D-6650 Homburg/Saar (p. 14)

Brion, J. P., Service de Radiologie, Cliniques Universitaires de Bruxelles, Hôpital Erasme, Route de Lennick, 808, B-1070 Bruxelles (p. 46)

Britton, K. E., Department of Nuclear Medicine, St. Bartholomew's Hospital, GB-London EC1A 7BE (pp. 261, 281)

Brooman, P. J., Department of Urology, St. Woolos Hospital, GB-Newport, Gwent NPT 4SZ (p. 158)

Carlet, J., Service d'Urologie, Hôpital Henri Mondor, 51, Ave du Maréchal De-Lattre-De-Tassigny, F-94010 Creteil (p. 185)

Carloz, I., Département de Médecine Nucléaire, Centre Hospitalier et Universitaire, Hospices Civils, F-67005 Strasbourg (p. 239)

Carmignani, G., Clinica Urologica Università, Viale Benedetto XV, I-16132 Genova (p. 197)

Charlton Edwards, E., Department of Urology, Manchester Royal Infirmary, Oxford Road, GB-Manchester (p. 256)

Chopin, D., Service d'Urologie, Hôpital Henri Mondor, 51, Ave du Maréchal De-Lattre-De-Tassigny, F-94010 Creteil (pp. 185, 225)

Cichero, A., Clinica Urologica Università, Viale Benedetto XV, I-16132 Genova (p. 197)

Constable, A. R., Institute of Urology, 172 Shaftesbury Avenue, GB-London WC2H 8JE (p. 246)

Coolsaet, B., Department of Urology, Academisch Ziekenhuis Utrecht, NL-3500 Utrecht (p. 53)

Cordonnier, C., Service de Radiologie, Hôpital Henri Mondor, 51, Ave du Maréchal De-Lattre-De-Tassigny, F-94010 Creteil (p. 185)

Cranage, R. W., Institute of Urology, 172 Shaftesbury Avenue, GB-London WC2H 8JE (p. 246)

Damascelli, B., Istituto Nazionale Tumori, Via Venezian 1, I-20133 Milano (p. 108)

Dardenne, A. N., Département de Radiologie, Cliniques Universitaires St. Luc, Université Catholique de Louvain, Avenue Hippocrate, 10, B-1200 Bruxelles (p. 1)

De Faveri, D., Divisione Radiologia, Ospedale Civile, Università di Padova, I-35100 Padova (p. 202)

De Leval, J., Service d'Urologie, Hôpital de Bavière, Université de Liège, Bd. de la Constitution, B-4000 Liège (p. 319)

De Meirsman, G., St. Raphael Clinic, University of Leuven, Kapucynvoer 35, B-3000 Leuven (p. 314)

Denis, L., Department of Urology, A. Z. Middelheim, B-2000 Antwerpen (p. 146)

De Sy, W. A., Department of Urology, Akademisch Ziekenhuis, University of Gent, De Pintelaan 135, B-9000 Gent (p. 83)

Elkhazen, N., Département de Gynécologie, Hôpital Universitaire St. Pierre, Rue Haute, 322, B-1000 Bruxelles (p. 127)

Engelmann, U., Urologische Klinik, Universität Mainz, Langenbeckstr. 1, D-6500 Mainz (p. 293)

Evans, K. T., Department of Urology, St. Woolos Hospital, GB-Newport, Gwent NPT 4SZ (p. 158)

Feinendegen, L. E., Institut für Medizin an der Kernforschungsanlage Jülich GmbH, Stettiner Forst, D-5170 Jülich (p. 301)

Felix, R., Strahlenklinik, Abteilung Radiologie mit Poliklinik, Klinikum Charlottenburg FUB, Spandauer Damm 130, D-1000 Berlin 19 (p. 121)

Feneley, R. C. L., Department of Urology, Norfolk and Norwich Hospital, Brunswick Road, GB-Norwich, Norfolk NR1 3SR (p. 326)

Fiegler, W., Strahlenklinik, Abteilung Radiologie mit Poliklinik, Klinikum Charlottenburg FUB, Spandauer Damm 130, D-1000 Berlin 19 (p. 121)

Fitzpatrick, J. M., Institute of Urology, 172 Shaftesbury Avenue, GB-London WC2H 8JE (p. 246)

Freundlieb, Ch., Institut für Medizin an der Kernforschungsanlage Jülich GmbH, Stettiner Forst, D-5170 Jülich (p. 301)

Frick, J., Urologische Klinik, Landeskrankenanstalten, A-5020 Salzburg (pp. 118, 143)

García Alonso, J. F., Dept. de Urologia, Centro Especial "Ramon y Cajal", Carretera de Colmenar Km. 9100, E-Madrid (p. 23)

Gil-Vernet, J. M., Dept. de Urologia, Clinica San José, Universita de Barcelona, Monegal 1, E-Barcelona (p. 87)

Giuliani, L., Clinica Urologica Università, Viale Benedetto XV, I-16132 Genova (p. 197)

Glen, E. S., Walton Urological Teaching and Research Centre, University of Glasgow, Southern General Hospital, GB-Glasgow G51 ATF (p. 304)

Green, N. A., Department of Urology, Norfolk and Norwich Hospital, Brunswick Road, GB-Norwich, Norfolk NR1 3SR (p. 41)

Griffiths, G. J., Department of Urology, St. Woolos Hospital, GB-Newport, Gwent NPT 4SZ (p. 158)

Grob, J. C., Département de Médecine Nucléaire, Centre Hospitalier et Universitaire, Hospices Civils, F-67005 Strasbourg (p. 239)

Haertel, M., Urologische Abteilung, Inselspital, Universitätsklinik, CH-3010 Bern (p. 193)

Hahn, K., Urologische Klinik der Johannes Gutenberg Universität, Langenbeckstr. 1, D-6500 Mainz (pp. 234, 293)

Hald, T., Department of Urology, Herlev Hospital, DK-2730 Herlev (p. 310)

Hall, M., Service de Pédiatrie, Hôpital Universitaire St. Pierre, Rue Haute, 322, B-1000 Bruxelles (p. 219)

Ham, H. R., Service des Radioisotopes, Hôpital Universitaire St. Pierre, Rue Haute, 322, B-1000 Bruxelles (p. 219)

Hendry, W. F., Department of Urology, St. Bartholomew's Hospital, GB-London EC1A 7BE (pp. 28, 261, 281)

Hill, J. T., Norfolk and Norwich Hospital, Brunswick Road, GB-Norwich, Norfolk NR1 3SR (p. 41)

Hofstetter, A., Urologische Abteilung im Städtischen Krankenhaus, Thalkirchner Str. 48, D-1000 München 2 (p. 113)

Hutschenreiter, G., Urologische Klinik der Johannes Gutenberg Universität, Langenbeckstr. 1, D-6500 Mainz (pp. 166, 234, 293)

Janson, R., Radiologische Universitätsklinik, Sigmund-Freud-Str. 25, D-5300 Bonn-Venusberg (p. 62)

Jiménez Cruz, J. F., Dept. Urologia, Centro Especial "Ramon y Cajal", Carretera de Colmenar Km. 9100, E-Madrid (p. 23)

Jones, C. H., Fertility Clinic, Chelsea Hospital for Women and Physics Department, Royal Marsden Hospital, GB-London S.W.3 (p. 28)

Köhle, R., Urologische Klinik, Landeskrankenanstalten, A-5020 Salzburg (p. 118)

Kolle, P., Urologische Abteilung der Medizinischen Hochschule Hannover, Karl-Wiechert-Allee 9, D-3000 Hannover 61 (p. 135)

Kuhn, G., Service de Radiologie, Cliniques Universitaires de Bruxelles, Hôpital Erasme, Route de Lennick, 808, B-1070 Bruxelles (pp. 73, 171)

Kunit, G., Urologische Klinik, Landeskrankenanstalten, A-5020 Salzburg (p. 143)

Lang, G., Urologische Klinik, Terrasse 30, D-3500 Kassel (p. 101)

Larde, D., Service d'Urologie, Hôpital Henri Mondor, 51, Ave du Maréchal De-Lattre-De-Tassigny, F-94010 Creteil (p. 185)

Laurini, L., Divisione Urologica, Ospedale Civile, Università di Padova, I-35100 Padova (p. 202)

Laval, K. U., Urologische Abteilung, Medizinische Klinik der Rhein.-Westfälischen Technischen Hochschule, Goethestr. 27/29, D-5100 Aachen (p. 301)

Lecudonnec, B., Service d'Urologie, Hôpital Henri Mondor, 51, Ave du Maréchal De-Lattre-De-Tassigny, F-94010 Creteil (p. 179)

Lembo, A., Divisione Urologica, Ospedale Civile, Università di Padova, I-35100 Padova (p. 202)

Marberger, M., Urologische Abteilung der Krankenanstalt Rudolfsstiftung, Juchgasse 25, A-1030 Wien (p. 293)

Mebel, M., Urologische Klinik des Krankenhauses Berlin-Friedrichshain, Leninallee 49, DDR-1017 Berlin (p. 221)

Melchior, H., Urologische Klinik, Terrasse 30, D-3500 Kassel (pp. 101, 265)

Methlin, G., Département de Médecine Nucléaire, Centre Hospitalier et Universitaire, Hospices Civils, F-67005 Strasbourg (p. 239)

Moncada, J., Urologische Klinik der Stadt, Klinikum Barmen, Heusnerstr. 40, D-5600 Wuppertal (p. 80)

Moretti, J. L., Service de Médecine Nucléaire, Hôpital Henri Mondor, 51, Ave du Maréchal De-Lattre-De-Tassigny, F-94010 Creteil (p. 225)

Msallag, M., Service de Médecine Nucléaire, Hôpital Henri Mondor, 51, Ave du Maréchal De-Lattre-De-Tassigny, F-94010 Creteil (p. 225)

Müller, P., Urologische Klinik des Krankenhauses Berlin-Friedrichshain, Leninallee 49, DDR-1017 Berlin (p. 221)

Musumeci, R., Istituto Nazionale Tumori, Via Venezian 1, I-20133 Milano (p. 108)

Navío Niño, S., Dept. de Urologia, Centro Especial "Ramon y Cajal", Carretera de Colmenar Km. 9100, E-Madrid (p. 23)

Nebout, T., Service de Nephrologie, Hôpital Henri Mondor, 51, Ave du Maréchal De-Lattre-De-Tassigny, F-94101 Creteil (pp. 185, 225)

Nimmon, C. C., St. Bartholomew's Hospital, GB-London EC1A 7BE (p. 261)

Oliveux, A., Département d'Urologie et de Médecine Nucléaire, Centre Hospitalier et Universitaire, Hospices Civils, F-67005 Strasbourg (p. 239)

Oosterlinck, W., Department of Urology, Akademisch Ziekenhuis, University of Gent, De Pintelaan 135, B-9000 Gent (p. 83)

O'Reilly, P. H., Department of Urology, Manchester Royal Infirmary, Oxford Road, GB-Manchester M13 9WL (pp. 205, 256)

Pagano, F., Divisione Urologica, Ospedale Civile, Università di Padova, I-35100 Padova (p. 202)

Papandreou, N., Medizinische Hochschule, Urologische Klinik, Karl-Wiechert-Allee 9, D-3000 Hannover (pp. 14, 135)

Peeling, W. B., Department of Urology, St. Woolos Hospital, GB-Newport, Gwent NPT 4SZ (p. 158)

Perez-Bustamante, I., Dept. de Urologia, Centro Especial "Ramon y Cajal", Carretera de Colmenar Km. 9100, E-Madrid (p. 23)

Pfeifer, K.-J., Urologische Klinik, Thalkirchner Str. 48, D-8000 München 2 (p. 113)

Picard, C., Département de Gynécologie, Hôpital Universitaire St. Pierre, Rue Haute, 322, B-1000 Bruxelles (p. 127)

Piepsz, A., Services de Pédiatrie et des Radioisotopes, Hôpital Universitaire St. Pierre, Rue Haute, 322, B-1000 Bruxelles (p. 219)

Piscart, R., Service d'Urologie, Hôpital de Bavière, Université de Liège, Bd. de la Constitution, B-4000 Liège (p. 319)

Pizzocaro, G., Istituto Nazionale Tumori, Via Venezian 1, I-20133 Milano (p. 108)

Preßler, M., Urologische Abteilung der Medizinischen Hochschule Hannover, Karl-Wiechert-Allee 9, D-3000 Hannover 61 (p. 135)

Pryor, J. P., Institute of Urology, 172 Shaftesbury Avenue, GB-London WC2H 8JE (p. 36)

Puers, B., Department of Physical Medicine, St. Raphael Clinic, University of Leuven, Kapucynvoer 35, B-3000 Leuven (p. 314)

Puppo, P., Clinica Urologica Università, Viale Benedetto XV, I-16132 Genova (p. 197)

Roberts, E. E., Department of Urology, St. Woolos Hospital, GB-Newport, Gwent NPT 4SZ (p. 158)

Romero Aguirre, C., Dept. de Urologia, Centro Especial "Ramon y Cajal", Carretera de Colmenar Km. 9100, E-Madrid (p. 23)

Rothenberger, K., Urologische Klinik, Thalkirchner Str. 48, D-8000 München 2 (p. 113)

Rupp, N., Urologische Klinik, Thalkirchner Str. 48, D-8000 München (p. 113)

Sanabria, E., Service de Médecine Nucléaire, Hôpital Henri Mondor, 51, Ave du Maréchal De-Lattre-De-Tassigny, F-94101 Creteil (p. 225)

Scheiding, U., Urologische Abteilung der Universität Mainz, Langenbeckstr. 1, D-6500 Mainz (p. 166)

Schindler, E., Urologische Klinik der Medizinischen Hochschule Hannover, Karl-Wiechert-Allee 9, D-3000 Hannover 61 (pp. 14, 135)

Schmoller, H., Urologische Klinik, Landeskrankenanstalten, A-5020 Salzburg (pp. 118, 143)

Schönberger, B., Urologische Klinik des Krankenhauses Berlin-Friedrichshain, Leninallee 49, DDR-1017 Berlin (p. 221)

Schoutens, A., Service des Radioisotopes, Cliniques Universitaires Bruxelles, Hôpital Erasme, Route de Lennick, 808, B-1070 Bruxelles (p. 217)

Schulman, C. C., Service d'Urologie, Cliniques Universitaires de Bruxelles, Hôpital Erasme, Route de Lennick, 808, B-1070 Bruxelles (pp. 46, 70, 73, 78, 127, 171, 219)

Shah, P. J. R., Department of Urology, Norfolk and Norwich Hospital, Brunswick Road, GB-Norwich, Norfolk NR1 3SR (p. 326)

Shields, R. A., Manchester Royal Infirmary, Oxford Road, GB-Manchester M13 9WL (p. 256)

Siewert, H., Urologische Klinik des Krankenhauses Berlin-Friedrichshain, Leninallee 49, DDR-1017 Berlin (p. 221)

Simon, J., Service d'Urologie, Cliniques Universitaires de Bruxelles, Hôpital Erasme, Route de Lennick, 808, B-1070 Bruxelles (p. 78)

Strangfeld, D., Urologische Klinik des Krankenhauses Berlin-Friedrichshain, Leninallee 49, DDR-1017 Berlin (p. 221)

Struyven, J., Service de Radiologie, Cliniques Universitaires de Bruxelles, Hôpital Erasme, Route de Lennick, 808, B-1070 Bruxelles (pp. 46, 73, 171)

Testa, H. J., Department of Nuclear Medicine, Manchester Royal Infirmary, Oxford Road, GB-Manchester M13 9WL (p. 256)

Unglik, A., Service de Gynécologie, Hôpital Universitaire Brugmann, B-1030 Bruxelles (p. 46)

Van Cangh, P. J., Service d'Urologie, Cliniques Universitaires St. Luc, Université Catholique de Louvain, Avenue Hippocrate, 10, B-1200 Bruxelles (p. 1)

Vasile, N., Service d'Urologie, Hôpital Henri Mondor, 51, Ave du Maréchal De-Lattre-De-Tassigny, F-94010 Creteil (p. 179)

Vela-Navarrete, R., Dept. Urologia, Fundacion Jimenez Diaz, Avda. Reyes Catolicos 2, E-Madrid 3 (p. 288)

Vereecken, R. L., Department of Urology, St. Raphael Clinic, University of Leuven, Kapucynvoer 35, B 3000 Leuven (p. 314)

Verhas, M., Service des Radioisotopes, Cliniques Universitaires de Bruxelles, Hôpital Erasme, Route de Lennick, 808, B-1070 Bruxelles (p. 217)

Vigo, M., Divisione Radiologia, Ospedale Civile, Università di Padova, I-35100 Padova (p. 202)

Von Seelen, W., Institut für Biophysik, Universität Mainz, D-6500 Mainz (p. 166)

Vyska, K., Institut für Medizin an der Kernforschungsanlage Jülich GmbH, Stettiner Forst, D-5100 Jülich (p. 301)

Wagenknecht, L. V., Urologische Klinik der Universität Hamburg, Martinistr. 52, D-2000 Hamburg 20 (p. 106)

Walz, P. H., Urologische Abteilung der Universität Mainz, Langenbeckstr. 1, D-6500 Mainz (p. 166)

Weißbach, L., Urologische Universitätsklinik, Sigmund-Freud-Str. 25, D-5300 Bonn-Venusberg (p. 62)

Wespes, E., Service d'Urologie, Cliniques Universitaires de Bruxelles, Hôpital Erasme, Route de Lennick, 808, B-1070 Bruxelles (p. 70)

Wessels, G., Urologische Abteilung der Universität Mainz, Langenbeckstr. 1, D-6500 Mainz (p. 166)

Whitaker, R. H., Department of Urology, Addenbrook Hospital, GB-Cambridge C32 5EH (p. 285)

Whitfield, H. N., Department of Urology, St. Bartholomew's Hospital, GB-London EC1A 7BE (pp. 261, 281)

Wickham, J. E. A., Department of Urology, St. Bartholomew's Hospital, GB-London EC1A 7BE (pp. 261, 281)

Zanoni, F., Istituto Nazionale Tumori, Via Venezian 1, I-20133 Milano (p. 108)

Zattoni, F., Divisione Urologica, Ospedale Civile, Università di Padova, I-35100 Padova (p. 202)

Zingg, E. J., Urologische Universitätsklinik, Inselspital, CH-3008 Bern (p. 193)

Zöckler, H., Urologische Abteilung der Medizinischen Hochschule Hannover, Karl-Wiechert-Allee 9, D-3000 Hannover 61 (p. 135)

Zubicoa Espeleta, S., Dept. de Urologia, Centro Especial "Ramon y Cajal", Carretera de Colmenar Km. 9100, E-Madrid (p. 23)

Subject Index

MIX
Papier aus verantwortungsvollen Quellen
Paper from responsible sources
FSC® C105338

If you have any concerns about our products,
you can contact us on
ProductSafety@springernature.com

In case Publisher is established outside the EU,
the EU authorized representative is:
Springer Nature Customer Service Center GmbH
Europaplatz 3, 69115 Heidelberg, Germany

Printed by Libri Plureos GmbH
in Hamburg, Germany